Grace Flandrau
～ VOICE INTERRUPTED

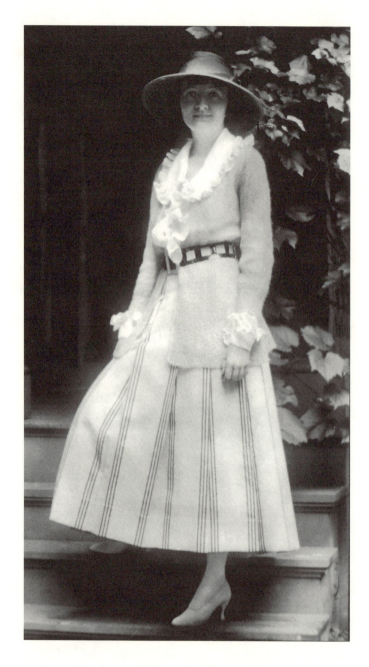

Grace Flandrau at Hill-stead, Farmington, Connecticut
ALFRED ATMORE POPE COLLECTION, HILL-STEAD MUSEUM

Grace Flandrau
∾ VOICE INTERRUPTED

Georgia Ray

EDINBOROUGH PRESS

2007

Edinborough Press
P. O. Box 13790
Roseville, Minnesota 55117
1-888-251-6336
www.edinborough.com
books@edinborough.com

The text is composed in Adobe Garamond Premier Pro and printed on acid-free
paper.

LIBRARY OF CONGRESS CATALOGING-IN-PUBLICATION DATA

Ray, Georgia.
    Grace Flandrau : voice interrupted / Georgia Ray.
        p. cm.
    Includes bibliographical references and index.
    ISBN-13: 978-1-889020-18-1 (acid-free paper)
    ISBN-10: 1-889020-18-4 (acid-free paper)
        1. Flandrau, Grace, 1889-1971. 2. Authors, American–20th century–Biography.
3. Journalists–Minnesota–Biography. 4. Minnesota–Biography. I. Title.
    PS3511.L265Z85 2007
    851'.1–dc22
        [B]
                            2007011645

Contents

Dedication

IN MEMORY OF MY PARENTS, Philip L. Ray and Berenice S. Ray—the two kindest people in the world—who always seemed to believe in me while never letting it go to my head, and my two darling grandmothers, Genevieve E. Ray, who indoctrinated me with her love of books and ideas, and Agnes H. Steuerwald, who taught me to respect domesticity, and in honor of my three way above average children—Alida, Donald, and Claire DeCoster—who are still raising me and hoping I will turn out all right.

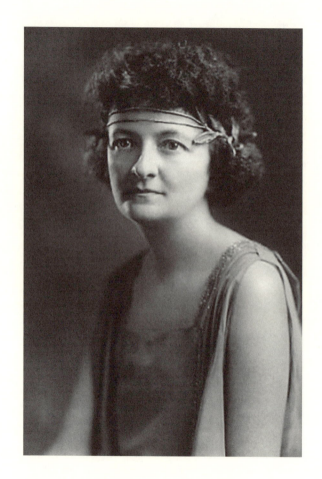

Grace Flandrau, ca. 1920
MINNESOTA HISTORICAL SOCIETY

Preface

EXPLORING THE UNIVERSITY OF ARIZONA CAMPUS on a trip to Tucson in winter 1983, I stumbled upon a handsome pink brick building called the Grace H. Flandrau Planetarium. I wondered at the time why Arizonans had named a major science building for a forgotten woman writer from St. Paul, Minnesota, my own lifelong residence.

Pursuing the answer to that question in both Arizona and Minnesota, and eventually in Connecticut and New Jersey too, I stumbled again, this time onto the never-told life story of a brilliant but star-crossed woman. I had expected to find and document a literary record and I did. Grace Flandrau was a widely read, much-praised writer, 1912–1955. What I had not expected to uncover, however, was the author's unusually poignant personal history, a narrative that begs for an audience to whom time and disconnection have given impartiality.[1]

After my discovery in Tucson I decided to write an article about Grace Flandrau for publication, but other work delayed me for several years. The mystery of the author's recognition in Arizona and her present-day obscurity in Minnesota, however, kept nudging my curiosity. I had no idea then what a controversial saga Flandrau's was.

Preliminary research between 1983 and 1987 revealed there was no way to write a quick piece about the St. Paul author. I found her record too extensive, with too much of it flying in the face of conventional opinion in Minnesota, for superficial treatment. For instance, the evidence that at least ten American anthologies, 1932 to 1952, included Flandrau's short fiction, that Hollywood filmed three of her six books, and that nearly a dozen editions of *Who's Who*, 1924 to 1969, included her name and accomplishments made her present oblivion decidedly puzzling. Much work lay ahead.[2]

Investigation for the biography that follows has focused on restoration of the author's literary record and finding answers to three main questions: was Grace Flandrau a good enough writer to merit resuscitation today, thirty years after her death in 1971? If she was, why is she forgotten or, worse, disparaged, in St. Paul, her birthplace? And why did she feel misunderstood and criticized "for all the wrong reasons" when she left St. Paul in 1955? Hours of research in eight archives in four states, numerous interviews with Flandrau relatives and friends and their descendants, a careful reading of her published and some of her unpublished works as well as those of her contemporaries—along with serendipity—have provided the clues to reconstruct the author's lost story.[3]

Before excavation of Grace Flandrau's buried saga began in earnest I assumed most of my research would be done at the Minnesota Historical Society in St. Paul. Minnesota was the home of the famous frontier pioneer, Charles Eugene Flandrau, Grace's father-in-law, and his family from 1853 until Grace's departure from St. Paul in 1955. Grace's own well-known forbears, the Hodgsons, also arrived in Minnesota Territory in the mid-1850s. Surely, I thought, most of the records about the author's literary career and personal life would be located in the state of her birth and longtime residence, but I was wrong. More surprises followed.

By 1984 I learned that Flandrau descendants in Arizona had just removed the Flandrau Family Papers (including those of both Grace Flandrau and her celebrated brother-in-law, Charles Macomb Flandrau, the essayist) from a vault at the Minnesota Historical Society and trucked them to the Arizona Historical Society in Tucson. Subsequently, I discovered that a Tucson resident named John S. Greenway, great-grandson of Charles E. Flandrau and great-nephew of Grace's husband, William Blair Flandrau, had inherited the papers from Grace, who died in 1971. It was Greenway's decision to move the Flandrau papers to Arizona permanently.[4]

The Flandrau Family Papers, consisting of more than 9,000 documents, include family members' correspondence with many of the great and famous in American and Minnesota political and literary history in the late nineteenth and first half of the twentieth centuries. Just a few examples of family correspondents are Theodore Roosevelt and Eleanor Roosevelt, Corinne Roosevelt Alsop, George Cabot Lodge, H. L. Mencken, Alexander Woollcott, Edith Wharton, F. Scott Fitzgerald, Maxwell E. Perkins, and other Scribner's editors, Stephen Vincent Benét, William Rose Benét, Frederick Faust, Kay Boyle, Brenda Ueland, and Meridel Le Sueur.

The massive collection includes family correspondence of Charles E. Flandrau, founder of the Minnesota dynasty, his two wives, his four children, Grace Hodgson Flandrau, and her father, St. Paul businessman Edward J. Hodgson. The volume of Grace Flandrau's papers is slightly larger than that of Charles Macomb Flandrau's.

John Greenway, a lawyer and literary buff himself, personally directed the cataloguing of the collection, now permanently housed at the Arizona Historical Society. As I launched my investigation in Tucson, it was obvious that

Greenway should be my first interviewee, but I didn't know quite how to approach him. Then luck came to my assistance.

A Minnesota friend with whom I had discussed the problem, the late Barbara Hannaford Bakewell, referred me to a Tucsonan she knew named Louise ("Deezie") Manning-Catron. Manning-Catron, who, I discovered, was a childhood friend of John S. Greenway, arranged my first meeting with him in 1987 at breakfast in his home at the Arizona Inn. There I saw but did not investigate the Flandrau Family Papers in their new cartons on Greenway's porch.

John Greenway's late mother, Isabella Flandrau Selmes Ferguson Greenway King, the thrice-widowed only grandchild of Charles E. Flandrau, founded and ran the Arizona Inn in Tucson from 1930 to 1953. At her death, John S. Greenway assumed the Inn's management.

John S. Greenway ("Jackie" to Grace and "Jack" to everyone else) became keeper of the Grace Flandrau flame in his family. Although he was more than forty years younger than Grace, they were kindred spirits. Jack took care of Grace in her old age as a son would and became her faithful correspondent, attorney, and guardian in her lonely last years. Studying Grace's story after she left Minnesota in 1955 and reading correspondence between them, one concludes that Greenway probably saved his great aunt's life.

Other Flandrau kin of Greenway's generation—the late Martha Breasted (his half-sister), Saranne Neumann (his step-sister) and his niece, Patty Ferguson Doar—also befriended Grace in her late years. When I first met them in 1987, however, puzzlingly, none seemed aware that their elderly relative had once been a famous writer. Apparently Grace hadn't attempted to enlighten them either. They only seemed to know her as an exceedingly bright, dependent, and very rich old lady who gave lively parties with eccentric guests. These relatives believed, like many in St. Paul today, that Charles Macomb Flandrau had been "the *real* writer" in the family.

My conversations with Greenway about Grace Flandrau, which continued when I visited Tucson each winter between 1987 and 1994, opened with a penetrating question from him and closed seven years later with his emphatic summing up statement. His two phrases stand like bookends framing our interviews. At our first meeting in February 1987, when I asked him if he thought Grace Flandrau had been a good writer, Greenway responded: "Did you ever know James Gray?" Jack told me he had met Gray (a well-known St. Paul book critic and Flandrau family friend) shortly after Grace's death in

1971 and had heard Gray's opinion that, except for her travel writing, she had not been a good writer.

At our last meeting seven years later, after reading Grace Flandrau's drafted reminiscences, found during my research in her papers and now published as *Memoirs of Grace Flandrau*, Greenway said he found the work to be "distinguished prose" and suddenly blurted out, with resignation: "Charlie was really terrible." He did not elucidate and I did not probe further. Readers of the following biography will have to determine what he meant.[5]

Other serendipitous happenings gave wings to the task of research and illuminated Flandrau's story. On one of many research trips to Arizona I discovered that my old college friend, Ann Snow Rush, another Tucsonan, was also a childhood friend of Greenway's. Jack had introduced Ann, a young writer, to the elderly Grace Flandrau forty years earlier when the latter began wintering in Arizona. Ann gave me good descriptions of Flandrau in her last years.

In Minnesota and in the East I located some of Grace and Blair Flandrau's old friends and their descendants. Some refused to be interviewed but most did not. The late Kate S. Klein, her son Blair Klein (named for Blair Flandrau), Mary Griggs Burke, the late Barbara White Bemis, Constance Shepard Otis, Olivia Irvine Dodge, the late Frances Myers Brennan, the late David Daniels, Thomond R. O'Brien, Kate Klein Piper, the late Albert W. Lindeke, Jr., C. Richards Gordon, the late John L. Hannaford, Jeanne and the late Gordon Shepard, Lucy and the late Frederick E. (Ted) Owens, Jr., C. E. Bayliss Griggs, Pierce Butler III, and others were generous with memories of Grace and Blair Flandrau and St. Paul lore.

Making contact with Grace's relatives, the Hodgsons, was more problematic. It appeared to an outsider that the author must have been entirely estranged from her father's relatives since childhood, but I later learned that Grace connected with at least two Minnesota Hodgsons in her middle years. Nevertheless, I knew no way to locate her contemporary local relatives. Then luck intervened again.

At a 1988 meeting of St. Paul's New Century Club (a 115-year old women's study group in St. Paul of which both Grace Flandrau and I have been members), I overheard an older member speak about attending the funeral of "Corrin Hodgson's wife." Since Grace's full name was "Grace Corrin Hodgson Flandrau," I knew I had struck pay dirt. Whirling around, I broke through two rows of chairs and accosted the speaker, Julia W. (Mrs. Donald L.) MacGregor. When I explained my mission, she agreed to help me contact

Dr. Corrin Hodgson, a retired Mayo Clinic surgeon and widower, now in his late nineties. Corrin is Grace Flandrau's first cousin-once-removed. Next, MacGregor invited me to meet Ann Hodgson, Corrin's niece, who put me in touch with her uncle. Corrin Hodgson soon invited me to a family picnic at Greenvale Cemetery near the old Thomas Hodgson family farm outside Castle Rock in Dakota County.

I contacted Hamline University in St. Paul to familiarize myself further with Hodgson family history. Edward John Hodgson, Grace's father, and several of his brothers and their children received college educations at Hamline, both before and after the university's move from Red Wing, Minnesota, to St. Paul. I also found extensive material on Flandrau and Hodgson family members, including Grace, at the Minnesota Historical Society in St. Paul and at both the St. Paul and Minneapolis public libraries. Those records supplemented, not duplicated, what I found in Tucson.[6]

To study Grace Flandrau material located in Connecticut I visited both the Hill-Stead Museum in Farmington and the Beinecke Rare Books Library at Yale University in New Haven.

The Hill-Stead Museum, once the private residence of the late Theodate and John Riddle, wealthy step-in-laws of Grace Flandrau, possesses records of the author's years as the Riddles' frequent guest and part-time neighbor in Farmington. The Beinecke Rare Books Library at Yale holds the papers of Richard E. and Alice Lee Myers, close friends and correspondents for many years of Grace and Blair Flandrau, Charles Macomb Flandrau, and other twentieth century American celebrities such as Ernest Hemmingway, F. Scott Fitzgerald, J. M. Barrie, Sarah and Gerald Murphy, and Archibald MacLeish.

Finally, the following two discoveries are the most significant fruits of my research:

1. Two fat folders in Grace's personal papers in Tucson packed with her draft-typed but never finished, never published reminiscences of her childhood, her school years in France, and her honeymoon trip to her husband's coffee ranch in Mexico. Apparently drafted at the urging of Maxwell E. Perkins, executive editor at Charles Scribner's Sons in the 1930s, but never submitted to him (Perkins wanted autobiographical fiction from Grace, not memoir), these reminiscences have recently been published as *Memoirs of Grace Flandrau*. They represent Flandrau's mature prose at its best and are her only non-fiction account of her youth.[7]

2. The mysterious absence from Grace's papers in Tucson of about three-

fourths of her original correspondence from Maxwell E. Perkins in the 1930s. Carbon copies of all this important correspondence, however, including copies of all the missing originals, exist in the Charles Scribner's Sons archive at Princeton and in author's private collection. The latter collection includes over 200 letters between Grace and Scribner's editors in the 1930s, eighty of them between Perkins and Flandrau.[8]

Contemporary literary professionals in Minnesota assert that the amount of attention Grace Flandrau received from Maxwell Perkins and other Charles Scribner's Sons editors during the 1930s indicates they took her seriously as a writer. Therefore, the absence from her papers of a large segment of Perkins's original correspondence to her casts a sinister light on her story.

With her experience of surviving both triumphant success and humiliation, Grace Flandrau's life is a powerful lens through which to view not only a celebrity writer among her twentieth century literary peers but also human frailty and one woman's struggle to transcend it. And what she has to share with us is told in imaginative, often funny, always affecting prose.

The narrative and the truth of the following biography, therefore, depend heavily on Grace's sensible, humane voice and on the distinctive voices of Charles Macomb Flandrau, her brother-in-law, and of Blair Flandrau, her husband, as well as on the voices of their friends and other family members to reinforce the accuracy of my interpretation.

To separate truth from the harmful rumors that overpowered the author in middle age and to reestablish the reality of her literary career is the double purpose of this book. Grace Flandrau deserves resuscitation and a new generation of readers deserves to make her acquaintance.

CHAPTER I

Credibility at the Crossroads

"We have wanted to publish for you for many years."
Maxwell E. Perkins to Grace H. Flandrau, April 19, 1935 [1]

ON OCTOBER 8, 1937, a diminutive woman with a commanding voice addressed 5,000 listeners at the University of Minnesota's Northrop Auditorium.[2] She was the chosen speaker for "All University Day." With uncommon poise, she spoke engagingly to her sell-out audience about "The Congo I Can't Forget," describing a six-month-long expedition through the heart of Africa ten years earlier. Her documentation of that journey, *Then I Saw the Congo*, a book published by Harcourt and Brace, New York (1929), and G. C. Harrap, London (1930), had been an international triumph. At a time when few — and certainly few women — had undertaken such an adventure in that part of the world and written about it in such riveting detail, publishers on two continents considered Minnesota's Grace Flandrau an authority on Africa.[3]

Probably no one in the audience that night knew or could have guessed that the speaker, a well-known American author and radio personality, had never attended college. But the erudite St. Paul native had a talent for the tour de force performance. As a child spotlighted in her family for her precociousness, she had devoured the classics by the age of twelve.[4] Later she had been schooled during her adolescent years in Paris and had traveled widely in Europe and in the Orient. By the time she reached adulthood and had become a young society matron in St. Paul, the largely self-educated Grace Flandrau was writing for America's premiere literary magazines and book publishers.

The fashionable and worldly author—fifty-one in 1937—had always attempted to achieve beyond what was expected of women of her time and social status, and her literary efforts had brought her considerable remuneration and fame. *Scribner's* magazine sometimes paid her as much for her stories in the early 1930s as they paid Scott Fitzgerald.[5]

After her speech on Africa the author proudly wrote Charles Scribner's Sons executive editor Maxwell E. Perkins, with whom she corresponded in the 1930s. She wanted him to know that her Northrop audience had been exceeded only once before when Alexander Woollcott came in 1935 to the Twin Cities to speak at the same auditorium.[6] This evidence of Flandrau's broad following was no small achievement for a woman writer of her time—and she knew it. Perkins had been discouraging her from accepting public speaking engagements in order to concentrate her energies fully on writing.[7]

To her hometown critics and rivals—and she had quite a few—Grace Flandrau had undoubtedly seemed a trifle pretentious for years. Some could have found her zealous ambition a bit overweening. Because she never hid the fact she hadn't much formal education, her fluent French and sudden rise from obscurity to national publishing celebrity, 1912–1917, fostered skepticism. And her professional life—much of it conducted away from her home in St. Paul—naturally caused speculation. Nevertheless, Flandrau's unshakable self-confidence and undeniable success held local skeptics at bay for years.

When she enthralled her Northrop audience in 1937 this Minnesota author was at the zenith of her career with twenty-five years of solid literary achievement behind her. Her accomplishments included six hard cover books—two of them international best sellers—as well as numerous pieces of short fiction and historical journalism. By 1936 twelve of Flandrau's short stories had appeared in *Scribner's* magazine—at that time America's most admired literary monthly—and four collections of outstanding American short stories, 1932–1934, had included her work. Kay Boyle's *365 Days*, also published in 1936, presented nine of Grace's sketches of pre-and-post-revolutionary Mexico with short essays by other famous American authors.

Despite these successes, in 1937 Grace Flandrau's career was at a crossroads. She had achieved early fame because of her skill in handling writing genres of the past—sketches, the short story, and Mannerist novels. In spite of her journalistic coup in 1929 with *Then I Saw the Congo*, Grace seemed unable to produce the modern novel Perkins had been trying to coax out of her since 1930. She began turning her career toward public speaking, radio, and print journalism rather than struggle to live up to his expectations. Whenever she was in residence in St. Paul after 1935 Grace wrote columns for the *St. Paul Dispatch* and after 1936 she wrote scripts for her own radio show on local station KSTP.

Correspondence with Flandrau in the early 1930s from both Perkins and Kyle S. Crichton, associate editor for *Scribner's* magazine, reveals their high regard for her work. In 1930 Perkins called "One Way of Love," the first short story *Scribner's* magazine bought from her, "magnificent."[8] In 1932 when Grace agreed to offer a full-length book to Charles Scribner's Sons, Perkins wrote her:

"We have always been interested in your writing ever since your first novel."[9] After reading her moving manuscript, "The Happiest Time," published by *Scribner's* magazine in 1932, Kyle Crichton's praise was effusive: "We are so keen about your work here.... You belong with the very first of American writers. I want you to get that feeling about yourself very strongly."[10]

The perceptive Maxwell Perkins probably sensed that Flandrau had an unusually compelling personal life story. Having launched F. Scott Fitzgerald's career with publication of *This Side of Paradise* in 1920, perhaps Perkins was convinced that another St. Paul author was capable of a similar achievement.[11]

By 1933, however, Crichton had left *Scribner's* to become associate editor at *Collier's* and Maxwell Perkins had turned down Grace's first attempt at a modern novel.[12] The book, based on her father's life, was published instead by Robert Haas and Harrison Smith in 1934 as *Indeed This Flesh* and did not sell well. In addition, a collection of Flandrau's previously published African stories, presented by Charles Scribner's Sons in 1936 as *Under the Sun,* failed commercially. Grace was devastated. Perkins had strongly advised against coming out with a collection of her old stories before she produced a new novel, but he and Charles Scribner himself had finally yielded to her insistence and had gone ahead with the collection against their better judgment.[13]

Correspondence between them about Thomas Wolfe's triumphant new novel, *Of Time and the River,* 1935, however, demonstrates that in late 1936 Maxwell Perkins renewed urging Grace to go back to work on a new novel for Charles Scribner's Sons. Seeking the famous editor's advice Flandrau began drafting segments for the book between fall 1936 and fall 1937. Their letters in late 1937 about the work-in-progress, however, disclose that Grace and Perkins began to differ on one essential point. She wondered if she shouldn't handle her story in the first person, as memoir, but Perkins advised her to write it as fiction. Heeding his preference for fiction was an unfortunate turning point for the St. Paul author.[14]

Rather than protest his advice again as she had earlier with bad results, Grace gave up entirely on the book. Although extensive chunks of it turned up in her papers as unpublished reminiscences, she never completed the work and never attempted any other full-length book. The heart-wrenching irony is that, although she had Perkins's full attention, Grace never showed him her memoir drafts, although they represent her mature prose at its best.

By late 1937 the health of Grace's husband, Blair Flandrau, was deteriorating rapidly and she, setting work aside, remained in St. Paul for most of that year. A letter from Perkins to Grace dated November 8, 1937, indicated he knew it was a difficult time for her. He wrote, "I do hope you will come East, and I hope this time you will be willing to have lunch with me, or tea or something, so that we could talk outside the office. If you do come, it will mean that things are better at home, too."[15]

Perhaps Grace took Perkins's invitation as the opportunity to explain in person why she wanted to write her story as memoir, not fiction, or why she decided not to write the book at all. There is no further correspondence about her novel. After sending his condolences on news of Blair Flandrau's death in late 1938, Perkins introduced Grace to New York literary agent Carl D. Brandt. *Scribner's* magazine ceased publication in 1939 and Perkins retired in 1944.

Dozens of pages of Flandrau's drafted memories of her youth remained undiscovered in her papers until research for this biography began. Yet readers will find that Flandrau's prose style reached its zenith of authenticity in the timelessly relevant *Memoirs of Grace Flandrau.*[16]

In her mid-fifties, Grace returned to the genre in which she had always excelled: short fiction. Carl Brandt continued to represent her for the next twenty years. Stories in *Harper's, Pictorial Review, Good Housekeeping,* and three *New Yorker* stories, 1937–1943, show her in top form, but five subsequent autobiographical stories in *Colliers,* 1943–1945, where Crichton was by then managing editor, are slight by comparison. After 1945 she turned entirely to journalism claiming she was "no longer interested in fiction and seldom read it."[17] Although a few of Flandrau's articles and reviews appeared in British and American magazines and she won several awards in the late 1940s, her days as a celebrated writer were over. *Holiday* presented Grace Flandrau's nostalgic last essay, "Minnesota," in 1955.[18]

During the peak years of her literary career Grace was a social favorite in the Twin Cities and on the East Coast. Her marriage in 1909 to William Blair Flandrau, a member of Minnesota's wealthy pioneer aristocracy, had propelled her to prominence in St. Paul's high society and given her powerful connections nationally—connections that doubtless opened publishing doors for her. With her charismatic personality, polished French, and sophisticated—often outrageous—wit, Grace was as popular a hostess and guest in Minnesota, Manhattan, Connecticut, Mexico, and France as she was an author. Her friends always counted on her to entertain them. "Grace Flandrau lit up a room," recalled a St. Paulite recently about her parents' friend.[19] But

Grace was also a femme fatale who threatened other females' egos. "Men adored her and women were jealous of her," remembered a once-intimate St. Paul associate two decades after Flandrau's death in 1971.[20]

After they married Grace quickly charmed Blair's friends, but an air of mystery seemed to envelop her animated persona. Over the years St. Paulites noticed that in her personal life she seemed almost entirely dependent on Flandrau connections and detached from her own kin, residents of California. She did not visit or speak of her late father's relatives in Minnesota.

The author's high-profile double existence—in wealthy society and in the literary world—was a candle that burned brightly at both ends for thirty years. Its apex was from 1916–1946. Such a life was emotionally and physically exhausting because it demanded constant role-playing. The real Grace Flandrau—a natural scholar and cultural analyst—was usually in disguise in her social life. During her thirty-year marriage she suffered nervous exhaustion and depression more than once, but each time rededication to writing restored her to health.

A vivid description of the author appeared in *Golfer and Sportsman*, a Twin Cities social and cultural magazine, in fall 1934. In the article reporter Brenda Ueland, Flandrau's good friend and fellow writer, portrayed a powerful woman at the crest of her fame:

> How does she look? She has warm brilliant green-topaz eyes set remarkably far apart above wide cheekbones that should be Slavic but are not, and she is perhaps a little near-sighted. (People complain that she does not recognize them on second meeting.) She is feminine, elegant. She has slim shanks and aristocratically pointed feet and her walk always makes me think of the drawings of Little Lord Fauntleroy coming over polished floors. She has a very beautiful voice, rich, gay, full of vitality, excitement, ardor, flamboyant adjectives, laughter, derision, jeers, mimicry, earnestness, affection, ribaldry, truth. Intermittently, she laughs uproariously, becomes comic and refers to herself ludicrously as 'auntie' and no sobriquet could be more inapropos. She says 'darling' as often and exuberantly as a Russian. I have never heard her say anything that is not exciting, arresting, witty, alarming. To hear that voice and laughter through a roomful of shouting tea drinkers sets the corpuscles dancing with curiosity, excitement, amusement and it is downright pain not to be allowed (because of politeness) to go and hear what she is saying.

Privately, however, Ueland knew that Flandrau's charismatic public persona hid a troubled woman, someone who had suffered in childhood and had difficulty relating to others. Brenda's diary entries, written a few weeks before her profile of Grace appeared in print, reveal this awareness: "Read G. Flandrau's novel. It is so remarkably good; . . . such warmth, humor . . . Nobody has said anything appreciative of her book. How strange . . . a prophet in her own country?"

A subsequent diary entry confirmed that another friend of Ueland's "didn't like Grace Flandrau's book. Nobody does and it seems to be because they do not like Grace. But this is mistaken of them I know, I am sure."

The following spring Ueland's diary noted her continuing but unsuccessful efforts to penetrate Flandrau's façade:

> Grace is a curious person. . . . She is emotional and rich and affectionate and says darling very much—and yet elusive and far away; I keep expecting warm contact; can't get it; she withdraws from it . . . she doesn't want to be alone with anybody at all. She wants excitement, diversion. Communists, gangsters, society people, wits, literary lights all together.[21]

The death of Blair Flandrau in 1938 threw Grace into torments of despair, abruptly changing her life. Although she continued writing throughout the 1940s, her output diminished.

By 1950, Flandrau, at sixty-four, was on her way to obscurity, often lonely and ill, seldom living in Minnesota and seldom writing. As she aged, the private person—described as "dependent and scatterbrained" by St. Paulites who knew her—made the public persona of Grace Flandrau—the celebrity–author seem increasingly implausible. "We thought of her as kind of a joke," admitted a once-close friend in Minnesota. Doubtless, Flandrau's habitual secrecy and many absences had contributed to her loss of credibility in her hometown.[22]

In 1955, after having the old Flandrau house in St. Paul razed, the aging author moved permanently to Farmington, Connecticut, where for many years she had kept a second home—the Gundy house—as a secluded retreat for writing. Without children or husband, Grace was isolated in St. Paul. She had been estranged from her Hodgson relatives since childhood, and after Blair's death, no Flandrau kin remained in Minnesota. In the East she had many friends in the publishing world and adored theatergoing in Manhattan.

At seventy-eight, Grace Flandrau made her final public appearance in the state in August 1962, when the Minnesota Historical Society invited her to give a speech about her late father-in-law, Judge Charles E. Flandrau, at the society's annual meeting in New Ulm.

The author spent her last years in near seclusion, surrounded by servants, pets, and her beloved books. Correspondence with a few old friends and occasional visits from neighbors or Blair's Arizona relatives sustained her. Dividing her life between Farmington and Tucson, she seldom returned to St. Paul. On rare visits to the city of her birth she attended meetings of the executive council of the Minnesota Historical Society (of which she was a member for many years) or stockholders' meetings of Saint Paul Companies (formerly, Saint Paul Fire and Marine, Inc.). Blair Flandrau, who had inherited it from his older brother, Charles, left Grace a sizable legacy in Fire and Marine stock. As the years passed, that legacy became a large fortune.

Grace Flandrau died at eighty-five in 1971 and is buried in the Flandrau family plot at St. Paul's Oakland Cemetery. Had she not left her private papers to Blair Flandrau's great-nephew, John S. Greenway, her cherished friend and lawyer in her old age, the story of this Minnesota author's difficult youth and the record of her literary achievement would have been buried with her.

The late Jack Greenway—Yale-educated attorney and bachelor, a life-long resident of Tucson, and Charles E. Flandrau's great grandson—adored "Gracie." Although forty years separated their ages, the two were equally young at heart. They both detested hypocrisy, scoffed at smugness, and relished toppling icons. Greenway's intelligence, care, and persistence have made it possible to reconstruct his great-aunt's forgotten literary story and long-repressed personal history, for he is the one to whom she turned in her fear and loneliness, bared her heart, and left the record of her life and her literary career.

There are puzzling aspects to Grace Flandrau's disappearance from Minnesota's literary memory, discrepancies that demand clarification. Her demise seems to be more than the usual fading into obscurity that occurs after the death of most famous authors—at least temporarily—when they cease working or the genre in which they work goes out of style or the issue they address becomes history or their books go out of print.

Why have Minnesota writers Scott Fitzgerald, Brenda Ueland, and Meridel LeSueur been revived and Grace Flandrau left in obscurity when the stories of all four were published simultaneously in anthologies of the best short fiction in the 1930s? Why have Minnesota women authors Margaret Culkin

Banning, Wanda Gág, and Maude Hart Lovelace survived here but not their more famous contemporary, Grace Flandrau?

Why do some insist in St. Paul that "Grace Flandrau wasn't a good writer," seeming unaware that her work was praised by leading American and British publishers, editors, and critics as well as by other esteemed writers?

Why did contemporary descendants of the Flandrau family and Grace's own relatives, the Hodgsons, seem unaware of her one-time fame and publishing success when I interviewed them?

To present-day St. Paulites even Flandrau's financial generosity to worthy local causes as well as to needy relatives, servants, and friends is widely unknown. For example, the belief shared today by many St. Paulites who knew her is that Grace, who inherited a fortune made by her husband's father in Minnesota, left nothing to the state. But in reality a number of agencies in St. Paul alone shared bequests totaling around $3,500,000 from Flandrau's estate.[23]

A decade of research has unearthed the undeniable truth that by 1955 when she left Minnesota, Flandrau had become a pariah in her hometown. She had suffered a fall from grace of such magnitude that her literary reputation gradually eroded too. Why?[24]

Complex questions don't have simple answers, and complexity—compounded of secrecy, sensitivity, and myth—describes the aura surrounding Grace Flandrau's name today. Recovering her essence and reestablishing the reality of her literary contribution have required painstaking detective work. Passing years and layers of misinformation—or lack of information—skepticism and bias have further obscured the biographer's path. Grace's occasional lapses into exaggeration verging on prevarication have presented additional obstacles to understanding.

There are other explanations for Flandrau's demise. Meridel Le Sueur, Grace's one-time friend, described her former colleague as "double," an apt description of the rebellious social critic hiding inside the high society matron, Mrs. Blair Flandrau.[25] Many readers will recognize in these Carl Jung-influenced times that being "double" means the shadow side (or hidden side) of a personality is unusually strong. Grace understood and eventually acknowledged her doubleness. (Charles Flandrau, James Gray, Brenda Ueland, and Meridel Le Sueur—all key figures in Grace Flandrau's life story—may have been described by their contemporaries as "double" too.)[26]

Other factors shed light on the author's disappearance from literary memory. Stripped of its undeniable glamour and achievement, Grace Flandrau's story illustrates familiar proverbs about the malignant consequences of converging ego, fame, and jealousy. "Pride goeth before a fall." "If a nail stands out, pound it down." "A prophet is not without honor except in his own country."

The following quote makes the point. When one of Grace's early best-selling novels, *Being Respectable,* received a cool reception from the St. Paul press in the 1920s, Tom Boyd, a local literary colleague, consoled her: "Remember, in Thomas Hardy's village, the booksellers will not carry his books."[27]

Examples of disaffection from the famous abound. The boyhood friends of St. Paul's Scott Fitzgerald were openly disdainful of him and his youthful antics prior to and even at the peak of his international fame. Their disapproval of his personal behavior undoubtedly contributed to Fitzgerald's difficulty finishing his work in the late 1920s and 1930s, helping to sideline it and him for at least twenty years until his posthumous revival began in the 1950s, led by scholars mostly outside of Minnesota or not originally from Minnesota.

This is not to overlook or excuse any artist's selfish or loutish or otherwise indiscreet behavior that might provoke disaffection. It is, instead, to defend the artist's work, separating the latter from the former. The job of cultural historians is to salvage the artist's contribution from the wreckage of the artist's life.

Artists—this includes writers, musicians, dancers, poets, painters, all whose creative angst compels them to express themselves in some artistic form—are usually self-absorbed and often neurotic. Perfecting artistic expression always requires prodigious communication with the self and quantities of solitude—as well as uncommon self-confidence. Outstanding artists seldom win popularity contests, especially with their families and close friends.

Writers' comments about their own personalities and the stresses they inflict on their relationships illuminate this point. Novelist Georges Simenon, quoted in *View from the Loft,* a Minnesota writers' magazine, observed: "Writing is not a profession, but a vocation of unhappiness." The same article offers John Gregory Dunne's pessimistic view of writers' personalities: "Writers do not make easy friends of one another; they are professional carpers, too competitive, mean-spirited and envious for the demands of lasting friendship."[28] In his book about friendships between authors, *Love Without Wings,* Louis Auchincloss echoes and expands on these thoughts: "It is rare for writers of the first rank to feel no jealousy of each other."[29]

Jealousy of and between writers of the first rank is at the heart of Grace Flandrau's mysterious disappearance as is the automatic jealousy of both men and women toward any fellow being of such extraordinary natural gifts and self-empowerment. With the combined attributes of Margaret Mead, Anne Morrow Lindbergh, and Beatrice Lilly—to say nothing of Colette and Becky Sharp—Flandrau was probably too formidable a competitor on both the social and literary scenes to be tolerable. These factors no doubt have contributed to her absence from the contemporary roster of nationally-published Minnesota writers.

Withal, however, the brilliant Mrs. Flandrau must share blame for her fall from grace. Research and many interviews have revealed that, with her self-promoting personality and tendency toward opinionated outspokenness, the proud Grace had a knack for inviting rejection. The saying, "People who live in glass houses shouldn't throw stones," holds special relevance for a woman who always lived in a "glass house"—that is, she had both a high profile and high vulnerability—because she had the self-defeating habit of throwing stones. Retaliation was inevitable.

Although all who agreed to be interviewed for this biography spoke of Flandrau's intelligence and charm, some saw the author as self-absorbed and spoiled, an ambitious, calculating woman who manipulated her devoted husband for her own ends and satirized his friends in her books. Pretension and a strong ego dominated the public persona she projected at the height of her career, a mask that thwarted intimacy with all but a small and—after her husband's death—a diminishing circle of associates.

But Flandrau was a skilled actress as well as writer. Her veneer of sophisticated charm and formidable self-confidence had most people fooled. Inside, Grace was a frightened child. Only a few intimates recognized her vulnerability and those few loved her. A former St. Paulite, who knew the author as a good friend of her parents, said of Grace and her faults: "I forgave her as I would forgive a member of my family."[30] The daughter of another close friend said: "The women in my mother's crowd almost worshipped Grace Flandrau."[31] The daughter of a third intimate said: "I absolutely adored her."[32] Jack Greenway described Blair Flandrau's widow as "a great lady."

In the end, Grace Flandrau's is a story of transformation. The humbling loss of status she suffered in middle age fostered self-analysis and ultimately led to maturity. In the 1950s, Grace wrote her old friend Sylvia Beach, owner of the famous Shakespeare and Company Book Store in Paris, confessing: "My own strange fate . . . has been to grow old without growing up."[33] She profited from that kind of frankness and the response she received. She learned to depend less on public recognition and began caring more about personal relationships. When she returned to the Twin Cities in 1962 at age seventy-six for her speech at the Minnesota Historical Society's annual meeting, a *Minneapolis Journal* story said of the author in her own words: (Mrs. Flandrau) "distrusts ambition as mere vanity, a painful strait-jacket which may, especially in women, inhibit the flowering of the personality as a whole."[34]

During the author's struggle toward maturity the courage and ironic sense of humor she acquired during a difficult youth never deserted her, and her last years were spent in relative health and intermittent contentment. To a degree her creative gifts were reaffirmed and she gained moderate revenge against her discreditors. In summary, Grace Flandrau's is a courageous—but also a heartbreaking—story.

A building named for the author honors her in Tucson, but no sign of remembrance for one of its most famous authors exists today in St. Paul. In the city's Historic Hill District—the Flandraus' neighborhood for many years—a recent program to erect plaques commemorating well-known local writers included Zelda Fitzgerald but omitted Grace Flandrau. (Zelda published one book, *Save Me the Waltz*, and lived in St. Paul for one year.) A few copies of Flandrau's six books exist in Minnesota public libraries, but all are out of print. Dozens of magazine stories with her strongest writing lie buried and inaccessible in old bound copies of no longer published periodicals in the remotest sections of only the largest urban libraries.

Today even local historians and the few Minnesota readers who remember the author's name usually haven't read her work, having the vague impression she is a second-rate, dated writer. Yet, many readers would find that, in much of her work, this local author's point of view is entirely up-to-date and would recognize that she was a prophet in her own time. Now, one hundred and twenty years after her birth, it is time to revive Grace Flandrau's story.

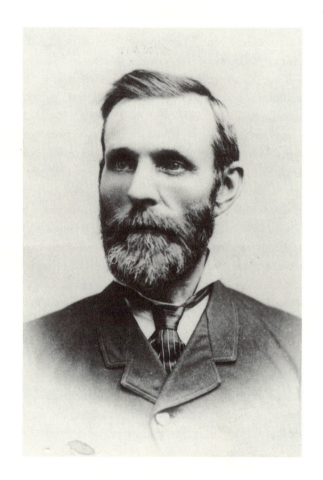

Edward J. Hodgson, ca. 1890

CHAPTER II

An Anomalous Childhood

"A little child is vulnerable. He can't defend himself against other folks' example
or something an older person wishes on him. But courage is what counts."
from "Palm Beach Soldier" by Grace Flandrau, McCall's, December 1944.

GRACE'S FATHER dominated her childhood and shadowed her life. To
understand his influence a brief reconstruction of his and his parents' stories
is necessary. Flandrau's novel about her father, *Indeed This Flesh* (1934), her
unpublished reminiscences and correspondence, and Hodgson family records
and memories are the main sources of information about this mostly undoc-
umented history. A careful reading of the author's autobiographical fiction
yields additional clues. The complexity of the Hodgsons' story led a Flandrau
descendant to comment recently: "We never got it straight."[1]

Grace Corrin Hodgson, born in 1886, was the illegitimate daughter of
Edward John Hodgson, a successful, prominent St. Paul lawyer and businessman, and his mistress, Anna Redding Hodson.[2] Edward's parents had immigrated to the mid-American frontier from the Isle of Man in 1843, bringing
two-year-old Edward and his baby brother, Thomas Corrin.[3] Anna, who
was born in Saratoga, New York, in 1853, was the young widow of William
Hodson. Both may have been distant relatives of Edward's from the Isle of
Man.[4]

The adult Edward Hodgson had most likely contacted Anna on one of his
business trips northwest of the Twin Cities. She came to St. Paul for Grace's
birth and remained briefly at Edward's home as the baby's wet nurse, apparently returning to her home (probably in North Dakota) soon afterwards.[5]
Nevertheless, rumors that the Hodgsons' cook was Grace's real mother
persisted in her family's Hill District neighborhood throughout Grace's
childhood. Edward was forty-four at the time of his daughter's birth. Anna
was thirty.[6]

Although Edward had dalliances with other women, Anna, with whom he
shared a passion for literature, was the love of his life.[7] In 1892 Edward and
Anna had a second child, William, also born out of wedlock. Anna brought
up her son alone, undoubtedly with intermittent visits from Edward.[8]

Edward and his legal wife, Mary Staples Hodgson, who was barren, raised Grace from infancy in their St. Paul home at 518 Dayton Avenue, along with an older foster daughter, Lucile. (Lucile was a child apparently left in their care by Mary's cousin and her husband, missionaries in Africa.) Edward may have had Mary's blessing when he fathered an out-of-wedlock child they could raise with Lucile, but she probably did not know her husband's liaison with Grace's mother continued for nearly two decades.[9]

In 1900 Edward sent Mary, Lucile, and Grace to live in Paris during his recovery from severe financial reverses brought on by the bank panic of 1893. Americans found it cheaper to support a family in Europe than in the United States.[10] With Hodgson's other family in France, Anna Hodson and her son William moved to Minneapolis in 1901.[11] Grace's younger brother was then nine years old. But Edward's second family lived near him only a short time before he became ill with cancer. When Mary and the girls returned from Europe in fall 1903, Edward had recovered solvency, but he was dying. Probably only then did Grace learn that Mary was not her birth mother.[12]

Edward Hodgson died in September 1903, the same year Alexander Ramsey, Minnesota's first territorial governor, and Charles E. Flandrau, a territorial supreme court justice and prominent attorney, died. (All three men were memorialized in a joint tribute in the October 1903 minutes of the St. Paul Chamber of Commerce.)[13] Within a few weeks, Lucile married Ralph Willis and moved to Connecticut.[14] Grace briefly entered Mrs. Backus's School in St. Paul, but as soon as Edward's estate was settled, Mary Hodgson fled Minnesota, taking Grace, age seventeen, with her. In the following six years of travel they barely visited St. Paul, where Mary still owned and rented out the Hodgson home.[15] In that long interval away from home Mary and Grace became practiced in the art of dissembling. For many years—even long after Grace married Blair Flandrau—neither woman revealed their true relationship.[16]

Before his death Edward's relatives in Minnesota became aware of Anna and William's existence but did not seek acquaintance with them. The Hodgsons, who had been close to Grace during her early childhood, apparently distanced themselves from Edward's widow, Grace, and Lucile after his death too. Such was the disgrace of illegitimacy in the early twentieth century.[17]

Although Anna Hodson and her daughter evidently never sought to know each other, Hodgson relatives may have taken Grace to visit her mother in North Dakota as a child. She didn't meet her brother William until 1932, when she was approaching middle-age. By then William Hodson was a nationally known lawyer, social worker, and advocate for children's rights, living and working for the Russell Sage Foundation in New York City.[18]

Grace felt bitter and betrayed as a seventeen-year-old when she learned of her father's mistress, but she came to understand the stress in his marriage and to forgive him.[19] Although she had adored him in childhood, as an adult Grace never spoke about him. Many years after Edward's death, however, she began writing about him.[20]

Grace's drafted "memoirs" reveal that Edward Hodgson was a power-ful—and unchallenged—influence in his daughter's upbringing as well as the source of her inspiration as a writer. His thirst for knowledge and his broad familiarity with world literature thoroughly imprinted Grace's youthful psyche.[21]

Motivated by her father, Grace became an outstanding student. Edward habitually read aloud to her in childhood, inspiring her to memorize and recite long passages of English poetry.[22] Her younger brother, William, must have benefited from Edward's influence too. He evidently settled money on Anna to educate their son, enabling him to graduate with honors from the University of Minnesota and from Harvard Law School.[23] Edward Hodgson's love of learning and ideas was exceeded only by his zealous quest for wealth and position.

Photos of Edward Hodgson in mid-life present a man with a high, domed forehead, full beard and intense, confident gaze. He had the appearance of a scholarly professor and, according to Grace's description, he was a tall man with an ardent, ironically humorous and temperamental disposition. By the time she wrote *Indeed This Flesh*, in 1934, (a fictionalized account of Hodgson's life), however, Grace knew that Edward's life had been a tragic fail-ure. While she was working on the book she described the hero in a letter to Scribner's editor Kyle S. Crichton as "a sensitive, naively ambitious, and terribly misplaced man of an essentially noble and perhaps even spiritual char-acter."[24] The real Edward Hodgson, however, disdained organized religion.[25]

Edward's attentive parenting had negative aspects. As a freethinker who was familiar with the most avant-garde social theories of his time, he held unconventional ideas about human behavior. These attitudes, as well as his indulgent treatment of his precocious daughter, had unhealthy consequences. Grace's reminiscences reveal her adult understanding that the favoritism she had received in childhood and her unusually strong bond with her father had contributed to her adult torment:

In our family I was the pet, the spoiled darling, the royal favorite. My father was the Victorian patriarch, the tyrant, the ruler by divine right, and I was subject to no discipline except the sudden, unreasonable lightnings of his uncertain temper.

I read from morning to night, uninterruptedly, and at night he reads aloud to me. It is understood the others may listen if they care to, but the reading is for me alone. I sit on his lap with my arm around his neck, my head on his breast, divinely happy and secure.

He drives up one day in a handsome hired carriage, with prancing horses and silver chains. I am invited to drive with him into the country. No one else is invited. This seems natural and to be expected as my mother and sister are to stay at home.

My violin teacher sends word that there is grand opera in Chicago, that she is going, and it would be good for us to go along. I am sent, but not my sister, though she was the natural musician. But that was as it should be, part of the tradition which went back to earliest childhood.

Searching for the source of her recurrent depression and sense of separation from others in middle age, Grace continued her reminiscences:

This then must be one of the threads, this favoritism, this suppression of the rights of others, the subordination of the pleasure of others to me alone, must be one inexorable part of the pattern. Perhaps you shudder already for the man who is going to marry the spoiled darling, and I do not blame you.[26]

Her father's blatant favoritism toward Grace must have stemmed from her status as his biological child, which Lucile was not. Harsh consequences for both women resulted from this unequal treatment. For one thing Edward's spoiling of his younger daughter earned her the nickname "Graceless" among his relatives.[27] For another, Edward's indulgence possibly turned incestuous.[28]

Hodgson's workaholism imprinted his adoring daughter too. Like him, Grace Flandrau as an adult put her work ahead of all other considerations—personal, physical, and social. She was conditioned to live and work—mostly alone—in perpetual "overdrive" as her father had.

Much of Hodgson's influence on his children derived from his Manx cultural heritage, but it also reflected the drive immigrants often exhibit in overcoming perceived disadvantages of birth and status. Edward's relatives of his generation in Minnesota and their children were as highly motivated achievers and parents as he and Anna Hodson. In his case, however, there was extra incentive to succeed financially and gain status, for Edward, like Grace and William, strove throughout his life to recover for his mother and himself their lost position in society.

Edward's siblings, four boys and two girls, were the children of Thomas Hodgson and Charollet Corrin Hodgson, residents of the Isle of Man until they immigrated to mid-America in 1843. The five younger Hodgson children were born in the United States, but Edward John, the eldest, and the second son, Thomas Corrin, were born on the Isle of Man in 1841 and 1843, respectively. They were the sons of two different fathers.

Indeed This Flesh clearly reveals that Edward was not Thomas Hodgson's son but the child of Charollet Corrin and her sickly young husband, an English aristocrat who died about the time their child was born. Charollet quickly married Thomas Hodgson, a mining superintendent who, Grace's book intimates, was somewhat beneath her station. They proceeded to have a large family and a hard life. In Grace's book, Pearson (Thomas Hodgson) raises his stepson, Will Quane (Edward Hodgson). Will grows up to disdain farming and, with his stepfather's encouragement, attends college, studies law and becomes a businessman.

Grace's paternal grandmother, Charollet Corrin, whose family in real life claimed descent from the ancient Viking kings of Man—called "Thorrin"—was a member of the landed gentry on the Isle of Man. Over the centuries, "Thorrin" was changed to "Corrin." Grace's great-great-grandfather Corrin built "Corrin's Tower" (also known as "Corrin's Folly"), a landmark on the Isle of Man outside the fishing village of Peel.[29]

Edward's stepfather, Thomas Hodgson, was born in Westmoreland, England, in 1805.[30] In 1840 he settled on the Isle of Man. Although trained as a miner and builder, he went to work on the Corrin family farm, "Knochaloe Beg," and soon married Charollet. Hodgson was a big, rugged extrovert; Charollet Corrin was tiny and patrician.[31]

In the United States, Thomas and Charollet (changed to "Charlotte" in America) settled first in Galena, Illinois, in 1844, where he worked as a miner and builder of housing for miners. Perhaps influenced by rumors of pending land grants to homesteaders, Thomas and Charlotte moved to Minnesota Territory in 1855. They acquired land among other Manx immigrants near

Castle Rock in Dakota County and resumed farming for the remainder of
Thomas's life. He died in 1874.

According to family records, Thomas was a sensitive man with a nice use of
language. Although he was educated, he never rose above manual labor after
his immigration to America. Having struggled to make a living after arriving
in Illinois, he was used to adversity. He was homesick, but he "stuck it out" in
America. In *Indeed This Flesh*, Pearson (Hodgson) became lazy after his boys
were old enough to manage the farm.[32]

Thomas and Charlotte, however, inspired their children with ambition.
Four sons attended Hamline University and three of these—Edward, James,
and William—became lawyers, the latter a judge.[33] The second son, Thomas
Corrin Hodgson, became a prominent educator, lay preacher, and farmer in
Grant County, Minnesota. Other descendants of Thomas and Charlotte in
America became professionals in medicine, journalism, and social work.[34]

The particulars of Thomas Hodgson's disability are unclear. While
Flandrau's novel *Indeed This Flesh* portrays Carlotta (Charlotte Hodgson)
as a strong, spiritual woman whose face and hands are a permanent, weath-
ered brown from doing outdoor farm chores, her husband, Pearson (Thomas
Hodgson), the stepfather of Will Quane (Edward Hodgson), is called a
drunkard. Nevertheless, Pearson recognizes his stepson's ability, urges him to
aim high in life, and sees to it that he receives some college education.[35]

In real life Thomas Hodgson managed to send Edward to Hamline
University (then located in Red Wing) for two years. After serving briefly
in the Civil War, Edward received a medical discharge for a throat ailment
in 1863. Following his discharge, he traveled for two years in England and
on the continent.[36] During those two years the scholarly, intense young
American was undoubtedly introduced to some of the ultraradical ideas then
sweeping mid-nineteenth century Europe, particularly the philosophy of the
utopian socialist Charles Fourier. The widely influential Fourier professed
that completely uninhibited sexual behavior was a panacea for human ills.
Thereafter, Edward's outlook and the future conditioning he gave his daughter were essentially European.[37]

Upon Edward's return to Hastings he read law in a judge's office. After
setting up practice in Red Wing, Edward first lived with and then married
Mary Staples, one of the blooming, sweet-tempered daughters of a prosperous
dairy farmer and horse-breeder. She too was a Hamline University student.

Edward had first encountered Mary when he was a young, shy, penniless student in Red Wing.[38]

For thirteen years Edward practiced law and worked as a real estate broker and land speculator in Goodhue County. He gradually built up an income by buying government, Indian, and other vacated public and private lands cheaply, reselling them for small down payments to new settlers and businessmen, and holding mortgages on the balance.[39] He became adept at speculating where entrepreneurs would build future towns and railroads. Old-timers remember that the Hodgson Real Estate Company introduced the railroad spur into Goodhue County to the lasting benefit of local farmers. Hodgson Street in Red Wing honors Grace Flandrau's father today.[40]

In 1876 Edward and Mary moved to St. Paul, where he continued a career that led to prosperity for a quarter-century.[41] He was able to assist his younger half-brothers and a nephew with housing and employment in his law office at the start of their careers. A Hodgson family letter describes Edward as "proud and selfish," but he was also an ambitious and versatile achiever.[42] His career expanded into speculation in residential construction and even into architectural design. He became president of both the St. Paul Chamber of Commerce and the Real Estate Exchange Board of the Commercial Club.[43]

Hodgson, who was a public-spirited man and a populist, was a member of the Republican Party. He wrote prolifically and spoke frequently on tariffs, financial panics, taxes, agricultural production, monetary policy, and immigration. He strongly advocated the gold standard. Minnesota newspapers often carried Hodgson's columns on these subjects in the late nineteenth century, and throughout his adult life Edward was a regular contributor to the best British magazines.[44] In 1880 he established the Hodgson Prize at Hamline University, with annual stipends of fifty dollars to the winners of rhetorical and essay contest.[45]

Edward's zeal for politics, his love of literature, and his talent for self-expression are manifestations of his Manx heritage. Over centuries of isolated island living, the Manx people, whose culture derives from ancient Celtic, Scandinavian, and Gaelic influences, developed a strong oral tradition. All kinds of communication—storytelling, recitation of poetry and historic events from memory, singing and playing musical instruments, debate—played an important role in daily life.[46] Edward Hodgson's siblings and their descendents revered their Manx heritage. Grace, who was exposed early to its influence, described it in her reminiscences:

You see a thin, small, high-strung, emotional child, with big shining eyes, broad forehead, surly, self-indulgent lips, a pointed chin. Intensely loving, hot-tempered, too full of laughter and too easily hurt. I sing, I recite, I play the violin, I speak pieces.

The house is full of company. I am lifted high above their heads and made to stand on top of a big iron safe, an empty safe, one kept for no known reason in the corner of the living room. Perched up there above them all I recite long poems, dramatically, with gestures, to which relatives and guests are compelled to listen. I have a fabulous memory for verse. It seems natural for me to be up there above everybody else, speaking pieces with all the faces lifted to me. There is only one person to whom I am not superior, and this is my father. I am the royal mascot.[47]

Edward's mother, Charlotte Hodgson, was also an influential figure in Grace's young life. Charlotte, who was widowed in 1874, remained on the family farm in Castle Rock with hired girls until 1886, the year Grace was born. That year she moved to Edward and Mary's home in St. Paul, where she lived until her death in 1901.[48]

Grace's novel *Indeed This Flesh*, depicts Carlotta (Charlotte) as a small but impressive old woman with a leonine head of white hair, who knits, humming old Celtic airs and mumbling passages of poetry to herself in a rocking chair by the fire. She had strong religious faith. Surely, Charlotte Corrin Hodgson, the descendent of Viking kings and wife of an immigrant farmer, must have inspired her sons to rise in the new world.[49]

In *Indeed This Flesh* Grace revealed the reasons for stress between her father and her sweet, insecure stepmother. Mary's obsequious devotion to Edward hardened him against her. She infuriated him when she consulted fortunetellers to remedy her barrenness and ran up staggering bills during his worst period of financial stress. Once he resorted to buying newspaper ads to disclaim responsibility for her debts. Her father's rages at Mary's naiveté provoked Grace's childhood tantrums.[50]

During Grace's early years the Hodgsons enjoyed a financially secure family life, but Edward made frequent trips away from home. Their residence, which was originally built by Mary's family, the Staples, after they moved to St. Paul from Red Wing, was a sturdy, three-story frame house in the early Queen Anne style. Edward and Mary occupied it in 1876 when the Staples moved to California. The St. Paul City Directory for 1876 lists "lawyer, real estate, loans" after Edward's name.

Hodgson's entrepreneurial instincts must have convinced him that the city's St. Anthony Hill (known today as "Summit Hill") was on the threshold of a building boom. Within the first decade after the Hodgsons' move to the city, the Hill District was denuded of its oak forest, streets were laid out, and hundreds of houses were built in the largest construction spree in St. Paul history. Huge mansions designed by some of the nation's leading architects sprang up along Summit Avenue, the newest and one of the grandest residential boulevards in the United States. Squadrons of skilled craftsmen and mechanical workers, American and foreign, converged on the young capital city to work on lavish residences for the new tycoons, building their own more modest homes in the blocks north of Summit Avenue.

The year Grace was born, 1886, was the peak of the building bonanza. Two hundred million feet of lumber and $28 million worth of real estate transfers fueled the construction frenzy (purchases and loans amounting to $600 million in 1999 dollars).[51]

In the 1880s Edward Hodgson joined Charles Wallingford and Allen Stem in the design and construction of two large houses on Summit Avenue.[52] He also collaborated as an architect with Stem in the design of a railroad station and residence in Montana. Recognizing the need for speculative capital, he steered his career toward mortgage banking. In 1886, Grace's father, with European and English partners, organized the London and Northwestern Mortgage Company.[53]

In 1890 Hodgson founded the Security Trust Company, a mortgage bank, in St. Paul and became its president. He remained in that office until his death in 1903.[54] Security Trust, however, nearly failed in the bank panic of 1893, and Hodgson suffered severe financial reverses. After paying off his creditors and customers, Edward narrowly escaped personal bankruptcy. The severely reduced circumstances of her family after the bank's temporary collapse and throughout the 1890s profoundly affected Grace's childhood. She never overcame her dread of poverty.[55]

Describing her family's precarious financial circumstances after 1893 and the bravado exhibited by her ambitious parents, Grace wrote many years later:

> There was the tradition in the household that although there was generally not enough money for the barest necessities, there was always enough

for the luxuries. When we had not food enough to eat or money to pay for warm clothes and coal to heat the house, we had nevertheless a French governess. When my father was staving off the bank we gave a large dinner for the governor of the state. When we had visitors from England my father drove them about in a hired brougham, and my mother ran up incredible bills for fine linen at the best department stores.

We were poor. My father drove himself as no galley slave has ever done to fend off bankruptcy to which he would under no circumstances resort. But "I'm ruined," he would cry, driving the blood from my heart. "The game is up. We'll all starve to death. We're going to the poor house."

But at other times he would talk suavely and like a rich man. How he would buy fine horses and especially statuary. He preferred, he said, statuary to painting. He would build a mansion on the bluff, with stained glass windows and a porte cochere.

That we should be about to starve and also about to buy mansions and statuary seemed as plausible as anything. And at the time when we were poorer than any other, when my father came home at nine or ten o'clock at night, white, exhausted, with a look of anguish on his beautiful thin face, suddenly it was announced that he was sending all three of us to Europe to Paris to school. A perfect French accent, he said, was the indispensable attribute of gentility.[57]

CHAPTER III

A Young American Turns French

*"Human beings may be and often are, at one and the same time, ignoble,
false, greedy, cowardly, vile and also noble, tender, aspiring, good."*
Grace Flandrau, Golfer and Sportsman, fall 1934

GRACE FLANDRAU ONCE DESCRIBED her stepmother, Mary Staples
Hodgson, as "gentle, innocent, timid, adventurous."[1] Those qualities were
apparent when Mary, Lucile, Grace, and Aunt Jennie (Mary's unmarried sister)
went, under Edward's edict, to live in Paris in 1900. Before money began to
arrive from home, the four barely knew where their next meal was coming
from or whether the girls' school tuition could be paid. For their very survival,
Grace and Lucile were dependent on Mary's pluck and resourcefulness, and
she did not fail them.

Among Mary's ideas for stretching their meager funds were subletting rooms
in their rented Paris flat, upholstering fruit crates for furniture, and altering
the girls' clothing as they grew. She was a competent seamstress who loved
fashion and social life. Somehow she managed to get them all invited, suitably
dressed, to the gatherings put on for Americans during the Paris Exposition of
1900. Mary also was able to finance trips with the girls to England, Germany,
Italy, and the Isle of Man during school vacations. Her letters from abroad to
Edward are a marvel of optimism.[2]

Going further to make ends meet in Paris, Mary Hodgson allowed Lucile
to drop out of school while keeping Grace in classes. Grace was the better
student. She enclosed her report card and this note to her father in one of
Mary's letters to Edward: "My teacher wishes me to explain to you that this
is the highest recompense one can have. It signifies that I have never once
failed the first for three months."[3] But Mary sometimes had trouble handling
her headstrong stepdaughter, and sometimes her resentment toward Grace
became clear. According to Grace's accounts of her school days at a French
convent in Paris, Mary neglected to send her even a Christmas greeting at
school, while she, accompanied by Aunt Jennie and Lucile, traveled in Italy
over the holidays. Grace felt abandoned. She wore a threadbare uniform and,
although her tuition and board were paid, not one cent of allowance was

provided. A servant took pity on her, mended her underwear, and bought her soap. By contrast, to the lonely American teen-ager, the school's French students appeared to be exquisitely groomed and cared for by their affluent and accessible parents. The experience strongly impressed Grace and reinforced the acute dread of privation that had been her more-or-less constant companion since her father's financial difficulties began in the 1890s.[4]

Postcards sent by Grace from Europe to her cousin Drusilla ("Drusie) Hodgson in Minnesota at this time, however, reveal no sense of hardship or homesickness. Instead, they carry rapturous descriptions of a trip taken to Italy, visits to the catacombs, carriage rides in the Bois de Boulogne, and dinners and teas in swank Parisian hotels. Grace naturally emphasized the positive and hid the negative from a close relative her own age.[5]

But the experience was maturing as well. While Grace inwardly suffered humiliation, outwardly she succeeded. During her two years in the convent, the French she had learned at home became remarkably fluent. She often ranked first in her courses, all taught in French, and was the first non-French student ever chosen to play the lead in the Christmas play.[6]

Living in Paris made a profound impression on Edward Hodgson's brilliant daughter. During her long stay in Europe Grace developed insights and attitudes that would empower her future writings but would make her a cultural misfit forever in the American Midwest. For one thing she became a lifelong Francophile. For another, influenced by the spirit of nonconformism, self-indulgence, and gender equality that characterized fin-de-siècle French intellectual society, Grace became an ultra-liberated, willful young woman.

Radical anti-Victorianism prevailed in Paris at the turn-of-the-century, and among its reigning icons was Sidonie Gabrielle Colette, the celebrity journalist and music hall performer. By the time she was in her mid-twenties, Colette's libertine, bisexual lifestyle and uninhibited writing had captured the attention of Tout-Paris. Her risqué "Claudine in School" about life in a French convent school was a journalistic sensation during the years Grace Hodgson, aged thirteen to seventeen, lived in Paris and attended a French convent school herself. While Mary Hodgson, Aunt Jennie, Lucile, and Grace lived in France, newspaper coverage of the hedonistic behavior of Colette, her notorious literary promoter spouse, Henri Gauthier-Villars ("Willy"), and their avant garde friends in the publishing world was constant. The highly literary Grace, mature beyond her years, could hardly have failed to notice.

The tolerance of Parisians toward Colette was most likely more reassuring than shocking to the young American.

Recent publishing has brought new understanding of the sources of Colette's unorthodox sexual behavior. That the author's unconventional, intellectual mother, Adèle Eugénie Sidonie Landois Colette ("Sido"), strongly imprinted her daughter has been well known. What has not been clear until now, however, is the nature of the conditioning Sido herself received. An examination of her radical beliefs—shared by many European intellectuals in the late nineteenth century—will help us understand, if not excuse, Edward Hodgson's unorthodox behavior with his daughter.

A two-volume biography, *Creating Colette*, by two French authors, Claudine Francis and Fernande Gontier, asserts that "it is impossible to understand Colette without an understanding of the ultraradical cultural background of her maternal family. . . . Sido grew up with her two elder brothers (both prominent journalists, writers, and publishers) [in Brussels]. Their lifelong friend was Victor Considérant, the most active proponent of the philosophy of nineteenth-century utopian socialist Charles Fourier. . . . Sido, who extolled free love, expounded for her daughter an ethic as radical today as it was . . . over a century ago . . . She left no taboos unmentioned, not even incest and followed 'a law written by herself for herself.'"[7]

Avant-garde European mores such as these broadened Grace's outlook (as they had Edward's) in her formative years. Her future conduct as a young woman and her adult writings would project tolerance for the unconventional and intolerance for the straightjacket of conformity.

Although Edward Hodgson never joined his family in Paris during their three-and-a-half-year stay abroad, he wrote and sent money regularly as he and Security Trust regained solvency.

When notified of Edward's serious illness, Mary Hodgson returned to Minnesota with Grace and Lucile in late summer, 1903, just a few weeks before he died. After his funeral in St. Paul in October 1903, followed by Lucile's wedding to Ralph Willis and settlement of Edward's estate, Mary Hodgson embarked on an endless hegira over the next six years, taking seventeen-year-old Grace with her. The bizarre circumstance of being conditioned to a life of luxury while living in dread of poverty continued to characterize Grace's make-believe adolescence. Many years later, Flandrau described their almost constant travels in her unpublished reminiscences:

For my mother, as for so many other American widows, travel had become an avocation, an excuse and a change—almost a necessity. We went back and forth across the continent, to California, and on across the Pacific to Hawaii, to Japan and China and the Philippine Islands. The few intervening years before my marriage were spent chiefly on trains and boats.

All this went on although the family conviction was at all times that we were desperately poor.... When we got back from Europe, I begged my mother to send me to boarding school, but she declared we were so poor she could not afford it. "No, I really don't know how we'll manage," mother said, scaring me dreadfully. But the year she refused to send me to boarding school, she bought me a thousand-dollar Amati violin.

That year Mary also dropped Grace off in New York for a while to study the violin. The following year they resumed their travels together.

We set sail across the Pacific to Hawaii, Japan, and China, and to the Philippine Islands, and we traveled with a private courier who waited upon us like queens and served us exquisitely dainty meals in our private compartment in first class railway carriages.

A whole winter was spent in a house in Bubbling Well Road [in Shanghai], a winter of such ease and gaiety as I had not yet known, with number one and two and three and four houseboys, all costing less than one hired girl in Minnesota.

We had endless clothes made by Chinese tailors, because they were so good and so cheap, and we came back to America loaded with Japanese kimonos, Chinese lion skins, Korean rosewood chests, carved ivory, teakwood, and bronze jars.

Soon after we returned to St. Paul, mother was heard moaning, "I don't know what's going to happen to us. I think we ought to go to stay with Grandma in California for a year. I really don't know how we'll manage otherwise."

At Grandma's I had to fight off a trip to Alaska which mother suddenly decided she would like to take. Instead, I returned to St. Paul and got engaged.[8]

Some insistent inner voice must have told Grace that her destiny lay not in California with Mary's relatives but in Minnesota where she had lived as a child. At first she felt "queer and apart" from the other young people in St. Paul, not understanding their slang. Nevertheless, she cast her lot for a future among her girlhood friends from Mrs. Backus's School and her family's other friends in the Cathedral Hill neighborhood of St. Paul.[9]

In the summer of 1909 Grace reencountered William Blair Flandrau on his yearly visit home to Minnesota from his coffee ranch in Veracruz, Mexico. The two had met once or twice years earlier, but she was eleven years younger than he, so they had few friends in common. When they met again, Grace, twenty-three, had just returned to live in St. Paul, accompanied not by her stepmother but by a French chaperone. After years of travel in foreign capitals, Grace had become a worldly and exceptionally stylish young woman.[10]

Long after her marriage in candid writing about her girlhood, Grace described herself at the time she and Blair had courted:

> I was nineteen [family records indicate she was really twenty-three] and I had been in and out of love several times. Of what is called learning I knew nothing except the French language. I spoke French like a French girl, with a perfect accent and complete fluency. I knew something of the great books Father had read aloud when I was a child, and I liked to read—in a desultory way I had read a good deal. I could play the violin fairly well for an amateur. In no school, however, had I learned anything. Neither in school nor out had I received any discipline. I was idle, and I was spoiled. I was used to being amused and to be waited upon. I could not sew, and I could not even pack.

Continuing to look back at herself, Grace wrote:

> I was in every essential without what is now called character training. I was, it is true, companionable. I liked to laugh, and I laughed a great deal and talked even more. I was vivacious and fairly amiable. Then and now I never kept a grudge. I think that may be a confession of weakness. There are grudges I ought to have kept and could not.[11]

Blair Flandrau, in his early thirties in 1909, was nine years out of Harvard. He had spent five years managing his large coffee plantation in an isolated, mountainous region of Veracruz, Mexico. Without knowledge of farming or Mexico, in 1904 Blair had impulsively invested a significant portion of his future inheritance in this foreign property in the form of a loan from his mother, Charles E. Flandrau's widow, Rebecca. His future loomed uncertain and there was no turning back.[12]

After meeting Grace, Blair proposed to her almost instantly. Not many girls in St. Paul could have dazzled a scion of the sophisticated Flandrau clan as she did. With her French-boarding-school background and Chinese tailor-made copies of Paris couturier clothes, her broad travel and knowledge of literature and languages, Grace must have appeared to her suitor as the rare younger woman who might measure to the standard set by the fashionable, intellectual Rebecca Flandrau.

As for the bride-to-be, whose father had given his daughter every advantage he could afford, her conditioning had prepared her for just such an entrée into the world of culture, wealth, and style as the Flandraus represented. Grace described her youthful inclination toward luxury this way: "I liked elegance at that time, delicate living, soft voices, perfume and fine clothes. . . . I wanted no part of work or of simple, humdrum family life." And from the moment tall, graceful, blue-eyed Blair Flandrau fixed his laughing gaze on her, Grace's heart was lost. Blair, who had adored his mother and needed mothering, was irresistibly drawn to women and they to him. She accepted his proposal quickly. Much later she wrote:

> And it all came about that summer in a very few days. And I remember when he asked me to marry him, I didn't even say 'yes,' I only said 'when?' Blair had given me his brother's book [*Viva Mexico*! by Charles Macomb Flandrau], written from his large coffee ranch in Mexico, to read—whether as an enticement or a warning I don't know—and if anything had been needed—and nothing was—to make up my mind, it would have been this description of the place where I was to live.
>
> The marriage had to take place very soon, before the coffee was ripe, but there had to be time for the inevitable trousseaux. Mother came on from Grandmother's, protesting every mile of the way against this hasty and inexplicable purpose of getting married so suddenly and rushing off to a coffee plantation. I was too young to marry anybody, she thought.[13]

The pair had little time to learn about each other. No doubt Grace was bowled over by her suitor's charm and his family's social position in St. Paul. And because Blair was a man of thirty-four who had lived away from his hometown for some time, that he or others would have informed Grace about his playboy tendencies is unlikely. If they had, she probably would not have listened.

Blair's older, bachelor brother, Charles, however, privately revealed skepticism about his younger brother's readiness for marriage. In a letter written on the eve of Blair's wedding Charles described the groom as "a thoughtless, incompetent, and pathetic child."[14]

The mutual attraction between Grace Hodgson and Blair Flandrau was predictable and theirs seemed a true love match. But they and their families had only superficial acquaintance and there were information gaps.

One of these related to money. Family records reveal that both the Flandraus and the Hodgsons were concerned about the newlyweds' financial security, but circumstances prevented each family from knowing much about the affluence of the other. The Flandraus were worried about how Blair might support himself and a wife should his coffee ranch fail. Raising coffee in Mexico had proved to be risky, requiring frequent unexpected outlays of cash, and Blair's attempt to win a U.S. consular appointment in Mexico had failed. Love in its usual way, however, thwarted all opposition.[15]

Blair and Grace were married in St. Paul at 6 P.M. at St. John's Episcopal Church, on August 23, 1909. After the wedding Rebecca Flandrau revealed concern about the couple's financial future in a letter to her oldest son, John Riddle, Blair's half-brother.

> Well, it all passed off quietly . . . the reception at the Aberdeen [Hotel] where Grace and her mother are staying. The Hodgsons have a very nice house on Dayton, but they've traveled so much since Mr. Hodgson's death that the house is rented. . . . Goo Goo [Blair] of course was so much in love that all questions of Who's Who were scorned. We told Mrs. Hodgson that Blair was penniless and all about the difficulties of life in Mexico. She smiled seraphically and said that "They would be happy, and with love . . . etc., etc."

In the same letter Rebecca said of Mary Hodgson:

> She is a kind and generous woman, I think, and is so charmed with her new son-in-law. There is every indication of money, judging from many things. . . . Our neighbor S. told Charlie that they were well-off, and I only

hope and pray for Grace's sake that it may be so. I know you would like her. She is very companionable, very presentable, and when I think of the escapes from the [other young women's initials], I cannot be but grateful. They left immediately for New York and sail . . . for Vera Cruz.[16]

The Flandraus' belief in Mary Hodgson's means was not entirely inaccurate. Because of Grace's exaggerated lifelong fears about money, however, constructing a precise picture today of the financial climate of her childhood and her situation when she met Blair is difficult. What she wrote in middle age about her family's finances is not fully borne out by how well they lived—at least some of the time—when she was a girl. Her ambitious father seems to have been ambivalent about money, often feeling poor even when he wasn't, probably an indication of the burden of supporting two households. And as eldest son in a large family Hodgson's attitude undoubtedly reflected the financial concerns of his immigrant parents.

Nevertheless, by the time Grace became engaged to Blair Flandrau, she knew precisely the feelings both of being poor and of living luxuriously. There was no doubt which she preferred. Though her father had left a comfortable estate—$67,000 (about $1,500,000 in 1999) in real estate, stock, cash, and receivables—to his widow, Grace knew that Mary, who was fifty-six in 1903, had to live on that for the rest of her life. According to his will, Edward J. Hodgson was owed a considerable amount of money in receivables and unpaid land contracts at the time of his death. Whether his widow was able to collect on these debts is unknown.

And Grace wanted independence. Although Mary was content to live with her Staples relatives in California, her stepdaughter was not. The bride badly wanted a marriage of luxury and financial security, but she and her stepmother seem to have been sufficiently impressed by the Flandraus' place in the wealthy pioneer society of St. Paul to disregard Rebecca's warnings about Blair's situation. Both families were somewhat self-deceived.[17]

Infatuation blinded the romantic pair to everything but what was immediately visible on the attractive surface of each other's lives, blunting any inclination to know more. The Flandraus' crowd, however, including Blair's more devoted and hopeful girlfriends—who may have felt themselves more eligible than the mysterious Miss Hodgson—probably saw more.

Quite a catch for the bride, they must have agreed, in light of the Flandraus' position, locally and nationally, as well as the inheritance Blair would come into after his mother's death.

Indeed, in 1909, her marriage to William Blair Flandrau must have appeared a heaven-sent rescue to Edward Hodgson's ambitious daughter, and in many ways it was. But Grace's subsequent decision to work as a professional writer and the messages of her future novels indicate she found it something more.

Her reminiscences written many years after the wedding describe Grace's youthful premonition that the sadness of her father's life would be perpetuated in hers:

> The day after I became engaged I went to the country to visit my father's grave. And the feeling that took me there was a subtle, exciting, secret thing. The visit had a romantic overtone, the quality, indeed, of a romantic tryst.
>
> I had been, ever since I could remember anything, the ... little queen of the family. ... He was my father, mine, nobody else's. There was a curious and profound sense of proprietorship. He belonged to nobody in the family except me.
>
> As I sat there, with my back against his tomb stone, my awareness of the pity and love I felt for him filled me with an acute premonition of sorrow known usually only in dreams. I felt not only the confusion, the loss, the failure of my father's own life but the significance of it and how it was part of a time not quite passed, from which I myself had suffered and by which I felt myself throttled, stifled, and would suffer more in many simple and intricate ways.[18]

No wonder Grace felt throttled. How could she explain the story of her father's double life to her new husband and his powerful family and friends? The truth about the mother and brother she had never known had to be a closed book. She decided to become a Flandrau, joined by marriage to Blair's friends and relatives, probably separated forever from her Hodgson uncles, aunts, and cousins in Minnesota. They appeared to want no further contact with her.[19]

Thus did the bride lock herself—for the next twenty-five years—within the prison of her own compromising experience. At twenty-three the highly intelligent Grace Hodgson was already a formidable actress, skillful at presenting a façade. Having transcended her "anomalous" childhood, she had become a practiced survivor with all the attributes that term implies: acute awareness, steel will, single-minded ambition, unerring instinct about where her own advantage lay, resourcefulness, adaptability, level headedness, and considerable powers of persuasion. These qualities are much admired in up-and-coming young men: in young women, however, they are nearly always threatening. Ambition is usually thought more seemly in males.

Nevertheless, the bride possessed exceptional powers to keep challengers at bay. She had youth, style, and talent, and with her slender grace and wide-eyed ebullience, Grace attracted attention wherever she went.

With this union the dynamic within the aristocratic, fame-conditioned Flandrau clan changed dramatically. The cultivated bride not only raised Blair's status in the Flandrau hierarchy—a major surprise, especially to his dominating older brother, Charles. She rapidly became a power to be reckoned with in the extended family and among their many friends. In the process, Grace began to rival—even outshine—the family's consequential female members, at least for a time. Eventually she even challenged Charles's literary preeminence. The Flandraus were not prepared for this shift in family power in favor of someone they doubtless considered a parvenu.

Nor were St. Paul socialites prepared for the ascendancy of Grace Hodgson from her somewhat dubious origins in their midst to lofty heights in national literary and social circles. Over the next forty years Flandrau would become the most famous Minnesota woman writer of her day and a much sought-after public speaker, in the Twin Cities and around the United States.

CHAPTER IV

To the Santa Margarita and Back

"You are a great deal like mother . . . always right."
William Blair Flandrau to Grace Flandrau, 1912

THE BRIDE AND GROOM set sail for Vera Cruz, the capital of Veracruz, Mexico, no doubt filled with romantic illusions about each other and their future life. Inevitably, Grace had been drawn to the excitement of her husband's ambitious venture south of the border without knowing much about it. As her "memoirs" remind us, Grace was very accustomed to foreign travel:

> That my marriage should take me to a far-off land seemed, under the circumstances, nothing more than was to be expected, quite natural. To have just married and settled down in St. Paul, Minnesota, was so outside of my habit that it just couldn't have come to pass. The sign of Mercury [travel] had always been and still is upon me.[1]

The couple's first decade as man and wife revealed wide disparities in outlook and character. Indulgent parents and many friends and admirers of the opposite sex had spoiled both, but the spoiling had produced different results. On one hand, Grace's devoted, achieving father and her teachers had showered her with attention and praise and conditioned her to have exalted aspirations for herself and high expectations of those around her. On the other, the ease and good fortune of Blair's youth had not prepared him for the rigors of managing a large agricultural enterprise in a foreign country or a long-term relationship with an ambitious, intellectually talented wife. Their temperaments and goals were poles apart.

But the two were well suited in other ways. Both were witty, fun-loving extroverts who seldom failed to amuse each other and their friends. Also, no two Minnesota families could have been more literary than those of Charles E. Flandrau and Edward J. Hodgson. Passion for reading and published authorship were commonplace, even taken for granted.

Grace adapted well in her first years as a bride in spite of the boredom and isolation of life at the Santa Margarita. The ranch, situated in mountainous countryside three miles from the tiny Mexican village of Misantla, was a two-day trip by pack mule across a rugged mountain range from the nearest city, Jalapa. Blair's letters home were ecstatic. Two months after the wedding, he wrote his older brother, Charles Macomb Flandrau (always called "Charlie"):

> I am leading such a good, clean life, feel so absolutely fit and am so bliss-fully happy. It seems silly, the way I feel, to write to mother and try to tell her that I'm not drinking myself to death, losing my mind, etc. I'm simply mad about Grace. I can't begin to tell you what a good sport she is. She is perfect in every way and I never knew it was possible to be as happy as I am now.

On the subject of the hastiness of his marriage, Blair continued:

> You and mother probably thought that I was marrying Grace in the same irresponsible way that I always did everything, but nobody can know the agony of fear I went through thinking how she would take it down here. Now I know, and I'm about the happiest thing you ever saw. I tell you what, Charlie, if it comes to you, and you'll know when it does, don't miss it, no matter what, for it will never come again.[2]

Blair informed Charles and Rebecca about the improvements Grace made to his house, the maid and cook she hired and trained, the garden they put in, the beauty of the silver wedding presents on the sideboard, and Grace's efforts to entertain his neighbors. He said the ranchers turned into different people when "there is a nice woman about." Grace studied Spanish and, Blair reported, soon spoke it better than he. He reported she was reading Charles Dickens aloud to him in the long winter evenings and that she fed every stray dog that came around. They now had three dogs, a parrot, and a dove, and he was expecting a monkey any day.

A few months after the wedding, Blair thanked his older half-brother, John Riddle, for his wedding gift of $100 and wrote:

> Do you know the song "Oh, Gee, it's great to be married." Well, it is and I never was so happy in all my life. Of course it requires an awfully good sport of a girl to come to a place like this to live and unless we were very much in love with each other the results would be too terrible . . . but

Grace says, "Of course I don't like it and don't even pretend to, still I can stand it for some years."[3]

Blair explained to John that he hoped not more than three years would pass before the ranch would do so well he could be away six months a year.

The Flandraus were impressed by Blair's happiness, and, as a family, they weren't easy to impress. Blair's fussy, often critical bachelor brother, Charles, who was fifteen years older than Grace, soon admitted she was intelligent and appeared to be fond of her. After one of Blair and Grace's annual visits home to St. Paul from Mexico, Charles described the bride to his half-sister, Martha ("Patty") Flandrau Selmes. Patty was his older half-sister and closest confidante at the time:

> She [Grace] has works in her head . . . and I think Blair's salvation and future consist in Grace's appropriating and wearing 'the pants' . . . She is devoted to him and has nevertheless realized every fault he has . . . He can scarcely put on a different necktie without asking her advice.
>
> Her influence over him is entirely good. She and Mother got on beautifully together and Mother is very fond of her. . . . She is a nice person "to have around" . . . clever and appreciative and tactful, with a well-developed sense of social responsibility that causes her to be agreeable to and considerate of people however boresome they happen to be.[4]

Constant worry over coffee prices, debts, and increasing political unrest in Mexico, however, made short work of Blair's contentment The newlyweds had only three years of married life on Blair's coffee finca (Sp. "ranch"), 1909-1912, before the impending Mexican revolution drove Grace, for safety's sake, into exile. The risk of his investment must have become quickly apparent to her. Even before she left the ranch, she began developing her own career as a magazine writer. Finally, due to the dangerous isolation of the Santa Margarita, in 1912 Grace retreated to Jalapa.[5]

Fending off worry and solitude in Mexican hotels, Grace began writing fiction based on the Totonac Indians of northern Mexico. She engaged literary agent Paul Revere Reynolds of New York to represent her.[6] Her first short story, "Josefina Maria," appeared in *Sunset* in 1912. Next she began working on a novel during the long months alone, first in Jalapa, then Mexico City, and finally New Orleans.[7]

In 1913 and 1914, when skirmishes between government troops and revolutionaries occurred more frequently throughout Veracruz and along the American border, Grace gave up trying to return to Blair's ranch. In 1915 she headed back to St. Paul to live in the Flandrau family home with Charles to wait out the revolution. She worried about Blair's safety and repeatedly urged him to leave Mexico.[8]

Blair longed for his wife, and they corresponded constantly. His letters were full of beguiling humor such as: "I miss you more than 17 3/4 of them. 17 3/4 is all there are, you know."[9] Writing Grace shortly after she fled the ranch, he admitted: "You are a great deal like mother . . . always right."[10]

Near the end of her exile from the Santa Margarita, 1912-1916, when Grace lived in St. Paul with her brother-in-law, Charles Flandrau worked as a columnist for St. Paul newspapers. Because of their shared love of books and interest in writing, the two developed a fairly comfortable relationship. Still, Grace often felt she and Blair were imposing on Charlie's hospitality, and she worried that her living situation might look ambiguous to Flandrau friends. But there was no other choice. Renting hotel rooms was expensive, and Blair was deeply attached to his childhood home, redolent with Minnesota frontier history and the prestige of his parents and their famous guests.

In 1915 the Flandrau house at 385 Pleasant Avenue was in a once gracious but slowly declining neighborhood near downtown St. Paul, a three-block, downhill walk from the Cathedral, looming up overhead on Summit Avenue. The stately, somewhat forbidding frame mansion—a blend of late Federal classicism with Italianate detailing and a touch of early Queen Ann asymmetry—was built in 1871 in an era when Native Americans still roamed the dirt streets of St. Paul and often sat on Judge Flandrau's back porch waiting to speak to him. The judge, who died in 1903 and whom Grace never met, had been U.S. Agent to the Santee Sioux (Dakota Indians) during Minnesota's territorial days. Even though Flandrau was later commissioned to lead troops against them in the 1862 Dakota Conflict the Indians never stopped seeking his advice.

When Grace moved into Charles's home in 1915 she hired and trained two maids for him—Katy and Josephine—and he was grateful. In spite of the continuing presence of the family houseman, Richard Walsh, after his mother's death, Charles had missed having a woman in charge of his home. Both brothers had been devoted to their mother and Charles had been possessive of her. He continued to live at home with Rebecca after his father's death in 1903 and traveled a good deal with her until her death in 1911. The two had made annual trips to the Santa Margarita between 1904 and 1908 to visit Blair. After Rebecca died Charles had a nervous breakdown. Because she advanced Blair the money to buy his coffee ranch in Mexico, Rebecca left the Flandrau house and furnishings in St. Paul to Charles in her will.[11]

Rebecca had been more involved in her sons' upbringing than Judge Flandrau. During their boyhood, their father was often absent. In a biographical sketch of Charles Eugene Flandrau written in her later years, Grace Flandrau gave this description of her father-in-law's probable detachment: "Flandrau was not, I should say, primarily a family man. . . . He seldom seems to have admonished or even to have advised his sons. Perhaps he expected them at any age, however young, to be men and independent as he had been."[12]

The Flandrau brothers were very different from one another. Both had their father's worldly, twinkling blue eyes set in a deadpan visage always on the verge of collapse into laughter. And, like their father they were entertaining raconteurs, men who, like many males of all ages in Victorian society, rarely showed restraint in their drinking.

There the similarity ended. The elder brother was a complex intellectual who usually masked any tendency toward kindness with cynicism; the younger was lighthearted, optimistic, and kind. Charles, who was stocky and red-haired, was famous for his wit and debunking tongue—a celebrity figure with snobbish as well as misogynistic tendencies. Blair was good-natured, tall, and lanky—an athletic outdoorsman and a gregarious man's man as well as a great appreciator of women. He had superb manners.[13]

The Flandraus ranked among Minnesota's most prominent families. Charles E. Flandrau had received several U.S. presidential appointments during his early days on the western frontier. After serving as Indian agent during the 1850s, Flandrau had a distinguished career as a territorial politician and state Supreme Court justice and later as a prosperous St. Paul lawyer after the Civil War. He was a handsome widower with two grown daughters when he married the refined Rebecca Blair McClure Riddle of Philadelphia in 1871. Rebecca was a young widow with a seven-year-old son, John Wallace Riddle, when she moved to Minnesota in 1871. Soon two little brothers, Charles Macomb and William Blair, born in 1871 and 1875 respectively, joined young John in his stepfather's home. Rebecca had a way of coddling all her sons.

The Flandraus' powerful connections reached back to New York, where Blair's grandfather, Thomas Hunt Flandrau, had been the law partner of

Aaron Burr. The family had social contacts in Washington, D.C. too, for they had been friends of the Theodore Roosevelt family for many years. When Grace married into Blair's family, the news that his half-sisters, Patty Selmes and Sally Cutcheon (Flandrau's daughters by his first wife, Isabella Dinsmore of Kentucky), and half-brother, John Riddle, circulated with members of Manhattan's "400" no doubt impressed her. All Charles E. Flandrau's children and Rebecca's son, John Riddle, were on close terms with each other and communicated frequently as adults. Blair was the beloved baby in a distinguished family. Charles was still referring to him as "Goo Goo" and "Cuckoo" when Blair married at age thirty-four. John Riddle usually addressed Blair as "Pig Wig."[14]

Charles Macomb Flandrau, four years older than Blair, taught freshman English at Harvard after graduation and quickly gained a national reputation as a promising young essayist with his popular stories in the *Saturday Evening Post* and *The Bellman*. At thirty-seven, Charles became an international literary celebrity with his essay collection, *Viva Mexico!*

John Riddle, Charles's and Blair's older half-brother, was academically gifted too, especially in languages, and after a successful career at Harvard University and Columbia Law School, he studied diplomacy at the École des Sciences Politiques in Paris and Russian at the College of France. After this preparation and with the help of U.S. presidents Theodore Roosevelt and Grover Cleveland, he launched himself on a thirty-year diplomatic career. Riddle eventually held high foreign posts including those of U.S. ambassador to Romania, Russia, and Argentina.

As late as 1893, however, when John, age thirty-one, was beginning his career as secretary to the U.S. Legation at Constantinople, Turkey, his mother addressed him in letters as "Precious Baby." In 1908, fifteen years later, when John was appointed ambassador to Russia (where Rebecca and Charles went to nurse him during a bout of pneumonia), Rebecca used salutations such as "Dearest Don Bon" in correspondence.[15] At the time of Blair's wedding in 1909, John at forty-five and Charles at thirty-eight were still bachelors with a doting widowed mother. John didn't marry until he was well past fifty. In 1916 he finally married noted architect Theodate Pope Riddle, an extremely wealthy, socially prominent, middle-aged woman from Farmington, Connecticut, who more or less supported him for the rest of his life.[16]

Blair attended Harvard too, but his college experience differed from his brothers'. Although John and Charles excelled in school, Blair was always more successful at social life and sports. In boyhood, his family's position had protected him and his devil-may-care attitude in school hadn't made any difference. Judge Flandrau, nearly fifty when Blair was born, perhaps grew more lenient. Rebecca tended to overrule his attempts to discipline Blair.

Besides being the youngest in a brilliant family, Blair had the burden of trying to live up to the standard set by his father, whom everybody thought he took after. Like Charles Eugene Flandrau, Blair was tall, handsome, and a thorough gentleman, but he lacked his father's self-possession and independence. His youthful escapades and happy-go-lucky attitude concerned and angered his family. After sixteen-year-old Blair had a romantic adventure with the young wife of a Minnesota governor his parents hastily dispatched him to boarding school at Andover. Scholarship did not distinguish Blair at Andover, but he was popular and enjoyed boxing, playing the cornet, and meeting girls. When his debts and demerits infuriated his father and Andover threatened to expel him, however, Blair settled down and managed to get into Harvard. That was in 1896, when he was twenty-one. Charles was still an upperclassman at Harvard.[17]

Although Blair served as secretary of the *Crimson*, the college newspaper, and enjoyed life in Cambridge, renewed debts and bad marks plagued his experience at Harvard. He was too fun loving and sought-after to succeed as a serious student. He left Harvard in 1900 without graduating, and Judge Flandrau, grumbling again about $1,200 spent to settle his younger son's debts, dispatched him to Montana to train in the railroad business at "Jim Hill's Kindergarten" in Missoula. There Blair joined the ranks of other rambunctious young St. Paul friends of the Hills. One of these was Ramsey Furness, the grandson of Alexander Ramsey, Minnesota's first territorial governor. Ramsey had been Blair's fellow cut-up at Andover.[17]

In April 1900 soon after Blair's arrival in Montana his father sent advice on conduct toward employees, on taking care of himself, and on saving money:

> Keep in mind duty and its performance. . . . Don't go into debt. . . . Don't <u>drink</u>. Form resolutions as to what you ought to do, and live up to them, even so small a one as to write to me once a week on a certain day. If I find you are complying with this request, I will feel more comfortable about your success. Papee.[19]

On the whole, however, Judge Flandrau tended to be indulgent with his

wife and sons, and his attempts to discipline Blair were destined to be inef-
fectual. Other family correspondence reveals the judge's devotion to his somewhat delicate wife and his probable discomfort at crossing her.

Moreover, the senior Flandrau had been an unruly lad himself. He ran away
to sea at an early age, and, after reading law for a time in his father's office in
New York State, headed west at age twenty-five and never returned to the
East. One nineteenth-century biographer described Charles Eugene Flandrau
as "original, unique, picturesque, versatile, adventurous."[20] Another labeled
him a "cavalier of the border."[21] Like his younger son, the judge much admired
handsome women and was known to spend hours telling stories over drinks
with his men friends in St. Paul bars. Flandrau, a bon vivant, was chosen
Boreas Rex (King) of St. Paul's Winter Carnival in 1890.[22]

A tall, charming "cavalier of the border" like Charles E. Flandrau must have
been as appealing to women as he was to his male friends. Perhaps occasional
desire to distance herself from peccadilloes of the judge explains Rebecca's
long sojourns in Europe with her sons—but without her husband—in 1880,
1884, 1890, and 1892.[23]

Whatever the case, the couple clearly held each other in high regard. The
senior Flandrau wrote Charlie at Harvard: "Your mother is the wisest and
best woman I have ever known."[24] And Rebecca, writing John Riddle after the
death of her husband in 1903, said: "I can hardly realize yet that Papee is gone;
He was so splendid and different from other people."[25]

All three sons wrote Rebecca separately from their father. In typical fashion,
her letters to Blair in Missoula always began with "Dearest Baby," "Dearest
Deary," or "Dearest Goo Goo."[26] They usually concluded with a message such
as the one she wrote on August 21, 1900: "I love you a great deal dear Baby and
think of you a great deal of the time." Blair was twenty-five.

Rheumatism bothered Blair in Montana and was a key factor in the direction his future life took. He suffered intermittent back pain from a spinal
injury incurred on a canoe trip at age fifteen. When rheumatism plagued
him as well, he received medical advice to seek work in a warm climate. Soon
opportunity arose.[27]

At Judge Flandrau's death in 1903, his estate was valued at $158,000
($3,147,360 in 1995 dollars). His handwritten will specified Rebecca as sole
executrix and beneficiary of all his personal and real property except for a
legacy of $10,000 to his eldest child, Patty Flandrau Selmes, a young widow.
Flandrau had invested early in bank and railroad stocks and two pioneer Saint

Paul corporations—the Saint Paul Fire and Marine Company, Inc. and West Publishing Company, Inc. The latter two were destined to grow into huge national enterprises.[28]

After his father's death Blair quit his job with the Northern Pacific Railway in Missoula and returned to Minnesota to reassess his future. Once home, he applied himself briefly to the study of architecture in St. Paul with Beaux Arts-trained architect and Flandrau family neighbor, Cass Gilbert. In 1904, little more than a year after his father's death, however, Blair bought his coffee ranch and moved permanently to Mexico.[29]

Blair's unpublished autobiographical account described the circumstances leading to his investment. He explained that a former Harvard classmate introduced him to Fred Stevenson, an American sportsman and big-game hunter. Over dinner at the Chicago Club, Stevenson invited Blair to visit his coffee plantation in the state of Veracruz on the East Coast of Mexico. Favorably impressed by what he saw, Blair quickly decided to purchase the Santa Margarita, a coffee plantation not far from Stevenson's place. The owner was a Belgian named Siebelaner, an old rascal who had decided to leave Mexico.

His lighthearted account of his first business venture projects Blair as a daring, if not reckless, adventurer, a good sport, and a charming but naive gentleman. Siebelaner left the country with debts that Blair had to pay—just the first harsh lesson for the young adventurer from Minnesota.[30]

During his twelve-year stay in Mexico, 1904–1916, Blair worked hard and faced staggering frustrations. After Rebecca's death, he invested more of his inheritance to increase his ranch's size. He also borrowed money from both Grace and his mother-in-law, Mary Hodgson, who visited the Flandraus at least twice at the Santa Margarita. Blair also labored under a large debt to Arbuckle's, his coffee brokers in Jalapa.

Besides perennial debts and the uncertain price of coffee, Blair had an unstable work force to contend with. It took many hands to plant, thin, harvest, and dry the beans from a vast mountainside of coffee trees, and his crop frequently competed with Mexico's religious holidays, during which his workers would disappear for days. Mounting political unrest, however, was the worst problem.[31]

Grace described Blair's life in revolutionary Mexico in a sketch she wrote later for Harvard:

Long after the Mexican revolution made it impossible for most landown-
ers to return to their properties, Blair continued to spend the winters, as
usual, at the Santa Margarita. He was devotedly loved by all the Indians
and peons who had been in his employ and for that reason had little to fear
from the revolutionary leaders or the bandits who masqueraded as such. It
is true they carried away with them almost everything of value they could
find, but during their visits, they dined very politely at his table, spent the
evening sitting round the edge of the sala, their great hats beside them,
their belts bulging with firearms, listening respectfully to the phonograph,
and spitting gravely on the floor. Caruso was their favorite.[32]

In April 1914, on orders from President Woodrow Wilson, U.S. troops
seized and occupied the port of Vera Cruz for four months, helping turn the
tide toward constitutional government in Mexico. Blair witnessed and wrote
three articles about the event, published in *The Bellman*.[33]

But United States intervention made it increasingly dangerous for non-
Mexicans living below the border. Revolutionary bands roamed the countryside, jeopardizing the lives of foreign ranchers and threatening to cut off
the rail line between Jalapa and Vera Cruz. Late in 1915 Blair put the Santa
Margarita into the hands of his caretaker, Ramon, and moved to Jalapa.[34]

In fall 1916, after selling his last coffee crop, Blair came home to St. Paul for
good. He had lost more than a decade of work, and now a sizable portion of
his inheritance lay unyielding and illiquid in a foreign country. In late 1916 he
entered the bond business in St. Paul as a trainee.

CHAPTER V

An Uneasy Troika

"We are a wonderful little people, are we not?"
Charles M. Flandrau to Martha Flandrau Selmes, 1916

RETURNING UNEMPLOYED to his boyhood home, now owned by an older brother who had always outshone him, challenged Blair. A readjustment in family dynamics was inevitable. Charles's maddening habit of demeaning his younger brother while defending him and deriding him behind his back to Flandrau relatives, while claiming he loved him, threw the household off balance. What apparently began in childhood, as sibling rivalry over the affections of their mother, became a heavily disguised power struggle between two adult men. Blair's attractive, intelligent wife strengthened his side of the uneven equation but that didn't temper Charles's posture of superiority. He just co-opted Grace as his ally in managing Blair. While Blair had lived alone in Mexico, Grace and Charles ran the house in St. Paul and the three servants in apparent harmony. Now Grace had Blair to accommodate, but Charles couldn't conceive of deferring to his younger brother. Making matters worse was St. Paul's hero worship of Charles as an international literary celebrity. He was now writing an immensely popular weekly column for the Sunday *Pioneer Press*, "Flandrau Says," and reviews for the *Dispatch* and *Daily News*.

On May 2, 1915, a little more than a year before Blair's return to St. Paul, the Sunday *Pioneer Press*'s story, "The Singleness of Charles," had announced the launching of Flandrau's new weekly column of theater and music criticism. The biographical article, signed only "Pioneer Press Man," described Charles's "violet blue eyes, red gold hair, and ruddy skin," his education, opinions, and literary achievements. The doting piece, which referred to Charles's bachelorhood and speculated about his marital future, has the ring of female writing. The writer asked readers: "With the Right Environment Can Any Woman Marry Any Man?"*

---

* The author believes that Frances Boardman, a single, middle-aged woman and veteran columnist at the *Pioneer Press-Dispatch*, wrote "The Singleness of Charles." Boardman revered Charles's writing. Privately, Charles referred to her as "old Boardman" or "old blancmange."

Even though Charles's international literary reputation had faltered by 1916 and only his inheritance allowed him to live a comfortable dilettante's life as a slightly employed theater critic, Grace respected her brother-in-law's achievements and sought his advice on her own career. Charles's experience in and opinions about the publishing world would influence her for the next twenty years.

Brother and sister-in-law shared certain aspects of temperament. Both had sharp wits and cynical streaks. They took passionate interest in the contemplation of human nature in all its manifestations from the sublime to the ridiculous and both loved debunking sacred cows.

Although Grace and Charles's mutual admiration might have pleased him, Blair probably had mixed emotions about it. But his and Grace's self-interest required getting along with his temperamental brother. And Grace began to resent Charles's chronic demeaning of her husband; Blair's seeming acceptance of it no doubt disillusioned her. She responded by escaping into a blur of activity.

When Blair returned from Mexico in 1916, Grace had just finished her first novel, *Cousin Julia,* and won the following praise from Charles. He wrote Patty Selmes:

> Grace is as usual very busy with all sorts of things—too many I sometimes think. She has finished her novel which I have just read, and it is a remarkable production—interesting, clever and thoroughly professional. One really enjoys reading it both for the story and the extraordinary fashion in which she has told it. . . . We are a wonderful little people, are we not?[1]

Charlie's reports to Patty continued:

> Here all goes along about as usual except that Grace has been rehearsing for a play, "The New York Idea," in which she takes the principal part, and has worked herself into an appalling state of physical exhaustion and consequent nerves. The latter she has contributed to Blair who is in despair of seeing her in such a hectic condition, and I confess that much as I love them, it is difficult at times to keep the household atmosphere serene. Someone has to maintain a sense of proportion and a realization

that the world's destiny does not hinge on the presentation of a play by amateurs, and apparently I am it.

He added significant news: "You will be interested to know that Blair and I kissed the Cross and took the pledge. Nothing stronger than tea and coffee passes our chaste lips."[2] Patty, who couldn't have failed to guess whose influence was behind that commitment to sobriety, must have been impressed by Grace's fortitude in confronting the two confirmed drinkers she lived with and—at least temporarily—reining them in.

Charlie's letters confessed concern for Blair and Grace. He said that Blair, at the age of forty, admitted that he was not totally interested in the bond business, that he was depressed, and that he longed to be at his ranch picking coffee. "He feels that he isn't getting anywhere and that everything has been a waste of life and effort. I feel so sorry for him sometimes." He added:

> Then too, while he and Grace are devoted to each other and their marriage has been an unusually happy one, they are really not in the least alike. Intellectually they are far apart—Blair being like Father, only infinitely more so. In certain ways he is in fact typically "mid-Victorian" and Grace is anything but.[3]

In late November 1916 Grace went east to meet with D. Appleton and Company about her novel and to visit her married sister, Lucile Willis, in Connecticut. Grace planned to see Blair's and Charlie's other half-sister and brother-in-law, Sally Flandrau Cutcheon, and her husband, Frank Cutcheon, in Manhattan. Grace also had an invitation to stay with newlyweds, John and Theodate Riddle, at their estate, Hill-Stead, in Farmington, Connecticut.

Predictably, she charmed Blair's Eastern relatives and extended her stay over the holidays into January. Much of the time she was the Riddles' houseguest. Soon Grace became the childless Theodate's protégée.

In February Charlie again reported to Patty:

> Grace is still away, but we expect her day after tomorrow. She has been vibrating between John's and the Cutcheons and her sister's and no doubt will have serials when she gets back. She writes of prolonged sessions of bridge with the Admiral and old Caligula, who evidently took a fancy to

her, and I look forward to her cheerful gossip. ("Caligula" refers to Anna Roosevelt Cowles, the Riddles' neighbor in Farmington.)

Charlie had good news about Grace's book *Cousin Julia*:

> You may remember that I told you she was writing a novel? Well, I had it read by the D. Appletons, who publish my books, and they have accepted it. They want her to change the end, of course, as it ends the only way it could or ought to end, and all publishers are either fools or crooks. I hate to have her do it, but have advised her to make the concession, as having a book printed and out will be a great incentive to a person like Grace to go and write a lot more.

He confided that the book's royalties would be helpful to Grace and Blair's finances:

> It is entirely possible that she might strike a popular chord, and as she writes very rapidly and without any trouble to herself, it would mean much to her financially. They have something of course, but not by any means enough to live as they would like to even on a modest scale. Being with me seems to be about the only solution for the moment. They could take an apartment as most everyone else does, but Grace wouldn't like that. She prefers the house even with its various discomforts.[4]

Grace was still lingering in the East when she received this note from Blair. "Darling, I am so delighted about your book. I told you all along I thought it would be taken." His letter pleaded with Grace not to worry so much about money.[5]

Blair sent details of his social life in Grace's absence. He described his attendance at the Winter Carnival, where he shared a box at the St. Paul Auditorium with his friends Eddie and Florence Saunders and with Charlie and his date, Jannie Egan Ford. The latter two, Blair reported hopefully, fussed over each other with apparent mutual interest. He continued:

> I have never seen Florence [Saunders] looking so <u>lovely</u> as she does lately. She had on a dark green suit trimmed in coonskin and moccasins with fur around the top of them and a coonskin cap.

Everywhere I've been since I got home I always sit next to Florence, which certainly suits me fine. I never knew her so well before. She's a perfect darling. Saturday night I invited myself to Sunday night supper, and Florence said, "That'll be great. Eddie's going away and we'll be alone and sit in front of the fire and talk." A blizzard came up and Eddie didn't go away. I had an awfully nice time.[6]

Grace returned to St. Paul shortly. D. Appleton's, Charles's publisher, brought out *Cousin Julia* in August 1917. Reviews in New York and around the country were favorable, Edith Wharton sent a congratulatory note and Hollywood bought the screen rights.[7] *The Porcupine,* a Minneapolis literary newsletter, wrote a strongly favorable review.[8] In St. Paul a fetching photo of Grace ran with an extended caption mentioning *Cousin Julia* (but no review) in the society section of the *Pioneer Press* on September 9, 1917. Charles had bragged about *Cousin Julia* a week earlier in his column in the September 2, 1917, *Pioneer Press*: "My sister-in-law has just ... produced a 365-paged narrative that is at all times diverting, and often extraordinarily precocious and shrewd." Charles, however, never again published his views about Grace's writing until 1937, a year before his death. His other comments—mostly favorable—appear only in private correspondence with her.[9]

As his wife's talent, ambition, and discipline began to manifest themselves on the heels of his failure in Mexico and with his discontent in the bond business, Blair began to play more golf and cards. His nonchalance about his career aggravated Grace's inclination to worry. And, as Edward Hodgson's daughter, she disapproved of idle adults.

His older brother's lifestyle couldn't have been a good influence on Blair, whose circumstances were different. Although Charles's equity in the Flandrau house represented an amount roughly equivalent to Blair's original investment in Mexico and it too was illiquid, his owning it put a luxurious roof over Charles's head in a then-fashionable St. Paul neighborhood. And, having no wife or children, Charlie could spend his entire income on caring for himself in a style that included several servants, deluxe travel, club memberships, and, later, a car and chauffeur—all on his inheritance and his salary from a part-time job.

Continuing uncertainty over Blair's future and their financial security, dissatisfaction with married life at her brother-in-law's home, and concern that the brothers' relationship had long been destructive for Blair began to undermine Grace's health. Migraine headaches laid siege. By spring of 1917 she was in the early stages of a nervous breakdown in a doctor's care.

Charlie described the situation to Patty:

> Grace has been taking a kind of rest cure. She was very nervous and dreadfully thin, and her doctor said she ought to go to bed, have a nurse and eat seven or eight varied meals a day. So the big library side of the house has been turned into a hospital for several weeks.[10]

The sinking of the *Lusitania* in May 1915 provoked national outrage at German aggression, and within two years the United States declared war. Luckily for Blair and his marriage, at the age of forty-two, in spite of his old back injury, he obtained a position in army service.

Blair was intensely patriotic. He enlisted and was assigned in July 1917 to the U.S. Army's Commissary Department for building and equipping barracks at Fort Dodge, Iowa. It was his kind of work—physical, outdoors, and performed in the company of ordinary people. Once construction of the base was completed he was reassigned to the camp quartermaster, supervising the operation of the commissary. Blair kept the commissary books, learned to type, and won an award for his department. He enjoyed the camaraderie of army life.[11]

While in the army, from fall 1917 to spring 1919, Blair received monthly pay in sums from $150 to $200, and he also received dividends from St. Paul Fire & Marine in amounts from $500 to $1,100, sometimes monthly and sometimes quarterly. West Publishing provided dividends in lesser amounts.[12] Grace may have received a small income from her father's estate as well. The Blair Flandraus were not poor by any stretch of the imagination—except in relation to their much wealthier friends and relatives.

But migraines continued to plague Grace. Blair again begged her not to worry so much about money and once sent her $500 to buy a fur coat.[13] He kept hoping she would recover enough to join him at Fort Dodge and later at the army base in Norfolk, Virginia, but, except for one or two short visits, a lasting reunion never occurred. Throughout the remainder of 1917, all of 1918, and half of 1919 the Flandraus lived apart, corresponding affectionately almost daily in late fall 1917, Theodate Riddle, Blair and Charlie's wealthy strong-willed new sister-in-law, suddenly appeared in St. Paul, removed Grace from Charlie's home, took her East, and put her in the care of the Riddles' doctor. Grace spent the rest of 1917 and all of 1918 living in luxury with the Riddles in Farmington, Connecticut, or in neurological clinics nearby, all at Theo's expense. Grace's nerves were exhausted.[14]

The Riddles' colonial revival mansion, Hill-Stead, designed by the New York Beaux Arts architectural firm of McKim, Mead and White at the turn of the century, was a gathering place in the early 1900s for the eastern seaboard's social, political, and cultural elite. As a young, unmarried woman, Theodate had demanded a role in Hill-Stead's design and construction, a project undertaken with her father, Cleveland steel magnate Alfred Atmore Pope. (Upon graduation from high school in 1886, Effie Brooks Pope, only daughter of steel magnate Alfred Atmore Pope and Ada Brooks Pope of Cleveland, changed her name to "Theodate"—gift of God).The mansion's collection of Impressionist paintings and huge dinners with stringed orchestras were famous. Hill-Stead's sumptuous lifestyle and the celebrity of its guests attracted Grace the way light draws a bedazzled moth.[15]

Theodate Pope Riddle, a woman of indomitable determination and great wealth, was a progressive idealist and philanthropist who attracted power and craved intellectual stimulation. The Flandraus estimated her fortune at $30 million before the 1929 crash. In her personal life she was kind, generous, and, some thought, domineering. Theodate's intervention on behalf of Blair's wife, whom she barely knew, was the beginning of a long period of ill will between her and Charles Flandrau.[16]

Many years after Theo's forceful action, Grace described the incident in a character sketch. Beginning with an account of what an unusual married pair the Riddles were, Grace explained how Theodate's and Charlie's antagonism started:

> Theodate as a middle-aged spinster married the middle-aged bachelor who was Charlie and Blair's older half-brother, John W. Riddle. An incredible match—he being the most frivolous, worldly, fashionable, skeptical, conventional, and yet darling old thing that can be imagined. He'd been a career diplomat, cavorted about with dissolute grand dukes and gambled for high stakes—losing most of his fortune and greatly annoying the President [Theodore Roosevelt, who appointed Riddle to several high diplomatic posts].
>
> Nothing could be more fantastic than this marriage, and nothing stormier than Theodate's relationship with Charlie who hated to have anybody

get married and especially to people who dabbled in psychical phenom-
ena. [Theodate had attempted but failed to endow a chair in psychical
research at Harvard.] Their first and most memorable battle was over me.
I was staying with Charlie while Blair was away in army service at Fort
Dodge when she descended upon St. Paul and forcibly—and I mean forcibly—removed me from Charlie's and brought me to Farmington.[17]

Thus did Grace disentangle herself from Charles Flandrau's domination.
No doubt she had described her and Blair's plight thoroughly to Theodate.
Charles was stunned. Grace's defection challenged his leadership in the
extended Flandrau family, and he never forgave Theodate.[18]

Writing Grace in Farmington from Fort Dodge in early December 1917,
Blair complained: "Oh, kiddie, I don't see why you and I always have to be
separated so much." Shortly thereafter he learned that Grace had opened her
own account at the Guaranty Trust in New York City.[19]

Although they tried living together in rented rooms off the base after Blair
was transferred to Norfolk in 1918, Grace's emotional health was too fragile
for the visits to succeed. Their letters refer to fierce arguments and make it
clear they both knew Blair's drinking didn't help her emotional state.[20]

Another factor separating them was that Blair didn't enjoy Hill-Stead. He
said he couldn't endure the big shots and lions who thought they were confer-
ring a favor on you to speak to you.[21]

Cousin Julia's success and production as a movie thrust Grace into the
national spotlight. In spite of unsteady health and frequent migraines, she
continued to write and send off short fiction to Paul Revere Reynolds in
New York. In 1918 *McClure's* magazine purchased *The Stranger in His House*,
Grace's patriotic war story. She was in good company, as *McClure's* frequently
published fiction by Edith Wharton and Mary Roberts Rinehart in this
period.

A New York newspaper columnist in *Town Topics* candidly portrayed the
author and the dilemmas of her life on June 13, 1918:

> It is said in St. Paul that Mrs. Blair Flandrau, whose book, *Cousin Julia*,
> has had a succès d'estime, has received a flattering offer from Mrs. Edith
> Wharton to assist her in literary and practical work in France. Mrs.
> Flandrau's health has been very indifferent of late, however, and she has

been under the care of specialists in the East, and at present is the guest of her sister-in-law, Mrs. John Riddle (Theodate Pope), at the latter's old home in Farmington, Conn., where she is near Blair, who is working for Uncle Sam at one of the Virginia ports. The charming Grace is inclined to go beyond her strength. Musical, a fine violinist, with literary aspirations and a great social favorite, she goes with the cleverest people—of the exclusives—in St. Paul, which includes her brother-in-law, Charles Macomb Flandrau, the writer.[22]

In October 1918 Grace entered another therapeutic clinic recommended by Theodate's friends and within days her recovery was under way. Six weeks' care under the supervision of Dr. Austin Riggs, a psychiatrist, at the Purinton Inn (now the Austin Riggs Institute) at Stockbridge, Massachusetts, gave her self-understanding and survival skills that benefited her for the rest of her life. Among the important lessons she learned was that working hard at something one believed in was therapeutic for "nerves" whereas idleness and solitude were not.[23]

On November 1, 1918, World War I ended, and on November 18 Grace was discharged from Purinton. Just days later, she had made plans to take a short-term job in Paris with the Franco-American Committee to Protect War Orphans. Her boss in France would be August Jaccaci, former art director of *McClure's* and an old friend of both John and Theodate Riddle. Jacacci considered Grace a gifted writer.[24]

Grace's contacts with Auguste Jaccaci and Edith Wharton may have come through her work for *McClure's*, but the introductions more likely occurred at Hill-Stead and/or at the Sheffield Cowles' home in Farmington. Anna Roosevelt Cowles and her husband, retired Admiral Sheffield Cowles, were the Riddles' neighbors in Farmington and childhood friends of Edith Wharton's.[25] John Riddle and Auguste Jaccaci had met years earlier when the latter had worked for the Hills in St. Paul. (In the early 1900s Auguste Jaccaci produced decorative artwork for James J. Hill's Summit Avenue mansion and the Capitol building in St. Paul and thus became acquainted with Hill family friends, the Flandraus and John Riddle.)[26]

Grace's and Blair's relatives were skeptical when she announced she was departing for Paris a few days after leaving Purinton—Charlie was openly critical and thought she was neglecting Blair—but six months in France, working to reunite war orphans with their families, restored her to health.[27]

She excelled at composing sensitive letters in French to war victims and their families. August Jaccaci, who was extremely pleased with his assistant, asked her to write an article about the agency.[28] The mood in Paris was buoyant and Grace's fluent French brought her numerous invitations. A committee of French women seeking to influence the newly created League of Nations asked her to attend with them an historic meeting with French president, Raymond Poincaré, and his wife at Elysée Palace.[29]

Grace and Blair hoped that after the war he could find a job in Europe in some aspect of food distribution or construction work. He looked into opportunities with the Hoover Commission, and Grace wrote of possible future positions for them both with the Red Cross. She opposed their return to St. Paul. But post-war jobs for Americans in Europe were scarce. Just before Blair's discharge from the army in spring 1919, a business opportunity came up for him in St. Paul.[30]

Charlie Flandrau's chauffeur, William Dundee Clark (always called "Clark") wanted Blair to go into partnership with him in the auto sales and service business. Charlie, who would be his driver's financial backer, insisted it was all Clark's idea and that he, Charlie, would not interfere.[31] Blair confided the news that "Will Lightner was willing to buy Mr. Lindeke's lot, put up a new building and lease it to us [Blair and Charlie] for ten years." They were thinking it over. Although Grace was skeptical, she knew Blair longed to return to Minnesota.[32]

Before the Flandraus' reunion in St. Paul an exchange of frank letters revealed they had no illusions about the causes of stress in their marriage and knew what was needed to relieve it. Blair confided that Charlie had warned him that all his friends had so much money that he and Grace might feel uncomfortable. He said he replied that Grace's ideas had undergone a change and that "you didn't place as much importance on 'keeping up with the Joneses.'"

Grace feared they would be left out in St. Paul without their own home, but Blair wrote: "It is impossible that we should become obscure in St. Paul if we live in a decent way, which we can perfectly well do." All his friends, Blair went on to say, "are crazy to be amused, and anyone who is willing to make an effort is an asset." But Blair knew that Grace sometimes blamed her migraines on the expectations of their friends.[33]

He conceded that he sometimes lost patience with his old crowd and hoped he and Grace could avoid getting caught up in it. For one thing, he was tired of explaining why he couldn't return to his place in Mexico. No matter how many times he described the lack of protection in the Mexican countryside, the uncertainty of labor in those revolutionary times, the size of the investment needed to bring his ranch back, and the lack of a stable coffee market, his listeners never seemed to remember.

Blair admitted that he too worried about their future: "I feel that we will come out all right, but it will depend on the way we look at things. We'll have to pull together."[34] Grace's response from Paris must have relieved him:

> Some mysterious Providence made me come and made me see all this. I have achieved some real sense of value, something real that has turned me from a selfish monster of egotism and stupidity into a human being. Don't spoil me when I get back: don't let me be so self-centered, help me to be as big a person . . . as I want to be. But I haven't much stamina. I'm weak. You must not only be good to me, as you've always been, but good for me.

Asking forgiveness for her selfishness and silliness, Grace continued:

> I long for a home. I have no objection to going to 385 [Pleasant] for a while if you are sure Charlie wants us. There must be no doubt about that. I don't want to have the feeling I had before that we were imposing on him as it gets on my nerves. Explain this well to him.[35]

A few days after mailing the letter, Grace left Paris for America.

Now it was June 1919, and she was back in St. Paul, determined to continue her professional life, to be taken seriously as a published writer. Grace was glad Blair would be as busy as she, immune to the temptations of long lunches and card games at the Minnesota Club, to the endless invitations for rounds of golf and hunting trips his friends would shower upon her.

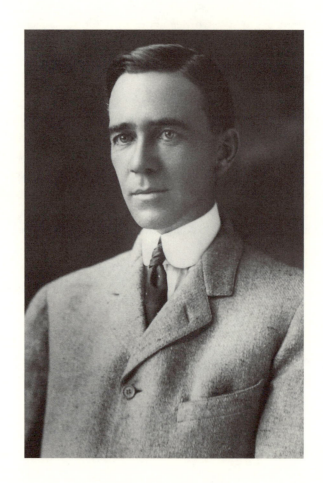

William Blair Flandrau

CHAPTER VI

Launching a Career

*"My hometown of St. Paul, Minnesota, has
been chiefly a place to go away from."*
Grace Flandrau, self-written profile, Saturday Evening Post, April 17, 1920

WHEN SHE JOINED BLAIR at his brother's home Grace found her misgivings
weren't exaggerated. The resumed ménage à trois wasn't destined to last. Charlie
had just taken a year's leave of absence from his columnist's job at the *Dispatch*,
and although Blair and Clark were planning the start-up of their business, they
were not yet working full-time.

Grace responded by renting an office away from home. After returning
from Paris, she resumed writing short fiction for popular magazines, renew-
ing her contract with literary agent, Paul Revere Reynolds. In summer and fall
1919 she took space in the New York Life Building (the location of Edward
Hodgson's last office) in downtown St. Paul. That winter she moved her office
to the Exchange Bank Building nearby. She began a productive and financially
successful period.[1]

Although she often told friends her favorite authors were those she dubbed
"the big boys"—European writers like Thomas Mann, Knut Hamsun, André
Gide, Romain Rolland, James Joyce, and Fyodor Dostoevsky, who probed
the deeper and more troubling aspects of human life—a strong desire for
commercial success motivated the young Grace Flandrau after World War I.
Having stayed abreast of the changing tastes of editors and publishers through
constant reading since childhood, she launched her career as an eclectic writer
whose style gradually evolved from genre to genre until she found her own
modern voice in travel writing, journalism, autobiographical fiction, and
memoir by the 1930s and 1940s. In 1919, however, the magazine market sought
entertainment and Grace provided it.

Magazine writing and illustration flourished in the decades between 1910
and 1940. Although circulation of literary periodicals began a slow decline
after 1900, many American readers during the infancy of radio and before the
days of television sought escape in the vernacular literature of popular magazines. Among writers and poets whose work appeared in these widely read

magazines 1915–1925 were Mary Roberts Rinehart, Edith Wharton, Robert Frost, William Faulkner, Edna St. Vincent Millay, G. K. Chesterton, Lincoln Steffens, Willa Cather, F. Scott Fitzgerald, Sinclair Lewis, Stephen Vincent Benét, Ring Lardner, Adela Rogers St. John, Arthur Payson Terhune, and Fannie Hurst.[2]

When she reentered the magazine field seriously after World War I, Grace's work appeared with these writers' stories in such periodicals as *McClure's*, *Ainslee's*, *The Smart Set*, *The Saturday Evening Post*, *Harper's Monthly*, and *Hearst's International*. Each of these popular periodicals projected a distinctive image. *The Smart Set* called itself "a magazine of cleverness"; *Ainslee's* was "the magazine that entertains"; *Sunset* was "the Pacific Monthly"; during World War I, *McClure's* became "the win-the-war magazine."

Grace's commercially profitable work in the immediate post-World War I period was light social satire. The emphasis was on sophistication, irony, and comic—sometimes slightly cruel—caricature. She often introduced irony and surprise. A steady market was available for her work.

Her earlier published writing, however, had revealed a more deeply feeling side. Grace's first published story, "Josefina Maria" (*Sunset*, 1912), is the touching portrayal of a young childless Mexican Indian woman longing to hold an infant in her arms again after her own baby has died. The story's message is that the power of maternal longing transcends all other yearnings women have for wealth, position, and domestic stability. In spite of some complex phrasing and too-long sentences the writer's deft handling of a poignant subject and the customs, speech, and dress of the Mexican villagers is unmistakable. Acute powers of observation and feeling are obvious in the haunting phrase: "The mysterious beauty of a sleeping child."

Grace wrote "Josefina Maria" in Mexico after reading Theodore Dreiser's *Jennie Gerhardt,* a novel that profoundly influenced her. The main figure of Dreiser's story, Jennie, is a single mother with a child born out of wedlock. Dreiser portrayed her as a virtuous, intelligent woman and an intensely loving mother—not as a trollop or fallen woman, the way many would.

Both Grace's first novel, *Cousin Julia* (1917), and her patriotic story, "The Stranger in His House" (*McClure's,* 1918), were serious responses to human dilemma. Although the skillfully crafted, lightly satirical stories she began turning out after the war were popular and commercially successful, Grace's early work had promised more humane and subtle gifts. Her later writing would reconfirm those gifts.

In October 1919, Paul Revere Reynolds notified Grace that he had sold her story "Dukes and Diamonds" to *The Saturday Evening Post* for $350. By November, Metro Pictures wrote asking her what she wanted for the screen rights. Although Reynolds went to work selling the film rights to Hollywood, he did not succeed. Nevertheless, the story continued to attract offers.[3]

"Dukes and Diamonds" is an intricately worked-out story about the accidental heist of a Manhattan jewelry store by a nonchalant, bumbling young titled Englishman named Terry, Lord Selwyn. Grace wrote and sold three stories in 1919-1920 about Terry and his adventures in America.[4]

The Terry stories are full of tongue-in-cheek observations such as: "Contrary to the great American creed that to be a poor nobleman is to be a fortune-hunting crook . . . " and "Terry, in some cloudy region where instinct did his thinking for him, felt that the depressing reports about his heritage constituted some sort of barrier between himself and Sylvia [an American heiress]." In the second Terry story, "Let That Pass," the unsuspecting Lord Selwyn is set up for a scam by an American con artist [Spangle] posing as a tycoon and his beautiful daughter, Yolanda. Grace's description of their encounter demonstrates her power to entertain and sure touch with detail. Readers feel sure the author has encountered these types herself:

> His [Spangle's] eyes stabbed into Terry's eyes and held them. Flashing, domineering eyes they were, that blazed out from under bushy eyebrows. Terry felt a distinct thrill when they bored into him. His many centuries of privilege and civilization had bred him back into almost as distinguished a barbarian, though of a distinctly different kind, as Spangle, whose race had never started away from the barbarous on the long circle back to it. Spangle was the real thing, and Terry had a flair for the real thing. Besides this kindred flash he was drawn to him as small boys are drawn to the ogre in the fairy tale. He held out his hand joyously, and Spangle with a sudden smile took it.

When Spangle takes Terry to his rooms for supper and drinks, "the talk was of the deliciously blood-curdling kind the Far West can produce when it lights upon innocence."

Describing two society matrons in the same story, Grace wrote: "Their bosoms were flawless toboggan slides, down which coasted pearls and diamond lavallières."

"Terry Sees Red," Grace's third story about young Lord Selwyn, appeared in the December 1920 issue of *Harper's Monthly Magazine*. (Why the *Post* didn't carry the last of the Terry series is unknown, but disagreement over price is likely.) The story conjures up intrigue to trick the naive British lord into attending a Communist rally and tries to maneuver him into making a speech denouncing the British monarchy. But Terry surprises everybody by vehemently defending his country and his beliefs. A riot erupts, Terry is hauled off to jail, newspapers carry the story, and Terry becomes a hero. At last Sylvia and her American family are impressed.

That fall Reynolds sold another of Grace's short stories, "Making Fine Birds," to *Ainslee's*. The magazine's editor, W. Adolphe Roberts, predicted the story—a sophisticated spoof of the fashion industry and its customers—would please women readers. After "Making Fine Birds" appeared in the January 1920 issue of *Ainslee's*, Roberts indicated he wanted longer stories of five to six thousand words. Although editors frequently asked Grace for greater length, her forte was writing sketches and the short, short story. Nevertheless, the quick success of "Dukes and Diamonds" and "Making Fine Birds" gave Grace and Blair confidence they could afford their own home. Reliable income from magazine writing seemed assured.

Blair and Clark's auto business, the Dundas Motor Company, opened in August 1919. Charlie simultaneously set off on extensive travels, saying he dreaded being drawn into quarrels between his brother and his chauffeur and didn't want to be in town during the shakedown period. When he returned to St. Paul after three months' absence, however, Charlie found the Dundas Motor Company operating well. He also found that Grace and Blair had moved out of his house into a residence at 548 Portland, a mile west up on Summit Hill. Their new home was in Portland Terrace, a Georgian brick townhouse row designed by Cass Gilbert in St. Paul's most fashionable neighborhood.

Charlie explained the move in a November letter to Patty Flandrau Selmes, a widow and single like himself.

> Grace and Richard hate each other. Richard [Walsh] is (quite inevitably) a "privileged" personality, "spoiled" would be the conventional verdict, set in his ways, no longer young, and at times somewhat blunt and ungracious. Grace naturally regards him as merely an uncomfortable "servant" as she has been in the family for only ten years.

But Richard has been in the family for over thirty years, and I, quite simply, cannot conceive of existence without him . . . he is about the only person with whom I still always feel like a young boy—which means a great deal, although it probably would take a May Sinclair or Arnold Bennett novel to elucidate. Grace (and I understand it perfectly) cannot apperceive Richard in this light, and they have had some unfortunate encounters. But I am supposed not to be aware of them.

Charlie told Patty he was glad Grace and Blair had stayed on good terms with him and described their new residence:

The house they have taken is lovely—one of the prettiest in town—and I know that after a very short time they both will realize how agreeable it is to have a place of their own and will wonder how they ever endured living in such an uncomfortable, antique and unfashionable locality as 385. They both look better than they have looked for years, and I think it is because I have been away for so long, and Grace has been able (in the language of the problem play) "to live her own life."

His letter added that John Riddle was planning to come, alone, to St. Paul for a visit with him and that by the same mail Grace had had a letter announcing that Theodate was coming to visit her and Blair for a few days. Charlie wondered whether John knew of his wife's plans: "If he doesn't know it will be a blow to him—or, at least, it would be a blow to me." Theodate didn't come; John did.[5]

Charlie's next acerbic comment described Riddle's visit to St. Paul in a subsequent letter to Patty on December 19, 1919:

[John's visit was] . . . a pathetic attempt to get away from Theodate's domination. . . . John, having exchanged the only things that make life worth living for three meals a day perfectly served in the middle of an infinite ocean of ennui, apparently finds himself incapable of suffering the ennui without several weeks' surcease. That is the only reason of his being here.

He added this smug comment:

> It often seems to me that Cousin Julia [Julia Dinsmore, the unmarried
> maternal aunt of Patty Flandrau Selmes and Sally Flandrau Cutcheon]
> and I are about the most nearly contented persons of my entire
> acquaintance.... Neither of us has ever had the slightest intention of
> getting married.

Charlie mentioned that Grace was speaking often of headaches and "nerves"
but was looking well. He said Blair seemed deeply interested in the auto business, was working steadily and well at it, and that he and Clark were getting
along fine so far.

While Grace was in the East that winter negotiating the sale of screen rights
to "Dukes and Diamonds," she again stayed at Hill-Stead with the Riddles.
Blair joined her briefly but returned to St. Paul for Christmas. He moved
to the Minnesota Club while Grace was away.The Flandrau brothers spent
Christmas Eve and Christmas Day of 1919 together. Blair's letters to Grace
over the holidays gave optimistic reports on the Dundas Motor Company.
He wrote that everything was "lovely as to the Charlie and Clark situation,"
and that Clark would be out selling most of the time. They had taken on a
line of trucks, had hired two salesmen, and had some serious prospects for
sales. A service manager, McLeod, had been hired "to run the floor mess and
mechanics.... We are going to be well-organized and I think things will go
well."

Blair urged Grace to tell Theodate he wanted to repay her for Grace's medical care: "We're not paupers by any means. If the worst comes to worst 'we can
work,' as Charlie says."[6]

Despite Blair's protests to the contrary, however, he and Clark were beginning to dispute the management of Dundas openly. Their conflict inevitably escalated into a rift between the two brothers. Predictably, Charlie took
Clark's side.

As the rupture deepened, Grace concentrated on writing and arranging
her new home. She worked on sketches for *The Smart Set*, the sophisticated
monthly magazine edited by H. L. Mencken and George Jean Nathan and
continued to send off short fiction to Paul Reynolds in New York.[7] In spring
1920, she moved her office to 442 Summit Avenue, a four-block walk from
her new home.[8]

Grace's profile appeared in the "Who's Who and Why" column of the July
15, 1920, issue of The *Saturday Evening Post*. Besides "Dukes and Diamonds"

the *Post* had published Flandrau's second story about Terry, "Let That Pass," the preceding April 17. (Hollywood later bought the rights to both "Dukes and Diamonds" and "Let that Pass" to use as one piece.)[9]

The self-written profile projects a cocky, witty, thoroughly modern young woman of unconventional temperament, the prototype of what cultural historians have since called the "New Woman". Readers can imagine Katherine Hepburn or Carol Lombard deadpanning these remarks to reporters.

> I received the first part of my education—there wasn't any other part—in a French convent in Paris. . . . My first stories were written about the Totonac Indians of Vera Cruz, and they were published in *Sunset* magazine . . . My tastes are not simple, but I do not like automobiles. Incidentally, I hate noise, live turkeys, gardening and Parlor Bolshevists.
>
> My ambition is to write stories of gloomy realism in the mood of Artzybashef's *Seven Who Were Hanged* and find an editor who will publish them. Up to the present moment I have found no editor who did not regard such attempts of mine with enthusiastic and unmitigated indifference.

The story concluded with Grace's provocative comment: "My hometown of St. Paul, Minnesota, has been chiefly a place to go away from." That frank statement and the disillusioned, pessimist-leaning paragraph that preceded it reveal Grace's identification with other avant-garde American writers—spokesmen for the "lost generation"—and the literary trailblazers who had influenced them. She began dropping four years from her true age.

By 1920, a sea change in American literary taste had taken place. Malcolm Cowley, a critic, poet, and for many years editor of The *New Republic*, described the revolution in his books *After the Genteel Tradition* and *Exile's Return: A Narrative of Ideas*. Cowley's foreword for *After the Genteel Tradition* (quoting Sinclair Lewis's famous Nobel Prize acceptance speech in Stockholm in 1930) described this literary Armageddon and how it came about. The revolt, Cowley explained, was against Victorian gentility, Puritanism, provincialism, Emersonian optimism, and the influence of the English literary tradition on American writers. The sweeping change had been coming on for some time.

"The real war against gentility," Cowley wrote, "had been fought in the decade before World War I. . . . Every new book was a skirmish with the conservatives." Instigators of the revolt were writers of realism like Theodore

Dreiser, Willa Cather, and Hamlin Garland. An example of the "rallying grounds of the rebel forces" was *The Smart Set*, the provocative magazine edited by H. L. Mencken and his partner, George Jean Nathan. The magazine, launched in 1908 and at its peak of influence around 1913, heralded the message that it was time to challenge the sacred cows of American culture. Literary rebels, ready for change, rallied to the cry.

The leaders of "the lost generation," Cowley wrote, were younger writers who, for the most part, had been born around the turn of the century and who, as a result of the social disruptions, disillusion, and worldliness brought on by World War I, had broken with the values and traditions of the past. They had not yet replaced the old values with new beliefs.

In *Exile's Return: A Narrative of Ideas*, Cowley, himself a young dissenter, wrote:

> The first rebellion of the "lost generation" was against the conventionality of their elders and the gentility of American letters; then it was against the high phrases that justified the slaughter of millions in World War I. Then it was against the philistinism and scramble for money of the Harding years.

Cowley explained that the ideas of "the lost generation" were social and economic before their expression in literature. The young writers were seeking "a new way to live." And when their thinking found expression in writing, millions of Americans, their readers, "who had never been to New York, were thinking and talking like Greenwich Villagers." Although she was a decade or more older than most of these young writers, Grace, strongly influenced by Dreiser, Garland, and Mencken, wholeheartedly endorsed their thinking.

But different genres of writing always run parallel, overlap, and blur into each other. Although the movement toward realism began before World War I, disillusion, cynicism, and anti-conventionalism did not until after the war become dominant themes in American letters.

Grace's first novel, *Cousin Julia* (1917), a story about the clash of youthful idealism versus mature pragmatism in a wealthy family, had come out of the late Victorian Georgian or mannerist tradition. But her newer short fiction pieces for *Ainslee's* and *The Saturday Evening Post* ("Making Fine Birds" and the Terry, Lord Selwyn, stories, 1919 and 1920, respectively), moved toward satire of the upper classes for their righteous attitudes and narrow point of view.

Two Minnesota writers, Sinclair Lewis with *Main Street* and F. Scott Fitzgerald with *This Side of Paradise*, both published in 1920, were in the vanguard of the change toward realism. When national attention focused on these two new authors, their place of residence, St. Paul, Minnesota, became a high-profile literary capital, attracting other writers to the state. Sinclair Lewis, who was awarded the Pulitzer Prize in 1926 (although he refused it), received the Nobel Prize for literature in 1930. He inhabited at least three residences in the Twin Cities in the 1920s before leaving for New York City. Scott Fitzgerald, who was born in St. Paul in 1896, grew up in the city's Hill District and continued to live there before and, briefly, after his marriage to Zelda Sayre until 1922. Their daughter, Scottie, was born in St. Paul.

Although Charles Flandrau was two generations older than these "lost generation" writers and by 1920 had ceased writing professionally, younger writers still regarded him as the reigning literary lion in Minnesota. Scott Fitzgerald looked to him as a mentor—but also as a has-been—and asked him to read his manuscripts for *This Side of Paradise* in 1919 and *The Beautiful and Damned* in 1921, prior to publication.[10]

Other writers active in St. Paul and Minneapolis in the early 1920s were Thomas A. Boyd and his attractive wife, Peggy (Woodward) Boyd. Both began their literary careers as columnists, and Charles Scribner's Sons published both Boyds' first novels in the 1920s. Tom Boyd also managed Kilmarnock bookstore at 84 E. 4th Street in downtown St. Paul with his Harvard friend, Cornelius Van Ness, the owner. Kilmarnock's was a well-known gathering spot for local writers, a place where Sinclair Lewis and Scott Fitzgerald frequently encountered the Flandraus. According to his biographers, Scott first established contact with New York literary agent Paul Revere Reynolds through Grace.[11]

Another literary gathering place in the 1920s was St. Paul's Nimbus Club, an informal group of local professional writers that met once a week at Kilmarnock's to discuss books and authors. Its membership included, among others, Charles Flandrau, Grace Flandrau, St. Paul mayor, sports columnist, and poet, Lawrence Corrin Hodgson (Larry Ho),* Tom and Peggy Boyd, and local journalists Frances Boardman, her younger brother, Lawrence Boardman, and a new young critic and literary hopeful, James Gray. By 1920

---

* Poet, columnist, and later St. Paul mayor, Lawrence Corrin Hodgson, "Larry Ho," was Grace Flandrau's first cousin. Whether they acknowledged this connection publicly is unknown.

Gray had succeeded Charles Flandrau as music and theater critic for the *St. Paul Pioneer Press-Dispatch*. Naturally, these literary activists held strong opinions on the merits and shortcomings of books and authors, especially those in their midst.

A number of these writers—the Flandraus, the Boardmans, the Fitzgeralds, the Boyds, James Gray and his bride, Sophie Stryker, and Sinclair Lewis—lived in the same neighborhood, St. Paul's picturesque Hill District. In a loose way, despite age and social rank differences, they were acquainted in the way neighbors are—especially neighbors who are all writers. Undoubtedly, it was generally known that the magazine writer, St. Paul's Grace Flandrau, had grown up on Dayton Avenue, on the declining north edge of the Hill District, and that compromising rumors had clouded her childhood. (Grace's birthplace at 518 Dayton was a block away from F. Scott Fitzgerald's birthplace at 481 Laurel.)

Perhaps rivalry between local celebrity authors, would-be authors, and their local critics explains why both the *St. Paul Pioneer Press-Dispatch* and *St. Paul Daily News* literary pages virtually ceased in-house review of books in 1915–1920 but instead published a weekly list of new works purchased by the St. Paul Public Library. (Charles Flandrau's 1917 review of Grace's *Cousin Julia* was an exception.) Inviting their readers or the City Librarian to review new books for their pages, running syndicated literary columnists, and serializing chapters of new fiction by out-of-town authors were the newspapers' efforts at neutrality in these years. H. L. Mencken, George Jean Nathan, and Louella B. Parsons are examples of syndicated national writers whose ideas often appeared in the *Pioneer Press-Dispatch* Sunday pages during the 1920s. By comparison to the paucity of coverage of new books, local theater and musical performance consistently received extensive coverage in St. Paul newspapers.

Newcomer Tom Boyd, however, with the help of his wife, Peggy, began a successful literary column, "In a Corner with the Bookworm," in the *St. Paul Daily News* in 1920 and continued it until 1924 when he and Peggy moved to Minneapolis and, later, away from Minnesota. Rivalry between the Boyds and Flandraus may have precipitated their departure. Unquestionably, her connection with the famous Charles Flandrau advantaged Grace over other aspiring writers and tipped the scales in her favor.[10]

On Sunday, February 15, 1920 Grace's picture appeared with those of four other local authors in a *St. Paul Daily News* story called "Breaking into the Magazines: St. Paul Writers Tell How They Put It Over." The story by Chester

W. Vonier described the recent works of Lily A. Long, F. Scott Fitzgerald, Emma Mauritz Larson, W. G. Shepherd, and Mrs. Blair Flandrau.

By 1920 Grace had begun to view her popular short magazine fiction as trivial, but agent Paul Reynolds disagreed. His comments on the cynicism and pessimism in her newer work in the summer of 1920 were by no means favorable. He criticized "Alone" because, although he found it well done, it was depressing. "One Afternoon" was "clever but not popular in type." He felt he couldn't sell them. And while he liked "Just Like Wally," he criticized its climax. In June Reynolds wrote that "Ludlow's Luck" was a "bully story" and that he expected to sell it quickly. He didn't succeed, however, and the story didn't find a publisher for three years. Later that summer Reynolds notified Grace again that he hadn't yet been able to sell the motion picture rights to "Dukes and Diamonds." He also returned her new story "Billboards and Buttercups," saying he couldn't sell it to any of six magazines. In September Reynolds returned "An August Interlude" with the comment that he tried but failed to sell it to four magazines.[12]

By this time, however, perhaps discouraged by the uncertainty of magazine income and feeling she had something more serious to say than her agent found acceptable, Grace broke her connection with Reynolds and began working on a new novel. She didn't contract with another agent for the next two years.

Meanwhile, Blair and Charlie's relationship was deteriorating, and Grace's health, always a sensitive barometer of prevailing pressures in Flandrau dynamics, worsened. At the end of December 1920 she had surgery in a St. Paul hospital. Writing a young friend, she treated her operation casually and did not identify the nature of the surgery.[13]

Grace's correspondent, Elizabeth (Betty) Foster, was the daughter of Minnesota pioneers Burnside and Sophie Foster of St. Paul. Betty and her mother traveled frequently to Europe, spending several months at a time in France and Italy while Betty studied art. Foster was a St. Paul native in her twenties and Grace was twelve years older when their correspondence began in the 1920s. Her letters to Foster over the next twenty years reveal intimate details of Grace's life.

On December 29, 1920, two days after she was released from the hospital, Grace wrote Betty in Rome. She described her new home and the status of her writing. A young, duty-bound housewife's nostalgia for her carefree youth surfaced: "The house is rather charming in <u>spots</u>. The library is nice and the parlor would be if I had enough of the right kind of furniture. But I shall have to wait twenty or thirty years before getting it."

Imagining herself in Betty's shoes in Italy, Grace wrote, "When spring begins to come in Rome smell the orange blossoms for me. I am thinking of the sun in those piazza steps and the baskets of flowers. As to the rest I think the small bronzes and marbles and Palestrina masses I envy you the most—especially the music—a boy choir in a cathedral."

Continuing, Grace said that she was not putting "pen to paper . . . and sometimes I think I never will . . . however economic pressure looms before me rather threateningly." She told Betty that, although the editors of *The Smart Set,* H.L. Mencken and George Jean Nathan, liked her short fictional sketches of society figures and wanted to see more, she didn't consider them serious writing: "There are so many things one would like to think about tranquilly and deeply without rushing into print with some half-baked nonsense."[14]

John and Theodate Riddle repeatedly invited Blair and Grace to visit them in the winter of 1920-21. Theo worried almost as much about Blair's health as she did about Grace's. "Blair must fatten up at intervals," she wrote to Grace. Both women fretted over Blair's being too thin and his chain smoking. When Grace visited Hill-Stead after Christmas, Theo wrote Blair: "She has violent headaches and suffers from extreme nervous fatigue. I am not bringing into the question her attack of influenza which has made matters worse."[15]

Theo feared continuing poor health would undermine her protégée's will to write. Although Mary Hodgson urged Grace to recuperate in California after her surgery, she felt Blair should not be left alone again. Mary Hodgson kept hoping he would move his business out west.[16]

The rift between the Blair Flandraus and Charlie reached its climax in the early months of 1921. Problems at Dundas were increasing, and relations between Blair and Clark had been deteriorating for a year. But issues more profound than business were at stake: family leadership and credibility among Flandrau siblings. Charlie finally admitted the severity of his rupture with Blair and Grace and his perception of its causes in a February 1921 letter to Patty Selmes. He confessed that one day a year earlier Blair had telephoned him "in great anger and excitement to say that he was done with me."

After that call, Charlie continued, he had written Blair a conciliatory letter. But Blair replied with a letter in which he declared:

All my life ever since we were boys I had plotted against him, tried to undermine him and do everything in my power to injure him.

Well, this letter I did not answer. It was merely the reckless emanation of a person, ill at the time, and also in a rather pitiful state of nerves from the combined circumstances of financial complications, an emotional, sometimes hysterical wife suffering from wounded vanity, and large quantities of whiskey. . . . But I have never seen either of them since, never communicate with them even on business . . . The trouble was that when Grace found out from Richard . . . that after half a dozen years of having my home turned into a combined cabaret and sanatorium, I had reached the point of wishing to live alone, her poor, shallow, artificial little nature received a blow from which it has never recovered. . . . She was spoiling for a chance to be dramatic and break with me. Her pathetic painted lips used positively to tremble and waggle with hate, and she seized on the first excuse . . . to goad Blair on.

The past year has been to me one of absolute peace and contentment. The mere fact of not having to live in an atmosphere of continual marital misunderstandings, hurt feelings, accusations of "selfishness" (poor Blair once in so often would tell me in despair and at length that he had never dreamed any human being could be as selfish as Grace—and of course I would have to deny it and rush to her defense) has been of infinite relief to me.

Grace, for all her cleverness and superficial abilities, has always been a victim of temperament and ungratified ambitions. She cares only for the rich and the hectically fashionable, but has to be a perpetual parasite and "hanger-on" because Blair has no money and has always been incompetent to make any. . . . Mother never liked her.

Charlie's letter ended with assurances that he would always be ready to "take up the thread where it was dropped. . . . I feel toward them both . . . as I always have."[17]

Although low in spirits and health that winter, Grace received professional encouragement. George Jean Nathan wrote her early in March 1921, accepting "Oh, Horrors" for *The Smart Set* and asking to see "a longer short story of 3–4,000 words."[18]

"Oh, Horrors" (later renamed "Rubies in Crystal") describes the beginning of an illicit affair between a beautiful, young, unsophisticated American woman, Lilly, and a dark, intense, young Italian politician, Diego. Lilly is the wife of a wealthy, older man, Skarth, who is a pillar of Scarsdale, New York, society and from a higher station in life than Lilly. When Skarth receives a diplomatic appointment in Italy as Chargé, he and Lilly move to Rome where they frequently encounter Diego. Telling descriptions of the highly charged emotions between two young adults about to engage in adultery build, step by step, to the inevitable climax.

CHAPTER VII

An Unorthodox Wife in the Roaring Twenties

"That's Charlie's way,"
Blair Flandrau to Grace Flandrau, April 15, 1921

TO RECUPERATE FROM SURGERY and distance herself from bitter feelings between the Flandrau brothers, in spring 1921 Grace made an extended visit to Mary Hodgson, Lucile and Ralph Willis, and the other Staples relatives in La Mesa, California. Over the twelve years of her marriage, as she once confided to Charles, Grace had found visits with Mary and her relatives less and less congenial. For this visit, however, Grace was absent from St. Paul for about two months.[1]

Her stepmother's faithful correspondence with Grace projects the image of an ordinary, gentle woman, someone whose days revolved around cooking, sewing, gardening, and weather reports, whose occasional outings to organ concerts, church services, picnics, and movies provided all the entertainment there was. Mary Hodgson's letters to Grace frequently mentioned fashions but never books. La Mesa was a far cry from Hill-Stead.[2]

Despite their increasingly artificial relationship, Grace continued to call Mary "mother" and to treat Mary's Staples relatives as her family. She apparently had no contact with her birth mother, Anna Hodson, or with her brother, William, or even with other Minnesota Hodgsons in these years. In the 1920s the Flandraus still believed that the Staples were Grace's blood kin. During her stay in California, Grace's main correspondents were Blair, Theodate Riddle, Betty Foster, and Brenda Ueland.

Blair's letters reported on his social life and the progress of Dundas Motors. An affair between a prominent man and woman in their crowd had everybody talking. Blair told Grace he missed her terribly and had had no rush of invitations in her absence. He was being "an awful good boy"—going to the movies and to "symphony nights"—and he confided that when their friends asked for Charles's whereabouts (on his travels), they couldn't get over it when he didn't know.

While in California, Grace visited Blair's half-sisters, Sally Cutcheon and Patty Selmes, wintering in Santa Barbara. Afterwards she wrote Blair that

Sally and Patty had urged them to patch things up with Charles, but in his next letter Blair exploded over what he saw as his brother's habitual two-faced behavior:

> The reason Patty and all of them love Charlie is because they literally never see him, and he writes them nice long letters all the time. . . . Patty wouldn't be so infatuated with him if she saw him much. He wasn't her darling Buddie when he kicked her out of the house [C. E. and Rebecca Flandrau's house in St. Paul]. . . . Of course John and Theodate would be nice to him. You must remember we heard much more about the "tragic situation" of John and Theo's marriage than John and Theo did. That's Charlie's way.[3]

Blair's letters described his many invitations to accompany single women to parties in St. Paul. Although members of the Flandraus' St. Paul crowd had become her friends too, Grace often said she had little in common with them. They seemed a whole generation older than she. When she doubted their acceptance of her, Blair vehemently disagreed: "Everybody simply adores you. . . . There isn't another girl so loved and sought after as you." He called her "the little home brightener" and said, "Oh, Keekie, how I wish you and I could just live together out there and just love. I know it is impossible for me to be away from you ever again."[4]

During Grace's absence Clark left Dundas Motor Company, and Blair changed the company's name to "Flandrau Motor Company." In that period, Theodate Riddle made Blair a business loan, most likely to buy out Charles's interest. The company became the Minnesota dealer for F.W.D. cars and trucks. Blair placed two sales agents on the Iron Range where Minnesota's burgeoning mining industry was generating need for new towns and roads. In mid-1921, however, the United States was in recession and little home construction or road building took place in Minnesota.

Another problem, according to Blair's letters, was that many customers didn't pay promptly. Although prices of the vehicles carried by Flandrau Motor Company had gone down, sales commissions had gone up. The company's profit margin was shrinking.

As manager of their finances, Blair went over all the household bills in Grace's absence. Both spouses contributed to a joint account for household and personal bills. Notifying Grace that she had $924 in personal bills, Blair requested she contribute $500 from her account at Guaranty Trust in New York to their joint account in St. Paul. He said he would take Flandrau Motor Company funds to pay bills when customers paid up.[5]

Grace remained in low spirits that spring. In April 1921 she confided to Betty Foster, who was vacationing in Italy:

> La Mesa is the most inappropriate place to get letters from Rome, Sienna and Florence. It is a large, sunny, windy, empty piece of nothing. You feel intensely that no one has ever thought here or suffered. . . . It's dreadful! It's inconceivable that anyone should open a book. They just plant mindless carcasses on the back seats of automobiles and roll endlessly from movie to cafeteria . . . and play the phonograph and talk about the climate and get old and die in the sunshine and get buried by a Methodist preacher who splits his infinitives. Even St. Paul from this angle has all the flavor of a Gothic cathedral.

Envy of Betty's carefree single life in Europe surfaced in Grace's letters. "I suppose you are now in Paris . . . 'Paris,' said she with a low moan." Commenting on Betty's latest romance, Grace wrote: "Your Mr. Berrill sounds remarkably nice. I wonder why you aren't in love with him. I was always in love with everybody."[6]

While in California, Grace also confided in Brenda Ueland, a young Minnesota writer. Ueland, who was living with her husband, Ben Benedict, a banker, in a walk-up apartment in Greenwich Village, was pregnant and leading a Bohemian artist's life. Like Foster and Flandrau, Ueland had the anti-conventional, avant-garde views of many young women in the Roaring Twenties.

Responding to one of Grace's morose letters, Ueland wrote: "Too bad California is such hell. Benjy said Los Angeles was terribly unpleasant—boa constrictors, cacti, acacea [sic], blossoms, sunshine. San Francisco is better. In San Francisco it is foggy and gray. Much better." With feminist bravado, Ueland continued: "I don't know what the Taylors are going to do this summer. Anne [Anne Ueland Taylor, Brenda's sister] threatens to go to France for a couple of months, but I think she is bluffing, and I have an idea she is unfortunate in not possessing a debonair independence of husband like yourself or me. We leave them lightly without a qualm—the Taylors cling to each other."[7]

Grace and Brenda were believers in the "modern" view of marriage, a cornerstone of the "Jazz Age" culture. "Flappers" in that iconoclastic period held the view that their conduct could be as independent of conventional marriage as men's had always been. Irreverence toward idealized marriage often surfaced in *The Smart Set*, the sophisticated magazine Grace and other "new women" admired.

Reminiscing about the period, F. Scott Fitzgerald described post-World War I social attitudes and behavior in "Echoes of the Jazz Age," published in 1945 in *The Crack Up*: "It was an age of miracles, it was an age of excess, and it was an age of satire. . . . The word jazz in its progress toward respectability has meant first sex, then dancing, then music."

Brian Gallagher, author of *Anything Goes*, a 1987 biography of Neysa McMein (a famous Jazz Age magazine illustrator and femme fatale), quotes the artist's daughter, Joan, to describe the prevailing attitude of females in her mother's Algonquin Round Table crowd: "They were dutifully to have the extramarital affairs that the twenties demanded as proof of emancipation, but the point of such affairs was supposed to be their casualness." Gallagher's book elaborates further on the mood of the post-World War I era: "New York sophistication around 1920 demanded, from most of its practitioners, a certain hardness."

Unquestionably, Grace Flandrau and Brenda Ueland affected this hardness in the 1920s and undoubtedly invoked harsh criticism back home in Minnesota. One feels sure that the emancipated lifestyles of earlier women writers such as George Sand, Colette, and Edith Wharton strongly influenced Jazz Age artists such as Flandrau and Ueland.

Although Grace professed freedom from conventional ideas about marriage and later admitted to having had three affairs during her and Blair's many separations in their early marriage, there is no evidence she was chronically given to casual relationships. No aura of promiscuity lingers over the story of her life, and, as she aged, she grew more circumspect about appearances. Grace undeniably captivated men and unfailingly projected toward them, but she had devoted women and couple friends too. When they were apart, as they frequently were, Blair and Grace corresponded almost daily over many years. Nevertheless, the Flandraus' unusual married life gave both partners the independence for affairs. This "arrangement" must have led to endless speculation and vehement disapproval in the conservative Midwest.[8]

While she languished, bored and idle in La Mesa, Grace stayed in touch with the Riddles. She admitted to Theodate that, although she was planning work in her head, she wasn't writing.

At first Theodate was sympathetic to her protégée's low mood: "Do not push your intellect, which is frightfully fatiguing and makes one downright sick," but she urged Grace to resume her work: "You have very keen sympathetic insight and everyone you come in contact with is grist for your mill. . . . Something surges up if work is founded in the emotional nature. It is then art. . . . Art is the result of thwarted passion . . . Art is restrained and honest expression."

Theodate's next letter to Grace was a stern rebuke: "It is a sickening thing to me to observe you from this distance wasting your life . . . throwing your great talents to the winds. I am assuming you could have health if you would, and I believe my assumption is a true one."[9]

In 1921 Theodate Riddle threw her considerable resources and energies into establishing a new experimental school for boys in Farmington, Connecticut. Named the Avon Old Farms School for Boys, it was founded on Theo's strongly held premise that physical labor stimulated and trained the mind. She donated land outside Farmington for the school's campus and launched it with a donation of $1 million. "Hully Gee, as John would say," was Blair's response to the news.[10]

After Grace's visit to Patty Selmes and Sally Cutcheon in Santa Barbara, the sisters continued insisting to Charles that he reconcile with Blair and Grace. But his animosity toward his sister-in-law was deep. He wrote Patty in May, saying that although he thought Grace still loved Blair, "Theodate is 'on' to Grace."[11] In a June letter to Patty, Charlie admitted: "Grace is really almost a brilliant person, but, in all sincerity, at the age of almost fifty, I no longer give a damn about brilliancy."[12] His assertions marked the low point in Charles's relationship with his brother's wife. No doubt Grace's increasing influence in their extended Flandrau family and over the younger brother he had once dominated severely threatened Charles.

Grace returned to St. Paul in early summer to begin another productive period. She polished her sketches for *The Smart Set*, revised rejected stories, and continued working on her novel. She wrote Betty Foster:

> Keep your eye on *The Smart Set* and write me what you think. . . . Mr.
> Nathan insists on calling the sketches "Rubies in Crystal. " It approaches

a little more nearly what I wish to do. He and Mencken have been quite flattering about wanting more.[13]

In spite of growing success as a writer, however, Grace remained down-hearted. When she wrote Brenda Ueland that the black French bull puppy Blair had given her for Christmas wasn't trainable and ran away constantly, she must have confessed how much she wanted a child. Ueland sympathized and offered to give Grace her baby: "I am resigned to a dull life till baby comes. What shall I name it? Certainly I will give it to you. I wish you could have one. You are wrong [however]. Children are just as deceiving as French bulls." Both Flandraus were animal lovers, and after 1920 they never again lived without pets.[14]

During the years 1921 to 1925, Grace worked steadily at writing, and eventually her professional success and their mutual passion for books brought a lasting reconciliation with Charles—at least outwardly. By 1923, the two had resumed their correspondence whenever either was out of town.

For one thing, both Charlie and Grace became interested in boosting the career of Scott Fitzgerald. The success of *The Beautiful and Damned* in 1922 was cause for celebration. Between 1923 and 1925, whenever the Fitzgeralds returned to St. Paul, Charles gave dinner parties at 385 Pleasant for Scott and Zelda. During the period in which the Flandraus and Fitzgeralds saw each other regularly, Charlie wrote Grace: "Scott (F.) is the most clever, attractive, really sympathetic creature I have run across in years."[15]

A modus vivendi between Blair and his brother came more slowly. They did not correspond between 1919 and 1921, and, although both began seeking reconciliation by mid-1921, their uncomfortable relationship did not recover until nearly the end of their lives. After 1920 Blair pretty much left it to Grace to communicate with his brother.

Once resumed, correspondence between Grace and Charles flourished until his death in 1938. After Rebecca's death, he had transferred his dependence to Patty Selmes, and after Patty's death in 1923, he transferred it to Grace, who appeared to become her brother-in-law's closest confidante. With her he shared his thoughts about family news and grudges, literary opinions, St. Paul gossip, impressions from abroad, pets, and complaints about his health. When he sent her colorful letters on his travels, Grace typed and saved them for possible publication. Personal correspondence became the Flandraus' writing practice. It also provided an indispensable bridge between two equally proud, volatile temperaments. Among Grace's notes is this posthumous description of Charles Flandrau: "[He was] a man who sees every smallest detail, with sharp immediacy and human involvement . . . detached, reflective . . . almost schizophrenic . . . aloof and elusive, prissy, almost a trifle smug . . . constrained by an acute awareness of his own sensibilities or it might be, nerves."

And Grace thoroughly admired her brother-in-law's writing. In her Notes she spoke of Charles's "wry continual flow of wit . . . light felicity of expression [that] all tend to conceal the close knit sequence of his thought. . . . The pattern . . . the use of simile and metaphor . . . returned to again with . . . perfection not unlike the announced and recurring theme in music . . . and . . . the lapidary elegance, under a casual guise, of his prose. . . . But they are not the things for which the great mass of readers turn to the written word or have the patience or the perception to find and take pleasure in. . . . There are other serious readers . . . who demand a dimension, which Flandrau did not touch. . . . Perhaps one might call it the tragic sense."[16]

CHAPTER VIII

Celebrity

"I write because I must."
Grace Flandrau, New York Tribune, February 25, 1923

GRACE SPENT CHRISTMAS OF 1921 and New Year's of 1922 at Hill-Stead with the Riddles. She expected to negotiate a publishing contract for her new novel with D. Appleton and Company after the New Year. Blair declined the trip because of business.

Separation over the holidays became a pattern for the Flandraus. Publishers in New York frequently scheduled meetings with Grace after Christmas, and Blair was always in demand for seasonal festivities at home. Undoubtedly his friends sympathized with him over his wife's holiday absences. His letters spoke of missing Grace: "The house is so still and meaningless without you in it. I think I need you more than you need me." He confided that Charlie seemed increasingly lonely.[1]

Blair spent New Year's Eve by himself, but he was never alone long. Both men and women called him and kept him busy. He was trying to curtail his drinking. After he went to the Jack Ordways' for dinner early in January he wrote Grace: "The highball I had was the first drink of any kind I've had in four days, so you see I'm at least trying to be a good and a careful."[2] He reported that although the ladies seemed to find him attractive and tried to engage him in conversation, he was only polite. He confessed he had a good talk at one party with a beautiful divorcée, Mary Griggs Barbee. Another woman friend at the party, Caroline Lindeke, had probed for information on Grace's whereabouts.[3]

Grace met with D. Appleton's after Christmas, but Harcourt, Brace and Company also wanted to read her manuscript. Following an appointment with Harrison Smith, a Harcourt editor, Grace wrote Blair:

> Harcourt, Brace adores my book. They haven't finished it yet, but so far, the man [Harrison Smith] seems to be crazy about it! He's determined to get me away from Appleton's. He said, "It's great work, Mrs. Flandrau. Real and not dreary...Sinclair Lewis is bringing out a book about St.

Paul [Babbitt] in the autumn and this will be the feminine counterpart."
He may change his mind or Mr. Harcourt may not share his enthusiasm,
but I tell you it was pretty jolly. Don't breathe a word of this.[4]

Two days later, when she had made up her mind to stick with Appleton's,
Harrison Smith protested again and, with much flattery, persuaded Grace
to give Harcourt, Brace the publishing rights to *Being Respectable*. Frank
Cutcheon (husband of Sally Flandrau Cutcheon), a New York attorney,
advised Grace on the publishing contract. Cutcheon escorted her to dinners
and plays during her stay in Manhattan.

Blair sent a congratulatory note: "Now your ambitions will be realized. You
will have an interesting, successful and important life. . . . Oh, Keekie, you,
you have everything." He told her he knew she was a "very exceptional person"
and that he had prayed for her success.[5]

Grace remained in the east through January and into February. The Riddles
loaned her their apartment at Carlton House in Manhattan for meetings with
Harcourt, Brace. Late in January Harrison Smith sent a positive note about
Being Respectable: "It is an honest, straight-forward novel without any of the
sentimentalities that is [sic] the curse of American literature. It is written with
clear insight into the empty, hectic life you have seen about you and yet it is
warm-hearted and kindly. In my mind it is the type of novel, as you are the
type of writer, that we want to publish and encourage to go on writing and on
whom we are founding our success."[6]

In February, while still in New York, Grace contracted with a new agent,
Harold Paget of the Paget Agencies, 500 Fifth Avenue. Their professional
correspondence took place between February 1922 and July 1924. Paget was
familiar with her December 1919 *Post* story, "Dukes and Diamonds." He told
Grace he wished she could turn out that kind of "young-love-and-humor"
story once a week and revived the idea of selling the screen rights to the story.
He suggested she try developing the piece more.[7]

Blair's January letters contained accounts of movies, symphony classes,
dinners, cotillions, prizefights, and bridge. He wrote that he particularly
enjoyed Mrs. Roger (Katherine K.) Shepard, whom he described as "a peach
of a woman." He also mentioned that everybody was talking about the houses
of assignation that were springing up in the Cathedral Hill area, still considered one of St. Paul's nicest residential districts.[8]

Flandrau Motor Company was working hard to sell F.W.D. trucks to Great

Northern Railway, Blair wrote, to grade beds for new tracks and service their feeder lines. He scheduled meetings with C. O. Jenks, vice president for operations of the railroad, and William Kenny, vice president in charge of traffic, both of whom he knew personally. He hoped to land a contract for the purchase of as many as forty F.W.D. trucks. Jenks and Kenny notified him the mechanical department would make the decision.[9]

Blair was also working late hours with his bookkeeper, Moran, to bring the company's outstanding accounts up-to-date. In early February he wrote Grace: "Just the garage bills alone amount to almost $1650, but nobody pays anything anymore—you and I included—and it's <u>awful</u> to get any money in."[10]

A bone of contention between the Flandraus that winter was that Blair had paid no interest or principal on his debt to Theodate. Grace said she felt increasingly embarrassed about it, all the more so because the Riddles, who had been so generous to her, knew of her recent earnings. She leveled with Blair:

> It is very awkward here for me with their knowledge of the movie money and the money from stories, etc.—which sounds more than it really is—for us to be paying no interest on your debt. I'm even ashamed of producing a good-looking dress. Now, if you will please write Theo at once and explain that I would be glad to try to pay some of it from my earnings but you will not permit it. Explain again that you are counting on the gas-railway stuff to put you in a position to pay interest and capital in a year or so, and if it doesn't, that the garage is paying for itself, that inside five or six years you will own a building and will instantly turn over to her an interest in that building equivalent to your debt and interest. . . . Is there anything I can say to insure your doing precisely this the day you get my letter? If you have any idea that she is casual about that or any other money you are much mistaken. She [Theodate] is extremely business-like and needs every bit of money she can get now for the vast expenses [of the Avon Old Farms School for Boys]. So please do this, dear, and do it just as I ask.[11]

Before she left for the East that winter, Grace hired and trained Mary O'Malley, an Irish cook. Blair reported that buttons were miraculously reappearing on his shirts and underwear, though he "sort of missed the safety pins." Mary O'Malley's presence in the Flandrau household would last five decades.[12]

Grace returned to St. Paul in late February, planning to devote most of the rest of 1922 to completion of her third novel, *Entranced*. Blair had been working on a novel too. Grace planned to show his work to Harcourt, Brace and Company on her next trip East.[13]

Disciplined as she tried to be in St. Paul, Grace, like Blair, had difficulty spurning invitations. She too was an extrovert who thrived on the stimulation of lively discourse, but she also needed solitude for her work. When the young author, age thirty-six in 1922, appeared with her attentive husband, age forty-seven, at the dinners, teas, and house parties they were invited to in Minnesota, the hosts and hostesses, usually a decade or more older than Grace, had on their hands an attractive, highly entertaining, and unconventional personality as well as a severe social critic in disguise.

Twin Cities' society was probably unaware of Grace Flandrau's ambivalence toward its lifestyle and values in 1922 since her novels, *Being Respectable* and *Entranced*—social satires of St. Paul—would not be published until 1923 and 1924. But Grace revealed her thoughts freely to her younger friends. Writing Betty Foster in the summer of 1922, Grace said she and Blair had visited close friends of Blair's at the Brule River and at White Bear Lake: "I am rather enjoying it strange as it may seem."[14]

October 1922 brought mixed news from the publishing world. Harold Paget had sold her story "A Path of Gold" (a.k.a. "Ludlow's Luck"), to *Cosmopolitan*, but he advised that, since Grace had not published in magazines for almost two years, she would have to accept just $400 for it.[15]

Within two months she turned to another New York agent, Carl Hovey. Hovey took the assignment and offered both praise and constructive criticism. One of his first acts was to sell "A Path of Gold" to *Hearst's International*, but the price was still $400. The story appeared in the magazine's February 1923 issue. Flandrau had sent Hovey a copy of "Billboards and Buttercups,"—still unsold—the previous fall. In December, he wrote that he found the story "perfectly charming—Edith Wharton more than Ring Lardner." He urged Grace "to dig down more into the feelings of people. Even in a humorous or satirical story something has to matter enough to rouse the feelings of our readers." But, Hovey added, "I am positive there is no limit to your capacity! Please try a more real, a more emotional story, but don't leave out the humor either."[16] A month later Hovey repeated his suggestion that Grace "deepen and broaden" her work. He said that he had an offer of $500 for "Billboards and Buttercups."[17]

In mid-November 1922 Alfred Harcourt of Harcourt, Brace and Company wrote Grace, offering her $3,000 for her share of the movie rights to *Being Respectable*.[18] He informed her that Scott Fitzgerald had been paid $2,500 for the film rights to *This Side of Paradise* and pointed out that offering her such a high amount before her book was out was a big gamble for Harcourt. A subsequent letter from Donald Brace sought Grace's permission to use her name on any forthcoming film of *Being Respectable* and its advertising.[19]

Meetings with publishers again drew Grace to New York over the holidays in late 1922 and well into 1923. She spent Christmas and New Year's at Hill-Stead, ill with influenza.

After recovering, Grace moved to the Riddles' apartment at the Carlton House in Manhattan early in January. *Being Respectable* had just arrived in bookstores. With its publication, Grace's aspirations for recognition and financial reward became reality. Her disillusion with conventional [late Victorian] society had provoked massive popular response. Jonathan Cape's British edition of *Being Respectable* appeared almost immediately. Hollywood screened the novel in 1924.[20]

Being Respectable is a satirical study of society set in a fictional Midwestern city, a novel of manners. It is a roman à clef that put St. Paul society in a dither of curiosity and fury over the perceived identity of the book's main characters. The novel features a wealthy family named Carpenter, whose scion, Darius, is a pillar of society in Columbia (St. Paul). Darius is a widower with three adult children; Charles and Lydia are conformists, and Deborah, the youngest, is a rebel. The novel puts all three and their spouses or lovers to various tests imposed by conflicts between ideals and realities, between human longings and the requirements and expectations of conventional society, and between generations in a rapidly changing American culture.

The work's subject matter is dated today, but the writing is distinguished by the deft portrayal of high-society Victorian "types" and their motives and by the use of telling detail in physical description. The nonconformist daughter, Deborah, is an admitted self-portrait of the author. Deborah is restless and discontent, always wondering what she wants from life.[21]

Reviewers around the country immediately compared *Being Respectable* to Sinclair Lewis's *Babbitt*. The book critic for *The World Tomorrow* said of the author: "Her eye is as keen as Sinclair Lewis's and her reflections are her own." Another critic referred to Grace Flandrau as "Mrs. Babbitt."

Isabel Paterson wrote in her widely read *New York Tribune* column: "It

[*Being Respectable*] is not only worthy of serious attention: it provides many pages of sheer delight for its wit . . . its essential if incomplete clarity. It is a most distinguished piece of work." To *Tribune* reporters interviewing her about her motivation to write, Grace replied: "I write because I must."

Howard Weeks wrote in the *Detroit Free Press*: "It seems doubtful that this book would have been written if Sinclair Lewis had not first written his impressions of some slices of our Middle Western civilization. However, *Being Respectable* is a better book, a more finely, clearly and intelligently written book than either of Lewis's last two."

Reviews from Minnesota and Minnesota writers, however, were decidedly mixed.

A St. Paul friend and recent literary celebrity himself, Scott Fitzgerald, ten years younger than Grace, wrote a two-page mostly favorable review in *Literary Digest International.*

> Grace Flandrau's *Being Respectable*—the book of the winter and in all probability of the spring, too—is superior to Sinclair Lewis's *Babbitt* in many ways, but inferior in that it deals with too many characters. . . . A thoroughly interesting and capable novel. The writing is solid throughout, and sometimes beautiful.[22]

Privately to their mutual friend, Tom Boyd, Scott gushed: "I reviewed Grace's book. I thought it was magnificent of its type. Better than *Babbitt*."[23]

Boyd himself was cautious. In his column, "In a Corner with the Bookworm" in the *St. Paul Daily News*, he compared Grace's writing to Sinclair Lewis's: "Mrs. Flandrau's manner of writing is strong, masculine, one might almost say . . . a style which . . . possesses a great deal of guts." In private correspondence Boyd gave Grace his opinion that *Being Respectable* would have been a better book if she had put in more contrast. "The book needed something beautiful in it," he advised.[24]

Boyd's criticism was mild compared to the caustic words of Frances Boardman, the *St. Paul Pioneer Press* critic. Boardman labeled the book "a lecture on the perils of respectability" and said that, although *Being Respectable* was not a dull book, "It solves nothing and brings none of its main currents together in dramatic confluence."[25]

Charles Flandrau's private comments on *Being Respectable* illuminate his personality as well as his literary views. He loyally asserted to Grace that female rivalry explained Frances Boardman's negative coverage of the book. Writing her from Palma, Majorca, in February, 1923, Charles admitted that the *Pioneer Press's* review by "old blanc mange" was "well-written but as criticism, it doesn't exist.... I naturally remarked her labored (and feline) detachment.... No greater lie was ever uttered than Lydia E. Pinkham's trademark: 'Women Can Sympathize With Women.' Maybe they can—but all my life I have noticed that they don't."[26]

Scott Fitzgerald's comment in a personal letter to Grace undoubtedly pleased her: "Edith Wharton wrote Charles Scribner that she liked *Being Respectable* better than any American novel in years. She asked him for all data concerning you."[27]

Some St. Paul readers sent complimentary letters, but hometown feathers were decidedly ruffled. Grace's realistic portraits had hit too close to home. Early in February 1923, she wrote Blair:

> "Do you know I have made a discovery? Men like my work better than women. John Alsop is crazy about it—I just got a box of gardenias from him and a line.... Men like it much the best. Old ladies don't like it at all.... Some people say *Being Respectable* is dirty and dull, that it is untrue and immoral, others that it is an insult to all sacred things, that I scoff at religion and marriage, etc. Write me what you've heard. Do you think I'll be cut on the street by these outraged old dowagers?... The St. Paulites here [in the East] who have read it love it but seem to think I can never go back. I am just crazy to have some reports from the front"[28]

Blair's response was predictably proud and supportive. He said that although St. Paul critics had panned the book, the Minneapolis critic had praised it. When he investigated sales at a Twin Cities book store Blair was told Grace's book was selling better than any book they'd had in a long time—two hundred in two days.[29] He wrote later: "You are quite a personage, Keekie.... I have such great, great faith in—not your ability, that isn't what I mean—but in just your you. Your marvelous cleverness and insight. You've got 'em all beaten a mile, Tudie."[30]

Hearing in New York about St. Paul's dismay over *Being Respectable*, Grace wrote Betty Foster: "Scott Fitzgerald's mother...was more shocked than anybody and never tires of telling people what a dreadful book it is."[31] Lucius

Ordway wrote Grace that St. Paul was evenly divided about her book—older people were outraged and the young loved it.[32]

Being Respectable's description of a women's luncheon at a fashionable residence in the fictional city of "Columbia" explains what irritated St. Paul socialites:

> There was a shrill uproar—the toneless clatter of voices talking together. There were butter colored jonquils; linen a frenzy of filet lace and embroidery; an odor of sachet, crisp lettuces, and early strawberries. And, when one of the swift waitresses, all dazzlingly black and white, slipped through a swinging door, a prophetic whiff of coffee. In a word, there was minutely everything that in Columbia [St. Paul] is understood to constitute a "luncheon."
>
> And, of course, women, lots of women. Lots of rounded forearms, vivacious eyes, white teeth, velvets, and laces. All the subtle tensions, too, the nerve-charged atmosphere women create—especially women whose occupation is pleasure. Watchful eyes; listening ears; observation sharpened to catch self-betrayals, gaucheries; to ferret out what each one wished to hide; to amass material for talk at other luncheons.
>
> Currents of malice, of kindness; curiosity, shrewdness, cleverness, stupidity, loyalty, disloyalty; an effort to please, to do one's part, to be amused and amusing. Women—intricate, dangerous, persistent—never more terrible than at play. Oh, women, to whom as to the Jews, oppression has given a deadly vigor.

Another passage describes the sheltered lives and self-satisfied indifference of the "respectable:"

> Looking about him as he walked down Summit Avenue, he thought: 'How clean are the windows of the respectable! If I had a house my windows would never be so clean.'
>
> But he didn't want a house. Or domesticity. Domesticity—who wanted that? Not Steven. Not yet, anyhow. Domesticity at its most complete and comfortable, perhaps, right here. Lots of babies in these clean, warm houses. Babies being accurately fed on spinach, beefsteaks, and good milk. Being bathed, exercised, and brought up with straight legs, sound stomachs, and a pretty good chance of believing the world to be a benevolent

playground, an amusement park spotted with golf links, tennis courts, colleges, clubs, water to sail on in yachts, banks to get money out of, churches to get married in. To be elaborately married in, attended by a gently virtuous mother in lavender, wearing orchids, by a successful father in striped pants with a handsome check in his waistcoat pocket. Churches also to be buried from when you were old and dead, your coffin heaped with floral offerings from your lifelong friends, friends who knew all about you, who liked you, criticized you, were kind to you when you were sick, loaned you money—with discretion—and forgot all about you when your bank broke. Life of the plutocracy in the big cities west of Buffalo, east of Denver, south of the Canadian border.

These words may remind readers of another critic of Victorian society—Edith Wharton. Flandrau's arrow seems to be aimed at the hard-hearted complacency of many powerful people, not just at women or society in general.

A Minneapolis literary newsletter, *The Porcupine*, made a favorable comment: "Mrs. Flandrau has achieved a piece of work in which we feel a great deal of local pride. Our eastern friends continue to write us admiringly about it. We fail to sympathize with the indignation of certain St. Paulites. We'd be as proud as peacocks if we'd been in it." This example of traditional Minneapolis-St. Paul sparring probably augmented hometown resentment at Grace.[33]

New York publishers wined and dined Grace throughout January, and Theodate honored her with a reception at the Carlton. Brenda Ueland Benedict attended, bringing a date whom Grace couldn't abide. Scott and Zelda Fitzgerald were invited but didn't show up.

A few days later, however, Scott Fitzgerald dropped in on Grace at the Carlton, and she wrote: "He is so nice when he's sober as he seems to be just now." Grace assured Blair she was trying to spurn callers and social invitations.[34]

After Brenda and Ben Benedict entertained for her, Grace reported to Blair that she had been terribly rude to "a rich, chinless, self-made male guest who was condescending to the Benedicts in being there at all."

The Benedicts, however, had been loud in Blair's praise: "What a gentleman you were, how handsome, etc.," Grace wrote. She continued: "You've got to show me how to be <u>really</u> dignified. . . . I tell you, Blair, I am a ferocious snob, but I don't think I am going to go on being a fool snob. I know that

I shall demand the best, the finest sort of people and violently <u>detest</u> all the others. . . . The more I see of other people—men—the more of a miracle you seem to me. It's so darn jolly living with you—you put such an atmosphere of lovableness and dignity and joy into life. . . . A man who has won such intelligent adoration from such an intelligent woman has had to go some!"[35]

During the excitement over *Being Respectable*, Grace learned that Harcourt, Brace and Company was interested in her next novel. She also showed Blair's completed manuscript to Harrison Smith. Although nothing came of it, Grace read and assessed her husband's work with a familiar comment. "It is written with clear insight into the empty hectic life you have seen and yet it is warm-hearted and kind."[36] By mid-January publishing fanfare and late nights had exhausted Grace and she was laid up again at Hill-Stead with trained nurses. Dr. Riggs repeatedly told her during occasional check-ups at Purinton Inn that the main advice he could give her was not to get too tired. She told Blair she couldn't sleep without him and begged him to join her.[37]

But Blair wrote that he was increasingly worried about business and couldn't leave St. Paul. Other dealers were bidding lower prices on trucks than Flandrau Motor Company could afford to without losing money.[38]

Blair's St. Paul social life had been active as usual over the holidays. He described in detail a boisterous progressive dinner given on New Year's Eve 1922. The guests had gone for cocktails to the Ted Whites', then to Lucius Ordway's basement, which was fixed like a side show. There were cages with artificial animals and in one cage, Papie Motter, "having more fun out of it than anybody. Louie was dressed up as a circus barker and was very funny." Other guests were dressed as snake charmers.

At the next party there were two clowns from the circus with a boxing kangaroo. Clover Irvine had put on the gloves with the kangaroo, and the kangaroo caught her in the stomach with one of its back feet and knocked her clear across the room into a heap against the wall. "Next we went on to the Mitchells, where the basement was fixed up like a Turkish bath."

Then the party had moved on to the McDonalds' where the food hadn't been too good. Somebody had grabbed a duck from his plate and had thrown it at Blair, who had picked it up and given it back.

"Then to Irvines for the wind up . . . I came home at five with Sam and Mildred—sober as a judge, <u>honest</u>." The next day Blair and the whole crowd had gone to Roger and Katherine Shepards' farm for lunch and skating.[39]

Subsequent letters from Blair mentioned movies with B. C. Thompson and

Alice O'Brien and more parties. There was a Yale concert and a dinner at the Hills'. The names of Blair's favorite women friends came up often in his letters: Anne White, Katherine Shepard, and Dibbie Skinner. Clover Irvine told him, "Blair, nobody could get mad at you, you could do anything and everybody would like you just the same."[40] Blair also reported that he had been playing bridge with the Ritzingers, Pattersons, Sidney Deans, and Agnes Kennedy and was "getting away with it."[41]

Grace's response was: "I am afraid so many parties will be bad for you." She kept begging him to come East, but he refused, saying they had too many bills already and owed $200. She insisted: "See what's left in the bank and draw it all out."[42]

Blair replied: "Holy Smoke! Tudie, it seems to me that would be perfect madness. If I draw it out we'll spend it, that's a cinch, and then we would literally have not one cent." He enclosed bills amounting to $846 owed by Grace, mainly for clothes purchased in St. Paul.[43]

In addition to worrying about bills, Blair wouldn't go east because he was considering a business deal with one or more new partners. If the plan went forward, the Flandrau Motor Company would drop trucks and take on the Franklin auto. "I would turn over the property to the new company, receiving stock in the company for my equity in the property for which I would probably receive a salary," he wrote Grace.[44]

Blair also remained in St. Paul to receive the Flandrau belongings just sent from Mexico six years after the government's confiscation of the Santa Margarita. Two trunks had arrived already, holding all their silver except for one big platter that would arrive in a third trunk. He had spent seventy dollars and made many visits to Customs at the St. Paul Union Depot, filling out forms to claim their possessions and get them delivered.[45]

Friends showered Blair with attention during Grace's long absence, and by early February he was insisting she come home to handle his social life. He had started accepting two invitations for the same night and decided "either to go nowhere, go everywhere or kick people in the face except the few places you want to go. The last is the best."[46]

Grace worried constantly about his health and his drinking and nagged him about it:

> Blair, it's too awful to be so dependent for all real happiness on one frail
> human.... I don't mind you're not coming so much but I very much mind

your going out every single night in St. Paul—drinking, smoking, getting insufficient rest, etc. You know it's precisely what the doctors forbade you.[47]

Blair responded angrily, saying he hated to have Grace worry about his health. He thought he took after his father, he said, who couldn't endure anyone thinking he wasn't well and furthermore couldn't endure anyone else being sick. (Blair and Charlie theorized that Theodate enjoyed having sick people to take care of.) "For the last thirty-five years, with the exception of this back and a touch of grippe two winters ago, I haven't been sick," Blair insisted. He said he was not drinking his head off and wished she would trust him a little.[48]

At last, late in February, Grace gave in and agreed to return home. She had been gone for almost three months. Besides worrying about Blair's health, their income, and the progress of his business, Grace had another concern. She feared that after the success of *Being Respectable*, the literary world would expect her to produce a masterpiece: "What if I've shot my wad? It makes me damn scared when I see what they expect of me. What if I can't do it?"[49]

Apparently publishers weren't worrying. In March 1923, Donald Brace wrote Grace in St. Paul, offering her a contract for the publication of *Entranced*. He reported that sales of *Being Respectable* were going well.[50]

In April Brace wrote again, offering Grace a royalty increase earlier in the sales of *Entranced* than had been offered for *Being Respectable*. Later that month he wrote again, this time about her share of royalties from a British edition of *Being Respectable*. Shortly thereafter, she signed a contract with Harcourt, Brace and Company for publication of her new novel, *Entranced*.[51]

CHAPTER IX

Breakdown and Recovery

"As the result of this chaos of self-delusion, I became violently ill."
Grace Flandrau's interview with Brenda Ueland,
Golfer and Sportsman, 1934

WHEN GRACE RETURNED TO ST. PAUL a congratulatory note from John
Riddle awaited her. Riddle had been in Buenos Aires and had just learned of
Being Respectable's success. He wrote, "I was so glad to get your letter of January
7th with its staggering figures of the fruits of your industry. I am so glad that
there is one Flandrau (even though an acquired one) who is a moneymaker!"

Riddle complimented Grace on her portrayal of the characters in *Being
Respectable.* He found them "Tolstoian or Chekhovian in their realism" and said
he recognized St. Paul matrons among the characters.

John had spent his boyhood and school vacations during adolescence and
college at his stepfather's house in St. Paul and visited there often before his
mother's death in 1911. Even though he had long resided elsewhere by 1923,
Riddle's brief immersion in Twin Cities society and Minnesota life had made
a lasting impression.

In correspondence with his St. Paul relatives, John used family nicknames and
in-family jokes. He loved Blair's famous spelling gaffes. (For instance, describing
his nationality on an induction form for army service in World War I, Blair had
written: "Of American birth and decent." When relatives kidded him mercilessly about his spelling, Blair would respond: "Have you ever seen the Lewis
and Clark papers?")

Receiving Flandrau letters from abroad, Riddle often responded, "I wisht
I wuz dar." When he liked a book or a play or someone's attire, he might
comment, "Pretty smood, don't you tink?"[1]

Grace loved these Minnesota colloquialisms out of the mouth of a debonair
diplomat, and they often appeared in her correspondence with Riddle. He
was a well-read world traveler with cultivated tastes like hers.

The immediate success of *Being Respectable* propelled Grace to celebrity in
her hometown. Everybody wanted to meet St. Paul's newest literary star. In
1992 Meridel Le Sueur, who lived in Irvine Park in 1923–1924, remembered

encountering Grace at literary receptions held at the Alexander Ramsey house in those years. Anita and Laura Furness, Ramsey's granddaughters, often invited local writers to speak informally.[2]

Opinions about *Being Respectable* in St. Paul were sharply divided. Many years after the book's publication in an interview with Brenda Ueland, Grace reminisced about the local controversy her novel had ignited. Ueland's story was published in her December 1934 column, "Among Those We Know," in the *Golfer and Sportsman*, a Twin Cities social magazine. In the interview Grace said of *Being Respectable*:

> There was a great local to-do over it. It came out a little before its time, so that it impressed people as being full of the most incredible wickedness. But today if you go over it with a fine-toothed comb you will find nothing in it that could possibly be construed as even indelicate. And yet at that time it threw the people I knew into a perfect stew. . . . I heard that everybody was furious at me and that I would surely be ostracized forever, but I never experienced any of this. Everybody was just as gentle and kind to me as they had always been.

Probably most St. Paul mavens disguised their feelings toward Grace, both in 1923 when *Being Respectable* came out and in 1934 when Ueland's interview was published. By 1934 Grace had achieved international status as a writer, providing that undeniable insulation from criticism that goes with power. After Blair's death and increased awareness in St. Paul of Grace's illegitimacy and her unorthodox childhood it would be another story.

In 1923, despite a certain amount of negative local reaction, Grace's professional achievement and her emergence on the national literary scene caught the attention of some powerful St. Paul business leaders.

Louis W. Hill, son of James J. Hill, and Ralph Budd, president of the Great Northern Railway, discovered, right under their noses, an ambitious St. Paul writer who could produce a series of pamphlets about Hill's railroad and its historic role in opening the Northwest for settlement. Shortly after publication of *Being Respectable*, these officials offered Flandrau the intriguing assignment. The Hills' and Flandraus' long friendship no doubt helped Grace land the job.

She hadn't tackled historical research and writing before and probably had little understanding of the scope of Hill's and Budd's expectations or of the promotional nature of the project envisioned. The railroad's proposal was flattering and the money and prestige offered by working with such a substantial client had appeal. Even though she hadn't completed the novel Harcourt expected, Grace accepted the job.

Ralph Budd, who was a dedicated history buff, had vast ambitions for the work. He loved Northwest and railroad history, and he undertook complete charge of directing Grace's research. Determined to give his author a thorough background in her subject, Budd made elaborate plans for her to travel extensively in the West, gathering historical data, interviewing regional experts, and soaking up local color. It would be a two-year assignment. Budd provided Grace with a cabin on Louis Hill's ranch in Glacier Park for the secluded isolation she needed for extensive historic research as well as continuing work on her novel.[3]

In summer 1923 Grace moved into Hill's cabin, taking books on geography and geology, voyageurs, Indians, and railroads. She also took her manuscript for *Entranced*. Blair, who was refinancing the Flandrau Motor Company, vacationed with her briefly in Glacier Park and then returned to work in St. Paul.

After a month at Glacier, Grace traveled to St. Paul and went on to Farmington. Letters between the Flandraus that fall disclose they were both worried about Blair's business. He wasn't getting to work until ten or eleven A.M., and Grace, as usual, was alarmed about his health. She wrote him a twenty-one-page letter from Hill-Stead, giving encouragement and stern business advice. Blair had turned negative about taking on new partners.

Grace's letter thanked her husband for the kindness, generosity, and care he had given her and said she wanted to reciprocate:

> How lucky, lucky I have been to have inadvertently—blindly—stumbled on an angel when I married a man. Of course it has spoiled me. I take much of it for granted until I notice the petty egotism that crops out in most other men. Then it comes over me overwhelmingly.

She cautioned Blair against getting his business into any worse problems than he already had, going into further debt, facing bankruptcy, the loss of the building, and so on. Blair didn't have enough capital, she wrote, to swing an automobile agency alone without using capital they needed to live on. She reminded him of the trouble he had had meeting the prices of his competitors. Then:

Now, Blair, don't be guided by mediocre minds when you're getting advice from a mind that is by no means mediocre. That sounds fatuous, but I mean it. I may not be prudent in small things, but I have got a mind that when it wants to can cut through to main issues and don't you fail to believe it. I implore you to get busy on this matter at once.

You hold the balance sheet too close to your nose. That's necessary but it's necessary <u>too</u> to look at the thing in terms of a year ahead and years behind . . . the main thing is to get out of this mess with as little calamity as possible. Then with your practical experience you can start afresh with a group of men back of you to advise, etc. You simply cannot run a business alone without advisers and men to consult with.

Now, Blair, for God's sake get down to 'brass tacks' in this matter. Be not optimistic (I know you're no longer that) but <u>enterprising</u>. Get a new slant on the whole game and make for safety just as fast as you can go. <u>SAFETY</u>. Do write me at length as I am most uneasy.[4]

By the end of September 1923 Blair had sold his majority ownership in the Flandrau Motor Company to a new partner, Charlie Rusch. He had hired an accountant to work out details, with Rusch taking possession of the property on October 1. Blair didn't think he would need to put more money into the partnership but would continue as a minority partner.[5]

That winter the Flandraus occupied Mary Squires's house in Dellwood at White Bear Lake, a suburb ten miles northeast of St. Paul. Because Grace planned to be at Glacier Park much of the next two years, they rented out their Portland Avenue home in St. Paul on a long-term lease. At White Bear, as at Glacier Park, Grace hoped she would find the isolation she needed to work on *Entranced*. The novel was going well, and she loved riding the horse stabled on the Squires property. Blair continued working in St. Paul for Charlie Rusch.[6]

After gaining national literary celebrity, Grace went through a period of fantasizing about romances with other men. Grace hinted at potential love affairs and current crushes in correspondence with Betty Foster. In the 1920s modern females were supposed to have or want lovers. She wrote Foster in Paris in December 1923: "What a good time you are having. I envy you all the nice French and English young men." Grace told Betty that she was receiving frequent letters from "our friend, Mr. Bissell. (That's a secret so don't speak of it. Nothing really wrong you understand.)" Richard Bissell, a playwright, was the author of *State Fair*.[7] In the same letter Grace mentioned that Scott Fitzgerald wrote her that his play (*The Vegetable*) had failed in Atlantic City.[8]

Grace frequently mentioned Reinold Noyes in her letters to Foster. Noyes was a St. Paul friend who, with his wife, Doria, enjoyed reading plays aloud with the Flandraus on Sunday nights. Noyes never failed to send Grace his opinions on each of her books. Grace confided to Betty Foster that she alternated between liking Reinold Noyes very much and being perfectly furious at him. "Probably that is a sign of a very flattering regard," she mused.[9]

She also wrote Foster that a bachelor friend of Blair's, George MacPherson, had given her a lovely police dog, a puppy five months old. Mary O'Malley had named him "Daisy."[10]

After Richard Bissell came to visit the Flandraus for two days, Grace wrote Foster: "I am tremendously fond of him."[11]

Grace radiated female confidence with men and males of all ages did not fail to respond. In addition, by late 1923, she was probably felt released from the likelihood of pregnancy. She and Blair had been married for over thirteen years with no issue. Not surprisingly, with her youthful, avant-garde ideas, Grace increasingly identified with younger, unmarried women, like Betty Foster, childless like herself.

Grace probably fantasized about romances more than she consummated them. In spite of her surface identification with the rebellious outlook of Jazz Age culture, Flandrau was a levelheaded, pragmatic woman, not inclined to inflict serious insult on her devoted husband or upset her own apple cart. In the novel she wrote during this period of temptation, *Entranced*, Grace brought her young, married heroine, Rita Robinson, to the brink of an affair, and then pulled her back.

Guests often visited the Flandraus at their White Bear Lake cottage during the Christmas holidays in 1923—too many, according to Grace. She complained to Foster about frequent interruptions and said that due to "the pressure of personality" she found it difficult to write. People were always coming out from town, sometimes uninvited, to visit. In frustration, Grace wrote: "I can't get it [her novel] written within 100 miles of St. Paul."[12]

Early in 1924 Grace delivered the finished manuscript for *Entranced* to Harcourt, Brace in New York. Again she stayed at Hill-Stead. After returning home, Grace wrote Foster in Europe, expressing her views about St. Paul women. She explained why Theodate Riddle so impressed her:

Theo has some amazing fund of emotional power that sets her apart. I suppose in some way she is a genius. . . . I can't tell you how dwindled, thwarted and curtailed the women here [in St. Paul] seem next to her. It seems to me there is an almost unbelievable timidity here and conventionality of thought—unawareness of the keen, salt, bitterness, swing and freedom of life.

Then, despite her supposedly liberated views, Grace admitted her own timidity: "Jonathan Cape [the British publisher of *Being Respectable*] said to me 'American women have been coddled, protected, catered to so much they're soft,' and I see what he means. I'm soft. I have no courage. No real independence and detachment. I'm afraid of suffering and of daring and of loneliness and old age and all kinds of things."

Grace ended her letter with another mention of Richard Bissell: "He is really a dear. Too bad he's so old because he's so good looking and such a peach and very intelligent." Grace was perhaps more conventional than either Brenda Ueland or Betty Foster, both considerably younger than she.[13]

When Grace stayed with the Riddles at Hill-Stead that winter she found Theo and John in the midst of a bitter quarrel. In spite of her professed admiration for Theodate, Grace took John Riddle's part in the argument.

Riddle had just accepted an appointment as U.S. ambassador to Argentina, but because of Theo's intense involvement with her new school, she refused to accompany him to Buenos Aires. John threatened to retire and move to Italy if Theo didn't go with him to South America. Grace found herself their intermediary. Both Riddles, like Blair, had begun to depend on her judgment. But that dependence, plus the heavy social schedule at Hill-Stead, weighed heavily on Grace. She described the hectic scene to Blair:

I am almost dead . . . A house party of 21 or 22 next week-end, 58 people at dinner last night, 17 the night before, always 20 or so for lunch . . . We have a stringed orchestra every night . . . I'm trying to keep Theodate up to the point of going down [to the Argentine] with John. . . . He almost lost his post in Argentina because of her refusal to go with him. The school is taking all her money and time. I don't know how it's going to turn out. . . . I swear I don't. There is, it seems, an almost irreconcilable breach. It is all perfectly insane. Dinner dances and then talks with her til three A.M. Sometimes she seems almost not quite right. . . . It's all a fearful strain on me. I feel as if I were going stark staring mad and nutty.

I wish you could come on and have a talk with her and with him. You are so sane and I am not. Oh, Blair, sometimes money is a curse, isn't it?

While visiting Hill-Stead, Grace observed that her new clothes were making quite an impression on the Riddles' friends. She told Blair she must always have lovely clothes because they made a difference in the way people responded to her. Theodate had noticed and was insisting that Grace help her select all her clothes.[14]

After delivery of her manuscript, *Entranced*, to Harcourt, Grace was free to concentrate on the Great Northern Railway work. Budd was anxious to get on with the education of his writer.

Late in March of 1924, Grace filled in Foster, still in France, about her assignment and her reaction to her employer:

> Mr. Budd . . . whom I adore, sent for me the other day and proposes to send me to the coast over the route of an old overland trail, now traveled by a new deluxe train. They're hiring me to put a few fancy literary frills [on pamphlets] they're going to get out. . . . I have never done any advertising work, but I think it will be a great lark to try. Also to work with the delectable and so fabulously intelligent Mr. Budd.[15]

The trip was delayed due to some kind of surgery that put Grace in the Mayo Clinic for a time in May. Surgery and stitches had been required. Budd, she wrote Blair, had called from Seattle every day and sent flowers. Very likely Grace had a hysterectomy.

While recuperating in St. Paul, Grace reported to Foster that she had received a flattering letter from Edith Wharton, who wrote: "May an unknown reader write you of her very great admiration for your book *Being Respectable*? It's too full of good things to be adequately praised in a few words."

Grace also confided to Foster:

> That English actor spent the afternoon with me then wouldn't go but ate his dinner on a tray and dashed down to the theatre after eight. Then very shortly another gentleman friend arrived. (Don't speak a word of this) and stayed til now. The actor was gay and naughty and the subsequent caller

absurdly earnest and business-like which was very darling. I forgot to say that Blair left for unknown regions at 6 this A.M. to shoot ducks. Home Sunday night.[16]

Was Grace, after a probable hysterectomy, convincing herself that men still found her desirable?

Her letter to Foster two weeks later mentioned that the complimentary words of Mrs. Kohlsaat about *Being Respectable* encouraged her to go on writing. (Mrs. Kohlsaat was a Chicago matron whose prominent daughter and son-in-law were Katherine and Roger Shepard.)

"As you know," Grace confided to Foster, "I never really <u>want</u> to write. It's not my vocation or a vocation. It's a form of self-defense, a means not an end. A something to fill a vacuum."[17] Because Grace routinely hid her feelings, probably few people besides Foster and Brenda Ueland knew what a deep disappointment their childlessness was to the Flandraus. Grace's letter included this description of Zelda Fitzgerald: "You have undoubtedly heard before now that poor Zelda was unbelievably poor in the show [the St. Paul Junior League Follies] and rather tight and that she was almost <u>drunk</u> at the supper afterwards. Unbelievable little people aren't they?"[18]

Her letter compared St. Paul to the fictional Midwestern city, "Columbia," in which *Being Respectable* was set: "Blair is waiting for me now to go for a walk on the River Boulevard . . . it's Sunday . . . and then tea at the Irvines and then to say goodbye to the Cap Thompsons, who are going to Washington, and then I hope to the movies. Now isn't that 'Columbia?'"[19]

That summer an English review of *Being Respectable* defined what had so angered St. Paulites about the book: "Miss Flandrau describes the family circle of the millionaires in the big provincial towns. It is a far from edifying picture . . . these people are overfed, over-monied, under-worked, destitute of moral principles, yet unable to be really naughty."[20]

By June, Grace was immersed in the railroad job. Budd's plans for her research included traveling all summer in the West, accumulating information on every aspect of its development. He provided private railroad cars for Grace's travel, planned her itinerary, and made advance reservations for lodgings. Budd, who put the Great Northern staff at her disposal, booked her for interviews, ceremonies, and demonstrations wherever she went. He kept in touch with her progress through William N. Graves, a Great Northern executive assigned to be her personal escort.

Grace mailed letters that summer from Seattle, Spokane, Glacier Park, Great Falls, Helena, and Fort Benton. She described Indian agencies, speeches, track-layings and other railroad operations, logging activities, horseback rides, interviews with old-timers, ranchers, Jesuit priests, and Indians, boat rides, and fishing.

Her days were long and often tedious. Although she often had "a devil of a headache," every evening the neophyte journalist roughly recorded facts and impressions of the day's excursion and corrected drafts written the night before. Mornings Grace arose at seven to work before setting off on another expedition. She frequently invited Blair to join her and often repeated how much she missed him.[21]

In one letter to Blair, Grace described an unusual church service in Glacier Park, evidencing unusually forward-looking empathy and uncommon powers of analysis. Those must have been the qualities for which Budd and Hill hired her:

> I went to the funniest church service tonight in the bowels of the hotel. The poor anemic, white-faced red-nosed preacher announced that Chief Two Guns White Calf would speak through an interpreter, Heavy Breast. Oh, it was a dreary bare room with some cane chairs and a whiny melodeon. We drawled out some hymns and then two darling Indians came up.
>
> Two Guns is the handsomest Indian I ever saw. Proud and straight with the most marvelous carriage of his head . . . They had magnificent deep speaking voices so different from the mushy voice of the preacher.
>
> Two Guns talked in Blackfoot and Heavy Breast translated. The old dear tried to talk about God, but he didn't have much to say on that subject and then began on himself and became very eloquent. How he had gone East to New York and Boston, etc., etc., and everywhere great crowds [gathered], as it was his face on the Buffalo nickel—and how many thousand he shook hands with, etc.—how his father Mute Chief owned all Glacier Park.
>
> Then Heavy Breast made a speech along the same pleasant lines and then I rushed away before the preacher got a chance to talk. It was a strange diverting sight. The Indians wore mussed business suits with blue shirts and necklaces of shells, enormous white shell earrings and their hair in long braids with red braid pleated in. Never did the ceremonies of the Christian religion seem more preposterous.[22]

By August, Grace was ready to start organizing her research notes. A room was booked for her at the Jennings Ranch at Glacier Park Station. She urged Blair to join her.[23] Blair, however, was not faring well in his new partnership. He probably wanted to quit his job altogether but wouldn't admit it to himself or to Grace. She most likely understood between the lines what he wasn't saying. His letters included only the usual news of his social life and of their pets, Pea, Pasha, and Daisy. Sometimes he mentioned dates with single women Grace knew. In a June letter he said that he had taken Marie Hersey to the movies.[24]

Meanwhile, Grace thrived in the fresh air, beauty, and quiet of Montana. From Jennings Ranch, she wrote Doria Noyes in St. Paul, displaying buoyant spirits and a contemplative mood:

> I go into a trance—a day dream—all the beauty of the past month rises up like a tide and bathes me and carries me off I don't know where at, as they say out here. . . . I've been riding as much as thirty miles a day and come back feeling more rested than when I went out! But Doria, the real chic is the amazing loveliness of the place. <u>You</u> know—big, windy blue sky and white clouds and pine trees and smells and mountain peaks and then, below, the plains. I think I like them the best—rolling on and on and on like a petrified ocean. It's so beautiful your senses get all mixed-up—the long mountain slopes sing and the murmur of the pine trees is suddenly a cool purple color and the exquisite odors of the clean grasses taste good. It makes me long to have lots and lots of children and milk cows every night and smell the hay and their nice breaths . . .
>
> I have been eating three meals a day in an enchanting ranch kitchen facing a long table of cowboys, trappers, farmhands, woodsmen . . . and I assure you my views of human nature have changed considerably. You <u>can't</u> classify. Among them are knights and chivalrous courtiers and gentlemen and rogues and bounders and cheap skates and idealists and poets and hogs. It's <u>not</u> environment and it's <u>not</u> station—within every class is a surprising and bewildering variety—that much is certain.
>
> Several delightful letters from John Riddle asking me to be sure to make Hill-Stead while he's there . . . But somehow Hill-Stead so suddenly after this will be too much. Then I will go stark staring mad with bewilderment. Back there is the me who writes pessimistic novels.[25]

When Ralph Budd learned how well the quiet, outdoor life of Montana agreed with her, he again offered Grace the use of a cabin on Louis W. Hill's ranch in Glacier Park, this time for the whole winter. Hill's gamekeeper's lodge was available, Budd said, and with a little work and some additional furniture, it could be just the right environment for her work.[26]

Grace wrote Blair about the tempting offer and suggested he join her there. His letters, she commented, didn't sound cheerful. Then she added, "Mr. Budd turned up with Mr. and Mrs. Walker Hines.... He very emphatically did not come to see me." Quite naturally, speculation about Grace Flandrau and Ralph Budd flourished in St. Paul.[27]

Grace persuaded Blair to join her briefly at the Jennings Ranch to celebrate their birthdays and their wedding anniversary in August. She wrote Betty Foster that they were taking long horseback rides and she was also enjoying riding alone or with "a darling cowboy with heavy chaps." Then her Montana-induced contemplative mood took over:

> Tonight it seems to me there are only three endurable ways for a woman to live—one is to marry at twenty a man physically right for her and live on a farm and have ten children rapidly ... and watch the calves grow and the horses and cats and dogs and chickens and live deeply in the physical heart of life; the next is to have definitely a career, stage preferably, or paint or write; third (a sad and burning way) to be definitely <u>wicked</u>—live and love and die when you're thirty. All other ways are half portions. Oh, Betty, life seems so fleeting and disillusioning.
>
> This, however, is no way to write to a pretty girl in what some people call the hay [sic] day of youth. I hope you have got a nice beau again and wish I knew something about your future plans. Blair and I take a most expensive outfit, which we can't afford, and go on a camping trip back into the Rockies for a few days tomorrow.

The letter concluded with a typically frank query. Referring to Betty's "young Frenchman," Flandrau asked: "Did he make love well?"[28]

Blair's business life was fading. Both Grace and Theodate sensed his discouragement. Writing Grace in Montana, Theo spoke emphatically: "Why doesn't Blair sell out? He is working too hard. We know that. Grace, do get him to do that—no matter at what loss—just get out and lead a healthy life on his capital." Then, knowing nothing about Budd's offer of the gamekeeper's lodge, Theodate proposed lending the Flandraus a cabin she owned at Avon, Connecticut. She asked, "Why don't you both come on this autumn? Blair could join the hunting club—on my property—and have a grand time. I wish to goodness he would."[29]

In fall 1924, Blair resigned his position at Flandrau Motors Service Company. A year earlier, with new management, the company's name had changed. Whether or not the new partnership bought out Blair's share is unknown. At age forty-nine he retired from professional life and from 1924 forward devoted himself to managing his and Grace's business affairs, their home, their pets, and his social life.

Warner Brothers' film of *Being Respectable*, starring Marie Prevost, Monte Blue, Irene Rich, and Louise Fazenda, premiered August 10, 1924. Directed by Phil Rosen, the picture was widely and favorably reviewed. Grace, paid by Harcourt, Brace and Company for the film rights before the novel's release, had no part in writing the screenplay, but the national press continued to interview her about *Being Respectable*. In one article she made this world-weary remark: "The spectacle of human life is very amusing and very sad."[30]

Grace's third novel, *Entranced* was published early in the fall of 1924. She went east for the promotional fanfare accompanying the book's release. *Entranced*, like *Being Respectable*, is a novel in the mannerist tradition. The author examines the conduct and motives of the main characters as they grapple with social and moral issues. The plot demonstrates Flandrau's observation that the rich and powerful, protected by their position, can get away with misconduct—even crime—while ordinary people cannot. The story seems simplistic today, but the characters are real.

Entranced's main characters, Rita and Dick Malory, brother and sister, come from a family very like Mary Staples Hodgson's family; there is a stolid, beautifully dressed, devout matriarch of a grandmother, surrounded by a bevy of widowed or spinster daughters. Rita (who is Grace) and her brother Dick, who are escaping this family and its conventional ways, both marry into the Robinson family, wealthy pillars of a Midwestern city like St. Paul. Rita's husband, Gordon Robinson, is a character much like Blair—a kind, uncomplicated, youthful man who occasionally drinks too much and often goes hunting. Rita and Dick both encounter extra-marital temptation, bad luck and other human dilemmas.

The first reviews of *Entranced* were generally good. *The Porcupine* praised Flandrau for her "keen insight and genuine love of the truth." The reviewer in the *San Francisco Bulletin* said, "*Entranced* is good though by no means great.... The young critic of life and manners is becoming more the understanding and sympathetic artist." The *Saturday Review* and the *New York Post* gave the book positive reviews. The *Pioneer Press* did not review the book.[31]

Although St. Paulites Milton Griggs and Reinold Noyes sent praise, other friends didn't like the book as well as *Being Respectable*. Alice O'Brien, a second-generation Flandrau friend, wrote Grace in detail:

> I miss the punch and verve that you always have in conversation and usually have in writing. Of course I can't help being personal about it, because I really believe that you can write a great book and I wanted this to be it and I am sort of mad at you because it isn't. Write your history quickly and then do a book, a cruel book about people. All intellectual curiosity is cruel, because it makes people so futile, but that terrible acidity of yours has a ring of truth to it that is compelling. You were too kind in *Entranced*.[32]

A decade later, when interviewed by Brenda Ueland for *Golfer and Sportsman*, Grace said that, under the influence of a puritanical friend, she had cut out the best part of *Entranced*: "It was after that that I became uncompromising. It was a good book before I did that. I knew it. You always know it." Perhaps the omitted part was Rita's affair.[33]

Grace persuaded Blair to join her for the winter of 1924 at Hill's Glacier Park cabin. By this time, gossip about the Flandraus' many separations and curiosity about Grace's activities away from St. Paul had undoubtedly discomfited her and Blair. Although both knew Grace had repeatedly invited him to join her during their separations, others didn't know.

Like most independent, achieving women whose professional ambitions take them away from hearth and husband, Grace was experiencing the harsh reality that nature abhors a vacuum, and in the absence of concrete information about people—especially, enviable people—others inevitably fill the vacuum with speculation. Next, perception, however erroneous, becomes reality. The Flandraus appeared to conclude, after fifteen years of marriage, that they were no longer willing to be perceived as leading separate lives.

While Grace was still in the east, Blair went west to ready Hill's gamekeeper's lodge for their occupancy. He stayed in a Glacier Park Hotel while making preparations. Montana affected Blair's health and spirits as it had Grace's.

Having enjoyed duck hunting, fishing, canoeing, hiking, and sports of all kinds since boyhood, he loved the outdoors. He must also have benefited from feeling useful, a necessary adjunct to his wife's career. Their correspondence that fall makes it clear that Blair was the manager, the list-maker, and the spouse who remembered details and organized the household. His letters were always dated; Grace's never were.

According to Blair's written instructions, when Grace came on from St. Paul, she was to bring a cook—a St. Paul woman named "Drake"—Blair's flashlight, shades for hanging light bulbs, and his Winter Carnival suit. The latter garment, indigenous to St. Paul, Minnesota, has never been excelled for a certain snug density designed to withstand the bitterest cold.

Blair related well to people from all walks of life. He reveled in companionship and story telling. In October 1924 he wrote Grace in St. Paul that he was making interesting new acquaintances in Montana: "Slippery Bill said Kalispell was the only town he ever saw where people drank as much as they did in St. Paul."[34]

Grace joined Blair at the cabin in October 1924, bringing Drake, Pea, Pasha, and Daisy from St. Paul. (Pea and Pasha were often referred to as "Big and Little Pees," for obvious reasons.) The Flandraus planned to stay in Glacier Park for two or three months while Grace finished her research, spending both Thanksgiving and Christmas in Montana while she worked. It was an unrealistic and self-sacrificial plan.

The Great Northern assignment was prodigiously demanding. The project involved condensing three hundred years of Northwest history—with all the people and circumstances impacting its destiny—into several pamphlets of stirring prose. Despite Grace's broad reading since childhood, her formal academic training had been limited, as she openly admitted. She was essentially self-educated. For the Great Northern Railway project she needed to reconstruct settings displaying familiarity with the history, geography, and geology of a vast area over an extended period of time—centuries. The task would have challenged any doctoral candidate to the maximum. Grace had set her sights as high as Ralph Budd's.

Her letters to Betty Foster in St. Paul provide the only record of the Flandraus' winter in Glacier Park (1924–1925). At first Grace wrote cheerfully that she and Blair had been snowshoeing or skiing every day. Eventually, feeling isolated and lonely, she begged Foster for gossip of St. Paul. Grace said she longed for an "accurate description of the clothes, looks, degree of intoxication and misdeeds of everybody."[35] In mid-November, Grace advised Foster, (who was giving art lessons to children in St. Paul), on how <u>not</u> to teach them. She described how she had once tried to teach Tommy Irvine the violin and had failed. She added that the Montana wind was howling and that Pasha, the cat, was sick. At Thanksgiving, Grace wrote Foster that she had been reading a lot about the fur traders. Brief Christmas greetings were sent.

By late December, Grace mentioned to Betty that she was very thin and that Ralph Budd was sending fresh greens and seafood from Seattle to perk up her appetite.[36]

Early in January, Grace left Glacier Park for the West Coast. Her work required research in archives available only in Seattle and Spokane. Blair returned to St. Paul in her absence. When she notified Blair about her declining health, he said it sounded to him like another case of oncoming nervous exhaustion. She may have confessed how overwhelmed she felt by the project she had undertaken. Blair responded that if she was fed up with the Great Northern job and wanted to leave Glacier Park, it was all right with him. He advised her to stay out of the hospital. While traveling on the West Coast, however, Grace collapsed and ultimately spent about six weeks—from mid-January to late February, 1925—in a Spokane hospital.

She entered St. Luke's Hospital in Spokane shortly after writing Blair. Communicating with Betty Foster from the hospital on January 15, 1925, Grace said she was too thin and hadn't been able to eat for a month because she had been so eager to finish her work for the railroad.[37]

Certainly, by 1925, both Flandraus were aware that Grace was a relentless perfectionist who had the tendency to drive herself beyond her strength. The standards she and Budd had set were unrealistically high. But, even if she was now admitting she had undertaken too vast an assignment and didn't even enjoy the kind of writing required, Grace wasn't a quitter.

Flandrau's nurse at St. Luke's wrote three letters to Foster, dated January 29, February 3, and February 10, 1925. She explained that her patient was seriously drained, had no appetite, and was not allowed to read or write letters. The nurse informed Foster it would take longer than they had expected to build her back up again.[38]

By the end of February, however, Grace was back at work in Glacier Park, writing Foster about the "acres of smooth, clean, purple snow."[39] Whether Blair met her there is uncertain, but, by early March, he was writing from St. Paul to Grace in Montana.

Blair, who was the supportive anchor every artist needs, had gone back to tending fires in St. Paul. He wrote of fielding Grace's fan and business mail, making arrangements for visitors expected later in the spring, and typing the Great Northern material Grace drafted and sent him. He reminded her whom to thank for notes and flowers received in the hospital and told her she wasn't to worry about the expense of her hospitalization. Blair also tried his hand at editing. In one letter he spoke of "rewriting Mrs. Thompson's manuscript."[40]

Grace completed several pamphlets for the railroad over the next two years, dividing her time between the cabin in Glacier Park and her home in St. Paul. The first four were published between 1925 and 1927: *Seven Sunsets* (1925), *The Verendrye Overland Quest of the Pacific* (1925), *Red River Trails* (1926), and *The Lewis and Clark Expedition* (1927). Eventually, she wrote a total of eleven pamphlets for the Great Northern. Her style in the series ranges from eulogistic public relations writing to fine descriptive, sometimes lyric, prose.

An example of the former is this quote from *Seven Sunsets* extolling James J. Hill and the Great Northern Railway:

> The Great Northern system was planned by a genius who felt as none other has the pulse and heart beat of American life and the direction its expanding forces must take. It is to that genius, to that system that much of the growth and vitality of this domain is universally accredited.

There is fine descriptive prose too. The foreword for *Red River Trails* displays the author's ability to invoke vivid physical imagery to describe complex geographical features:

> There is a certain hay meadow in southwestern Minnesota; curiously enough this low-lying bit of prairie, often entirely submerged, happens to be an important height of land dividing the great watersheds of Hudson's Bay and the Mississippi River. It lies between two lakes: one of these, the Big Stone, gives rise to the Minnesota River, whose waters slide down the long toboggan of the Mississippi valley to the Gulf of Mexico.

The eleven railroad pamphlets are notable for their meticulous historical research and colorful portraits of explorers, surveyors, and other key figures in the development of the West. Rare photographs, maps, and fine engravings accompany the texts. (See Appendix A for titles of the pamphlets.)

Although obscure diaries and historical documents are generously quoted and key sources mentioned in footnotes, annotation of the pamphlets is not up to modern standards. Nevertheless, Flandrau's research is sometimes cited in contemporary scholarship on the West.

In spite of her achievement in historical journalism, however, Grace was bored and drained by the long, isolating task. She was delighted to put it behind her. In her 1934 interview with Brenda Ueland for *Golfer and Sportsman*, almost ten years after she had started working for the Great Northern, she remembered:

> [It was] a period during which I did hack work for a railroad, which was the most disastrous waste of time from every point of view. I spent months and years on so-called historical research for which I was not fitted, digging out niggling details about the doings of fur traders, explorers, local big businessmen. A great mistake. Because really I hate the thought of all of them. Naturally![41]

That comment suggests an uncommonly forward-looking, anti-chauvinist point of view challenging the white male establishment's version of American history in the 1930s. No wonder Flandrau and Ueland found much in common; their shared insights into such issues as the conquest and subjugation of Native Americans and the eradication of Indian cultures would have put them squarely in opposition to the "Manifest Destiny" mindset of many Americans—especially industrialists and "empire builders"—of their day. Both women—misunderstood rebels in the 1920s and 1930s—held opinions that are much more widely accepted today.

In the mid-1920s Grace remained unfocused as to the kind of writer she wanted to be. The Great Northern job had satisfied her ego but had done little to further her career. In spite of the high standard of research and writing achieved in the perishable railroad pamphlets, few readers saw them except for railroad officials, their employees, and their customers.

Moreover, Flandrau in her middle thirties was still very much an actress, often masking her inner thoughts. Having been influenced by her hard-working, goal-oriented father and having undertaken the role of breadwinner, Grace had long suppressed her feminine side. Forcing herself to complete the massive task she had undertaken for the railroad was a lesson in the importance of staying in touch with your own feelings, though Grace didn't realize it at the time. Ten years later, however, speaking frankly about the tedium of the assignment, she admitted: "As the result of this chaos of self-delusion, I became violently ill."[42]

But there was good fall-out too. Ralph Budd and Grace remained friends for thirty years, corresponding about issues from history to unions. They continued to address each other in writing as "Mr. Budd" and "Mrs. Flandrau." It was only ten years after Blair's death that they began calling each other "Grace" and "Ralph." Although St. Paul gossips suspected a long clandestine relationship between the married Budd and Grace, the late Kate S. Klein, a Flandrau intimate for many years, scoffed at the idea of an affair. Speaking of the rumors, in 1993 Klein said of Grace: "It would have been out of character."[43]

An additional benefit was that the Great Northern task provided excellent discipline and training for journalism and other writing—fiction and nonfiction—Grace would produce in the 1930s, 1940s, and 1950s.

CHAPTER X

Becoming a Journalist

"Madame, soyez sérieuse." ("Madame, be serious.")
Carl Jung to Grace Flandrau, Paris, France, 1927

BETWEEN 1924 AND 1927 Grace was often ill with migraines, depression, or influenza. She began to wonder whether she was suited to writing. Despite her uncertainty, publishers, editors, and filmmakers seemed to believe Grace Flandrau was a marketable writer. Their demand for her work shored up her faltering confidence through completion of the tedious railway work.

Charles Flandrau encouraged her during bouts of self-doubt. By 1920 Charles had retired from his columnist's job at the *Dispatch-Pioneer Press,* and by 1922 he had also terminated his Sunday column for the *St. Paul Daily News.* Because he was traveling more often than not, he wrote his sister-in-law at least twice a month. Their letters during the 1920s provide a good record of family activities and opinions. When Grace confided her disappointment that *Entranced* wasn't a best seller like *Being Respectable,* Charles sent compliments on *Seven Sunsets* (the most lavish railroad pamphlet) and advised not worrying about sales of her novel.

Beneath his ridiculing, snobbish, increasingly alcoholic exterior, Charles occasionally revealed a surprisingly maternal—as well as childish—heart. As Grace and Blair's life among married couples moved in a different direction from his bachelor existence, Charlie grew more dependent on them. When he wasn't traveling he lived alone in his parents' home with retainers and pets. (Charles's pets included numerous dogs and a Mexican parrot, "Lauro.") Having lost his devoted mama but never having outgrown his need for mothering, Charlie behaved maternally toward Blair and Grace even as he expected to be mothered by them and his servants. Seeing his need and valuing his intellectual companionship, Grace accommodated him, while Blair vacillated between tolerance of and irritation toward him.

In a rare confession to the younger brother he had always put down, Charles wrote early in 1925: "I now and then wish that I had acquired the habit of matrimony—not that marriage is an ideal institution. It most distinctly isn't;

but as one grows older, and old, life contains a good many somewhat blank, lonely moments."[1]

Although single women—strangers and old friends—had pursued him for years, Charles consistently spurned their overtures. His letters to Grace record some of his most scornful words about women. They shared cynical views about the motives of many "society women." In one letter to his sister-in-law he referred to début parties as "letting out" parties. In another Charles cruelly described the guests at Mrs. Charles Furness's tea party: "[They were]...a bevy of tedious women I used to know as young girls who are now merely smug, complacent, almost senile sows—dilapidated old incubators, whose ideal of being entertaining is to tell you for ¾ of an hour how difficult and expensive it is to provide growing children with shoes."[2]

Although he could be outrageously funny in a black way, Charles's cynical tone, usually exacerbated by drink, gradually separated him from old friends. His young chauffeur, William Dundas Clark, [always called "Clark"] filled the void as the traveling companion, dutiful guardian, and best friend Charles needed in his middle-aged, eccentric loneliness. When Flandrau at forty-four went back to work as a columnist for the *Dispatch-Pioneer Press* in 1915 and needed a driver, he had hired Clark, twenty-three. For the next four years Clark drove him to theaters and concert halls and attended so many performances with him that Flandrau friends joked it was probably Clark who wrote the reviews.[3]

In 1919 Charles took a leave of absence from his columnist's job and, although Clark had a wife and young daughter at home in St. Paul, the two men often traveled together out of town, exploring the United States in a succession of elegant touring cars. Lawrence Peter Haeg, Charles Flandrau's biographer, wrote:

> His [Charles's] relationship with Clark renewed gossip in St. Paul society that he was homosexual.... The true nature of their relationship may never be known but Clark's devotion to Flandrau never faltered. The two had occasional spats caused mostly by Flandrau's moodiness. Clark would sulk occasionally, but they remained friends because of Clark's admirable sense of duty.
>
> His primary role was chauffeur, and he did it with what Flandrau could only call 'absolute perfection.' Clark became a different man around automobiles: solemn, reverent, sometimes pessimistic and a little owly. Cars

were his raison d'être, without one to care for he was melancholy. Flandrau
proudly outfitted him in standard chauffeur garb of the upper class, elegant
white Palm Beach linen and matching motor cap. Clark responded by
polishing the Hudson to a 'positively vulgar glitter' so it looked 'like quite
the biggest and most comfortable battleship extant.[4]

Occasional visitors to Charles Flandrau's house in the early 1920s were
younger writers who sought his cultivated conversation and hospitality.
Among them were Tom Boyd and Cornelius Van Ness (of Kilmarnock's
Bookstore), F. Scott Fitzgerald, and Sinclair Lewis. All left St. Paul within a
few years and none of the friendships lasted. By 1925 the Nimbus Club had
disbanded and Kilmarnock's bookstore had closed. Later, when Sinclair Lewis
tried to see him, Charles refused, referring to him as "that dreadful man."
Privately, Charles disparaged the writing of both Sinclair Lewis and Scott
Fitzgerald.[5]

In the late 1920s James Gray, the young drama and books critic who
succeeded him at the *Dispatch–Pioneer Press*, began cultivating Charles's
friendship. Gray, who was a University of Minnesota graduate almost thirty
years younger, idolized Charles Flandrau-the-writer and probably felt both
aggrandized and challenged by filling the shoes of his famous predecessor at
the paper. After Charles underwrote a European tour for Gray and his wife,
Sophie, in 1928, he earned Gray's undying loyalty. The Grays, although considerably younger, mingled with the Blair Flandrau's and Charles's social crowd.

Over the subsequent years the two critics spent many hours together over
drinks in the small library at the Flandrau house, discussing books, authors,
human nature in general, and St. Paul society in particular. Gray flattered the
lonely older author by repeatedly urging him to resume his writing career. Their
extensive correspondence reveals that Gray began to think and talk like his idol.
He was an aspiring novelist himself, with one novel to his credit by 1925.[6]

As Grace was winding down her Great Northern work, another journalistic assignment turned up. Late in 1925 editor Duncan Aikman asked her to
write a chapter for a collection of essays about the settlement of the West to be
published by Minton, Balch and Company. The book, entitled *The Taming of
the Frontier*, came out the same year.[7]

On April 23, 1926, Grace read aloud her chapter, "St. Paul, the Untamable
Twin," from *The Taming of the Frontier* to an audience at the Women's City
Club in St. Paul. She described the city's distinctive personality this way:

St. Paul, in spite of the advent of many important newcomers, is still, at the core and kernel, hereditary. The sons and grandsons of the sound merchant and banking class still give their stamp to the community—Griggs, Gordons, Saunders, Finches, Deans, Noyes, Ordways, Skinners, Lindekes and many others. The fortunes they have inherited were not made quickly or speculatively . . . a tradition of conservatism has been handed down with them . . . they are not Rotarians, not joiners at heart. They are individualists.

By 1926, after fifteen years of marriage, Blair and Grace appeared to be financially secure. Due to the boom on Wall Street, the market value of Blair's holdings in St. Paul Fire and Marine, West Publishing, and various bank stocks, plus dividends, apparently increased enough to support them without Grace's working professionally. Most of their St. Paul friends were living well off their capital during that frothy period, but, with her mixture of high material expectations and acute fear of financial reverse, Grace would have been uncomfortable living on capital. Nevertheless, not needing to earn money made it more difficult to justify working.

If Blair hadn't assumed the role of her business manager, Grace's literary career might have ended in the 1920s. But, with her husband and Mary O'Malley as her dependable financial and household managers, and in spite of unreliable health, Grace's career and social life continued in tandem.

Grace taught Mary O'Malley everything she knew about cooking. French cuisine was standard fare. The Flandraus excelled as hosts, and O'Malley prepared and served the elegant dinners the couple became famous for. Flandrau friends and relatives of all ages remember that Mary could transform even the cookies and sandwiches of afternoon tea into a gourmet meal.[8]

The Flandraus entertained informally and often invited friends for Sunday night supper followed by reading plays, poetry, and other books aloud. The household always included a menagerie of pets for Blair to superintend.

Blair's health, however, was declining. Chronic rheumatism of the neck and pain from a boyhood back injury had taken their toll. He had always been thin, almost malnourished-looking. By the middle 1920s, Blair was paying the price for decades of heavy smoking and drinking. Most likely he had depended for years on alcohol to ease his neck and back pain.

In mid-1926, at the age of fifty-two, Blair learned he had a prostate condition requiring surgery. Charlie wrote offering money to help pay for "dusting off the sacred organs of generation." Whoever paid for it, Blair went ahead with the operation and slowly recovered.[9]

As 1926 ended, Grace was at Hill-Stead for the holidays with the Riddles. Blair, declining as usual, had Christmas Eve dinner in St. Paul with Charlie and family friend Alice O'Brien. He wrote Grace the day after Christmas that he was worried about Charlie, who, according to the servants, was sick in bed and drunk.[10]

Grace and Alice O'Brien, about five years younger, probably became acquainted when both were students at the Backus School for Girls in St. Paul. Alice's grandfather, John O'Brien, was a pioneer lumberman in the St. Croix Valley when Charles E. Flandrau arrived in Minnesota Territory in the 1850s. Alice's parents, William and Julia O'Brien, and her brother, Jack, and his wife, "Cotty" [Katherine], were old friends of the Flandraus.

Alice was a wealthy, well-educated, and much-traveled unmarried woman when she began seeing Blair and Grace frequently in the mid-1920s. She was an art collector with exquisite taste and widely known for her shrewd business judgment. All the Flandraus sought her advice on financial matters. On many occasions she was the perfect addition to the small circle of Charles, Blair, and Grace.

Although very different, Alice and Grace developed an enduring friendship. O'Brien became an anchor-to-windward for Blair during his wife's many absences, looking after him on Grace's behalf. Alice understood and appreciated Charlie's wit while tolerating his ridiculing, cynical personality. With her, Charlie could be "in a darling mood," as she wrote Grace.[11]

During Blair's convalescence from surgery, O'Brien offered an intriguing opportunity to the Flandraus, who immediately accepted it. Her idea was a health tonic for both and led to career rejuvenation for Grace.

Alice O'Brien invited the Flandraus to accompany her on an extended trip across Africa, following the Congo River from its mouth on the west to its headwaters, then across Lake Tanganyika to Mombasa on the east coast. O'Brien longed to see the wild animals of Africa, and reading about the "Dark Continent" (much in fashion in the 1920s) had aroused her curiosity.

Charles E. Bell, a filmmaker from St. Paul, and Ben Burbridge, an experienced big-game hunter from Florida—a close friend of O'Brien's—also joined the party. As she and Burbridge planned the trip during the last months of 1926, Alice proposed that Grace keep a journal of the expedition as material for a book and film on Africa. The trip was to begin in late fall of 1927 and would take about six months.

The Flandraus decided to prepare their wills before making such a long journey out of the country. When Grace told Charlie what they were doing, he responded: "As far as my being your 'heir' is concerned (one of the few roles in which I have not so far visualized myself), I laughed aloud at the thought of being a hungry anticipant of your unfortunate demise. You must neither of you speak of such dreary things."

But Charlie admitted that, at fifty-six, he had given thought to his old age, anticipating that he would have to endure it by himself: "Mrs. Furness [daughter of Governor Alexander Ramsey] has a room reserved for me at the Home for the Friendless [later the Protestant Home], and for years I have kept up a chaste flirtation with the Mother Superior of the Little Sisters of the Poor [an order of nuns who ran a convent home for the elderly indigent in St. Paul]."[12]

While Blair and Grace made plans to go to Africa, Charles traveled extensively in Europe with Clark. He wrote affectionate letters and spoke of missing them and their pets. One of his letters from Paris included this characteristically acid observation of Americans abroad: "Ambassadors are merely mediocrities who have happened to marry unattractive, socially ambitious women with money. When one ignores persons like that at home, why should one seek them out abroad?" Probably no one quoted that remark to the Riddles. Charles's letter confided that someone had tried to buy his St. Paul Fire and Marine stock but, on Alice O'Brien's advice, he had declined.[13]

Preparations for the African journey were elaborate. The travelers studied Swahili and spent months outfitting the expedition. In October 1927 O'Brien, Bell, and Burbridge sailed for France, where they began ordering what was best obtained in Paris. The Blair Flandraus planned to join them there.

On June 22, 1927, before leaving the United States, Grace queried Maxwell E. Perkins, executive editor of Charles Scribner's Sons, proposing that *Scribner's* monthly magazine publish a series of her letters from Africa. She also wondered whether Charles Scribner's Sons would be interested in book rights to the material.

Perkins referred Grace's letter to a junior editor who responded negatively to the idea of separate articles but said he hoped Charles Scribner's Sons would have the opportunity to consider the book. Whether she queried Harcourt, Brace and Company immediately after this rejection is unknown, but, before arriving in France, Grace knew that the publisher of her last two novels—*Being Respectable* and *Entranced*—wanted her book manuscript on Africa.[14]

In Paris, still suffering migraines and depression, Grace arranged an appointment with Carl Jung, the famous Swiss psychiatrist. According to a family anecdote, after a short interview with the forty-year-old Flandrau, Jung, leaning across his desk and looking deeply into her eyes, said, "Madame, soyez sérieuse." After that advice, the author said, she committed herself to writing more seriously than ever and soon returned to good health. The interview with Jung reaffirmed Dr. Riggs's earlier advice to Grace at Purinton Inn: "Work hard at something you believe in."[15]

Grace's book *Then I Saw the Congo,* Harcourt, Brace and Company, September, 1929, documents the challenging trip across Africa made by Alice O'Brien, the Flandraus, and their companions from December 1927 to May 1928. According to her text, Grace wrote the manuscript on a typewriter "carried through the tall forest day after day on the round unwilling head of a black boy with a tattooed nose."[16]

Charles Bell brought enough film for three thousand still photographs and thousands of feet of movie film. At every opportunity he shot stills and movies of natives, their villages, animals, and African river and forest landscape. Grace's book and its subsequent serialization in the *St. Paul Pioneer Press* included four dozen photographs. A Hollywood film called *Up the Congo* also resulted from the journey.

The party of five sailed from Marseilles in December 1927, bound for Dakar, Senegal, then along the west coast of Africa to Matadi at the mouth of the Congo. From Matadi, by train and riverboat, they made their way to Stanleyville, where they purchased additional supplies and hired two hundred native bearers and other servants.

From Stanleyville, the party took a circuitous route through the jungle of the Ituri Forest to the heart of Africa. First traveling by car and truck and later by huge dugout canoes, each manned by twenty native paddlers, they stopped every day to set up an elaborate camp on a village clearing. After their return via the Aruwimi River to a point near Stanleyville, they proceeded by railroad, steamer, and truck to the port of Mombasa on the east coast of Africa, stopping at Lake Tanganyikana on the way. The trip covered seven thousand miles.

Supplies for the journey required a staggering amount of luggage according to Grace's description in *Then I Saw the Congo*:

Our baggage filled one entire little freight coach. From New York we had brought two moving-picture cameras, 28,000 feet of film, five complete camp outfits—tents, dining room fly, beds, baths, folding tables and chairs, medicines, powdered milk, canned tomatoes—six great packing-cases full in all. In Paris we added sixty-eight tin trunks in which our effects could be redistributed into fifty-pound loads—bedding, camp hardware, solera cloth suits with spine pads, helmets, mosquito boots. Nothing, we had innocently supposed, could be bought in all the Belgian Congo![17]

She wrote the following passage at the journey's beginning, just after the travelers had boarded the "Brazza" and set sail from Dakar down the west coast of Africa:

For three weeks we sailed south, then east under the great bulge of the continent, then south again. The ocean slept, breathing deeply, and the sun, blurred with humidity, made a path like moonshine on the oily swell. Sea turtles rocked on the waves and little fish like trout swam upward to the surface and flew and flew before the ship. Far away in the east, between the slowly swinging sea and heat-misted sky, was the dark, still outline of Africa. Below Dakar the blowy desert vegetation gave place to the great forest, which lay, unbroken and unending, upon the land; and palm oil, rubber, mahogany, and other products even more important to empire than peanuts, began.

This was the famous old, wicked old West African Slave Coast, and the very names, Gold Coast, Ivory Coast, Guinea, Dahomey, were rich with that peculiar glamour that attends an exceedingly evil reputation. History is sad reading—at least I find it so, although many, I believe, follow it unmoved or even with a certain exaltation at the forward march of the species. But I can never discount the cost, or refrain from getting angry at the heights of hypocritical ferocity to which our human kind so frequently rises. Even on days as indolent as those, when the "Brazza" lay peacefully at anchor in the shallow estuary of some sluggish river, one could not escape these shores—the exploiting, kidnapping, converting, that so merrily went on. Here the tall-masted slavers rocked at anchor, waiting, while everywhere, along all the inland trails, blazed, we read, by piles of human bones, down these rivers of anguish to the sea came the captives in thousands, in millions, led by the first Christian music heard here—the singing of whips, rattle of chains, weeping of mothers. All done in the names of their various Most Christian Majesties of Europe and later of our own most Christian republic.[18]

Publication of *Then I Saw the Congo* by Harcourt, Brace and Company in September 1929 attracted broad international attention. Groundbreaking for its time, the book is a detailed social, cultural, and physical description of central Africa in the mid-1920s and the adventures of the American group's visit there. Objective observation and original analysis, enlivened by the vivid narrative style of a humane writer, characterize the book. In *Then I Saw the Congo* Grace allowed her compassion for people and her passion for realism to flourish. Once again she challenged the premise of white supremacy. The publishing world took note.

Kermit Roosevelt praised the book in his column in the *Saturday Review of Literature* on October 19, 1929: "The book [*Then I Saw the Congo*) is a very real contribution to the literature of the no longer Dark Continent. . . . Among the most intensely interesting parts of her book are the constant thumbnail sketches of official and trader, and missionary and traveler."

G. C. Harrap brought out a British edition of *Then I Saw the Congo* the next year. Critics hailed it in London newspapers.[19] After translations appeared abroad, fan mail poured in from foreign readers and other writers.

The book caused barely a ripple in St. Paul. Charles Flandrau's only written comment to Grace was that the St. Paul Book and Stationary store was out of her new book and wasn't advertising it. *The St. Paul Dispatch* noted the book's release as a short news story on September 5, 1929, but did not review it.

On March 23, 1930, however, seven months after the book's appearance, the Sunday *Pioneer Press* began serializing *Then I Saw the Congo.* Not until 1936, however, seven years after the book's original release, did *St. Paul Dispatch* critic James Gray extoll the book as "one of the best travel books an American has ever written." This long gap in Gray's coverage is mysterious.[20]

A feature-length silent film called *Up the Congo* presented the visual record of the expedition. Only the strenuous protests of Flandrau and O'Brien, however, prevented Hollywood filmmakers from turning the documentation of people and places in Africa into a phony scenario featuring cannibal cauldrons and charging elephants. The film's production included translation of its subtitles into eight foreign languages. Showings of *Up the Congo* occurred all over the United States and received high praise. The author often lectured at out-of-state presentations after the film's release in 1930.

Twin Cities readers were impressed. Jack Ordway wrote Grace that Flandrau friends, including his mother and father, "who are as critical as the devil," were raving about the book.[21] Alice O'Brien told Grace that everyone she knew was genuinely enthusiastic about the African book and that she was completely satisfied with it herself.[22]

Recognition as a serious analyst of cultures propelled Grace to a new dimension of celebrity and credibility. Six years had passed since *Being Respectable's* big splash, and few readers had seen or heard of the Great Northern Railway pamphlets. Although Grace's short fiction hadn't appeared in magazines for almost a decade, now a broad-spectrum of periodicals, carrying both fiction and nonfiction, beckoned. In September 1929, *Travel* magazine published Flandrau's photo-journalistic essay, "Black Potentates of Equatorial Africa." In December 1930, *Contemporary Review*, a scholarly British periodical, carried her carefully researched nonfiction piece "What Africa Is Not." The latter article, an exposition of African history, geography, and colonial politics, solidified her reputation as a non-fiction writer.

Then I Saw the Congo is a rare example of modern travel journalism by a woman. A Minnesota historian, Eileen Michels, said of it as recently as 1977:

> Although no one in the party was a trained anthropologist, Grace Flandrau's *Then I Saw the Congo*, is a detailed description of their adventure written with sensitivity, knowledge, and humor. It was, as a matter of fact, a far more interesting account of travels in Africa than one written for the *New York Times* in 1927 by Martin Johnson, a well-known explorer of the day. Flandrau, an excellent writer, was particularly responsive to the often incongruous juxtapositions of indigenous old and transplanted new in equatorial Africa, to the shoddiness of much white colonial culture, to the brutality which often characterized treatment of black by white, to the nature of native villages and music, and to the style, dignity, and beauty of many native people, particularly the Mangbetu tribe—a group erroneously described at that time by the *Encyclopaedia Britannica* as extinct.[23]

CHAPTER XI

A Family Quarrel

"You see, the trouble with Charlie has always been that he was given
every consideration and he can't get over the feeling—way down deep
in his heart—that I was never given much or was entitled to any."
William Blair Flandrau to Grace Flandrau, from Seville, Spain, January 1931

AS GRACE BASKED in renewed public recognition, the collapse of the
American stock market in October 1929 brought an end to a decade of speculative frenzy and gave Americans of inherited wealth a rude awakening. Stocks
formerly counted on to appreciate and provide increasing net worth plunged
in value and reduced or stopped paying dividends entirely. Bonds defaulted as
corporations lost customers and income.

Following the financial catastrophe on Wall Street, the Flandraus, like other
Americans of reduced means, including many artists and writers, retreated
to Europe, where living graciously was less expensive. Blair estimated that it
cost a third less to live in France than it did to live at home. During their two
years in France Grace's literary career flourished. Charles Flandrau made the
first move abroad. After retirement from his columnist's job in 1920 Flandrau
often traveled away from Minnesota. His extensive correspondence demonstrates that by the mid-1920s Charles was making lengthy visits to European
capitols and the Island of Majorca, an enchanting place he described in vivid
letters and poetry to Grace.[1]

In spring 1929, on one of his frequent trips to France, Charles purchased a
manor house and farm in the Normandy countryside near Vernon, an hour's
drive northwest of Paris along the Seine River. He whimsically named it "Le
Petit Saint Paul" and invited family members and friends to visit him. After
the stock market plummeted in 1929 many took him up on his offer.

The address of Le Petit Saint Paul was 4, rue de Marzelles, Bizy-Vernon.
The Norman "cottage" is situated on a high wooded bluff in tiny, historic
Bizy—complete with ancient château and park that were formerly the fief-
dom of French royalty. It overlooks the modern town of Vernon and the Seine
River. Bizy-Vernon lies directly across the river from Givergny, the pastoral
village made famous by the painter and noteworthy gardener, Claude Monet.

Proximity to the ancestral seat of the Flandraus, his Norman Huguenot forebears, and to the colony of American artists and writers hovering about the elderly Monet attracted Charles to the area. Undoubtedly, the tolerant French attitude toward bisexualism made him more comfortable than he felt in the American Midwest. His surprising openness in that regard surfaced in a communication he sent from Bizy to an old American friend, Richard E. Myers.

Describing his first meeting with Ernest Hemingway, Charlie confided to Myers: "On the other hand, Ernest Hemingway's sex-appeal has devastated me. I can't for the moment recall whether or not we kissed each other good-bye. He is really almost as big and simple and unmasked as he professionally pretends to be. A man for whom men go mad."[2]

The Flandraus called Charlie's little French estate simply "Bizy." He maintained his residence there most of the time between 1929 and 1933, usually in the company of his faithful chauffeur, Clark, his French caretakers, and his touring car. Monet's ex-gardener began to work for him. Clark's wife, Virginia, and their little daughter, Elizabeth, who accompanied them to Europe, often toured by themselves or with Clark and Charles. Clark was strict with his employer about his drinking.

Charles's steady correspondence with his protégée in St. Paul, the young critic James Gray, provides much of this record. Gray's letters to Charles in the early 1930s repeatedly beseeched him to resume his writing career. In one note Gray wrote: "I will give up all other reading and devote myself to studying your letters." He confessed: "I could be reviled and hated of men and I shouldn't be very much concerned if I could occasionally have a little approval from you."[3]

During their extended stay in France, 1930–1932, the Blair Flandraus again rented out their home in St. Paul. When Blair occasionally returned to Minnesota during this period, he stayed at the Minnesota Club. If Grace came to America on business, she stayed at a Manhattan hotel or at Hill-Stead. In fall 1930, Bizy was the scene of a traumatic family quarrel.

In early winter 1930, Grace visited France alone, seeking seclusion for writing. She settled in for several months of work at a Paris hotel, using the Bankers Trust Company at 5 Place Vendôme as her mailing address. The literary world stayed in touch. In April William R. Benét, poet and friend of Grace's magazine-writing days, wrote asking to hear about her new work.[4]

Blair and Grace's arrival in France apparently augmented Charles's feelings of sibling and social rivalry. His monthly letters to James Gray in winter and spring 1930 hinted at his resentment. In January 1930, he wrote, "James, dear boy, I should like to see you and talk to you about a lot of things I cannot exactly write. . . . I realize that your family life . . . has been as superfluously complicated, as crowded with entirely undesired and disturbing underlying subtleties as my own."[5]

A month later he confided, "In late March or very early April "[he was] . . . turning this lovely, friendly place [Bizy] over to Blair and Grace and I'm not especially keen about it but for various reasons it has to be done." To Gray, Charles scoffed at Grace's interest in meeting his titled neighbors in the Vernon countryside.[6]

Blair, traveling with Mary Livingston Griggs (Mrs. Theodore) of St. Paul, and her teen-aged daughter, Mary, joined Grace on the Riviera in late winter 1930. Mary Livingston Griggs, a chum since Blair's youth, was the sister of his old girlfriend, Abigail Livingston. Blair and Grace expected to meet other guests from Minnesota at Bizy in early April.

In May, from Paris, Grace again queried editor Maxwell Perkins about whether he would like to read her six new African stories before they were published in book form. She told Perkins she wanted to finish mining the Congo episode before she began a new novel.[7]

In 1930 Charles Scribner's Sons and its monthly magazine, *Scribner's*, stood at the zenith of American literary publishing. Maxwell E. Perkins, executive editor, made his reputation and transformed Charles Scribner's Sons staid image with the publication in the 1920s and 1930s of the groundbreaking work of unknown writers like F. Scott Fitzgerald, Ernest Hemingway, Ring Lardner, John P. Marquand, Marjorie Kinnan Rawlings, and Thomas Wolfe. According to Malcolm Cowley's profile of the legendary editor in the April 1944 *New Yorker*, "Unshaken Friend," at Perkins's urging "the firm [Charles Scribner's Sons] took a sudden leap from the age of innocence into the lost generation."

By 1930, Perkins was overall manager of publications at Charles Scribner's Sons, both for books and *Scribner's* magazine. Alfred Dashiell was managing editor of the magazine and Kyle S. Crichton was associate editor. In the next seven years Grace corresponded often with these editors and she developed a close professional friendship with the intense, kind-hearted Crichton.

Charles Scribner's Sons' editorial staff had taken note of *Then I Saw the Congo's* success. Perkins responded to Grace's letter immediately: "We should certainly be very grateful for an opportunity to read these Congo stories . . . and we should like to see all of them." He advised that between seven thousand and fifteen thousand words was the least practical length for short stories.[8]

As she sent off the stories from Paris in mid-June Grace wrote Perkins again, thanking him and asking for criticism. Two of her stories, she said, were 15,000 words each, three were about 850, and one was about 660 words in length. Grace asked him to send any stories he didn't want to Horace Liveright, a rival publisher of emerging writers.[9]

On July 2, 1930, Perkins responded enthusiastically, complimenting Grace on her new work and offering $500 for her story "One Way of Love." He wrote, "Your stories came yesterday, and I read the two long ones last night. I think both of them very fine, but particularly "One Way of Love." That I think magnificent. . . . I have also glanced at the other stories, and although I should not speak of them without reading them all through, I must say I am very much impressed." Perkins added that "One Way of Love" fell into the category of a new genre for *Scribner's*, the long short story: "This one comes to the lower limit for that genre which we are trying to encourage. May we take this very remarkable story, and run it in the October issue?"[10]

Perkins assigned Kyle Crichton to work out details. On July 9, 1930, Crichton notified Grace officially that the magazine wanted to publish "One Way of Love" and suggested a few minor changes: "It ['One Way of Love'] is one of the most remarkable stories in years and we are proud to print it. It will be eligible for the $5,000 long short story prize which we are offering."[11]

In July 1930 Perkins offered to buy "Faith," another long short story of the African series, for $250. He said the Depression was affecting the prices publishers and the public could pay for books and magazines. Also, Perkins was more interested in publishing novels than short fiction.[12]

Crichton stayed in touch with Grace by letter and wire while she was in France that summer, continuing his praise for "One Way of Love," making sure Grace gave permission to enter the story in *Scribner's* annual contest, and commenting on D. H. Lawrence's problems with the U.S. Senate.[13] Grace accepted Crichton's changes, which he called "sensible," and added some of her own, which he labeled "simple genius."[14]

In September Crichton wrote that "One Way of Love" was "one of the finest things ever written by an American, not excepting *Ethan Frome*; I predict it is going to be an American classic."[15]

"One Way of Love" is an intense story contrasting the psyches of two white scientists in Africa. It subtly portrays the truth that bitter jealousy and even hatred often mask feelings of profound admiration and love. Walcott and Brant, the two main characters, are white scientists studying flora and fauna in Africa. Walcott, a temperamental entomologist, has more advanced training than Brant, but Brant —an uncomplicated, good-hearted man—always seems to make the key sightings and is more admired by the natives. Walcott, who mistreats the blacks, feels like a failure and is pathologically jealous of Brant, who, in spite of the mean-spiritedness of his partner, is kind and caring. Walcott, who becomes desperately sick and discouraged, finally plans his own death to impress Brant with his bravery and love. Although he has malaria, Walcott secretly stops taking his quinine tablets so Brant will have enough himself to survive.

The author tells the story of these two opposites and the dynamics of their partnership from Walcott's point of view—most likely inspired by her observation of Charles's and Blair's tortured relationship. Like all Grace's stories set in Africa, "One Way of Love" employs an infinite variety of the country's sounds, sights, smells, and climatic conditions to enhance mood. Its anthropomorphism endows inhuman objects with human characteristics, as in the following description: "Walcott raised the cup to his nose. He loved smells. He loved the cold-hot smell of the champagne. He drank his cupful down, restored by the sensation of its sly violence sliding through his veins."[16]

Charles wrote Grace an unusually complimentary letter in September: "I don't feel that the [*Scribner's*] editors in any way exaggerated in their appreciation of your story. It is really a beautiful study, beautifully—indeed perfectly—written, by which I mean ... that it is so 'all of a piece.' ... What I am trying ... to get at is my recognition and profound admiration of the marvelously skillful and harmonious architecture of the whole thing. ... Edith Wharton would have liked to write 'One Way of Love,' but she would have made a distressing, although readable, mess of it."[17]

His letter continued with news that James Gray had approached Alfred Knopf about publishing a collection of Charles's old *Pioneer Press* and *Daily News* columns, a revival of one of Tom Boyd's earlier ideas, but Charlie told Gray he would "wash his hands" of the entire affair.

"One Way of Love" appeared in the October 1930 issue of *Scribner's* and late that month Crichton notified Grace that letters from readers were "amazingly good. There are hundreds of them, and it is impossible to forward them to you. The readers were crazy about it!"[18] Charles Flandrau began addressing Grace as "the George Eliot of Ten Thousand Lakes."[19]

That humorous epithet, however, may have masked his inner turmoil about Grace's growing reputation in the literary world. Repeatedly beseeched to start writing again by James Gray, Charlie had finally resurfaced with "The Bustle," a light, nostalgic story published in the August 1930 *Harper's*, only to be upstaged by Grace's major coup with "One Way of Love" in the October *Scribner's*.

Gray, who undoubtedly recognized and probably shared Charles's not-entirely-hidden jealousy of Grace, wrote his idol a sympathetic letter: "I hope you'll forgive me for helping myself to a resentment I'm not particularly entitled to. But it has always seemed to me that since you were born Flandrau and since you had established the literary significance of the name long before it had been attached to works other than your own, you really had a right to the trademark."[20]

In late summer, 1930, Grace and Blair visited the Isle of Man, the ancestral home of the Corrins, Edward Hodgson's maternal forebears. Theodate Riddle probably urged Grace to make this sentimental journey, recognizing she needed connection with her own roots.

No record of contact between Grace and her father's half-brothers and sisters in Minnesota exists, but by 1930 one or two Hodgson relatives in St. Paul must have communicated with their increasingly famous half-cousin. Perhaps their conversations stimulated Grace's curiosity to see the island where her grandmother, Charlotte Corrin Hodgson, and step-grandfather, Thomas Hodgson, had lived in the early 1800s.

Grace wrote several long letters to Theodate from the tiny green Isle of Man, where she made acquaintance with her Corrin cousins at their country estate, "Knochaloe Beg," outside the fishing village of Peel. Describing the island, Grace wrote: "This is the cutest, most preposterous place in the world. The whole island is only thirty-three miles long and twelve wide, not counting an odd little islet off the south end known as the Calf of Man. And it's exactly like being at sea. The whole little green island is very much like a ship and when it's stormy, you're always suspecting it will spring a leak and sink."

She informed Theo that her great-great-grandfather Corrin, who built Corrin's Tower (still standing outside the village of Peel), had been a poet and a "ghostcatcher." Writing Kyle Crichton from the Isle of Man later in the summer, Grace said she was staying on alone to work. Blair had gone ahead to Bizy and would meet her there. Theodate and John Riddle were expected to join them and Charles at Bizy-Vernon for a visit extending into the fall.[21]

Although details are missing, subsequent family correspondence reveals that a severe quarrel erupted at Le Petit Saint Paul in late fall 1930. Letters suggest that after Charles lent Grace and Blair and their friends the use of his house, he made angry accusations about their misuse of it. In the aftermath Charles wrote Dick Myers that he had had enough of Blair to "do me for the rest of my life."[22] Grace wrote Myers that Charles was "simply impossible."[23] Blair later wrote Grace: "John's eyes have been opened at last as to Charlie. . . . It took a meat axe to do it."[24] As a result, the Blair Flandraus vowed never to return to Bizy.

Grace and Blair returned to Paris, then traveled to Spain, to stay at the Hôtel de Inglaterra in Seville. When Grace embarked for America, Kent Curtiss, a Minnesota teacher and close friend of Alice O'Brien's, joined Blair in Spain. Still smarting over the argument, Blair wrote Grace in New York from Seville early in January 1931: "You see, the trouble with Charlie is that he was always given every consideration and he can't get over the feeling—way down deep in his heart—that I was never given much or was entitled to any."[25]

Charlie was on the verge of leaving Bizy for the United States when he sent Blair a touching "cri de coeur," unmatched in tone by any other letter he wrote to his brother: "Dearest Blair. I care for you so greatly. I can scarcely see. You know of course that I love you and that is all I can say. I am going away in a few days."[26]

After deciding not to return to Bizy, Grace and Blair tried various hotels and spas in France. At times they complained of being broke and were considering an apartment rental in Paris, but doctors advised avoiding the cold winters there. By September 1931 they were staying in Aix-les-Bains where Grace sought a cure for her rheumatism.

In mid-September, traveling along the Riviera, they discovered a quiet inn in Menton, the Hotel Banastron on the Promenade du Cap Martin near Monte Carlo. The Hotel Banastron became Blair and Grace's European base in the months ahead.[27]

Menton is near Cap d'Antibes where Mark Cross heir, Gerald Murphy, and his wife, Sarah, entertained the Flandraus' St. Paul friends—the Scott Fitzgeralds, Oscar ("Colly") and Xandra Kalman, Jerome Hill—and the Richard Myerses at their seaside residence, the Villa America. Undoubtedly the Flandraus connected with these friends during their stay at Menton.

In fall 1931, Blair returned to Minnesota on business. He wanted to discuss his investments in person with those who managed them, Edwin C. White and Oscar Kalman.

Grace lingered at the Pont Royal Hotel in Paris into October and November. She was in a buoyant mood. "Faith," her serialized novelette about Africa, débuted in the October 1931 *Scribner's*, and Kyle Crichton sent word that William Faulkner, one of the judges, had pronounced "One Way of Love" the best in *Scribner's* annual short story contest.[28] Someone else won the prize, Grace wrote Blair, but Faulkner's comment meant a lot.

"Faith" is a long short story about profound human stresses in the lives of white officials and their families in Africa. The author exploited her considerable talent for physical description in the story, employing the African landscape as a potent character. Adjectives usually reserved for human beings describe elements of the African veldt and jungle, for example: "the singing green of the bamboos" and "the blond sky just darkened on the horizon by the even, somber line of the forest."

Grace indulged herself in Paris, setting aside fears about money for the moment. She lunched and dined with friends, attended plays and vaudeville shows with the Myers, and ran up bills at couturier houses.

Richard ("Dickie") and Alice Lee Herrick Myers, American residents of Paris from 1921 to 1932, were most attentive. Alice Lee had been a girlhood friend of Mrs. Tom Daniels (Frances) in the Chicago area, and, after marrying Richard E. Myers and moving to St. Paul with him, through the Tom Danielses, the Myerses became acquainted with many Twin Cities socialites, including Charles and Blair Flandrau. Dick Myers, who attended Yale University with Louis W. Hill's sons, worked briefly for the Great Northern Railway after graduation from college.

Myers, who was a portly bon vivant, dilettante, and connoisseur supreme of wine and food, was European editor of the *Ladies Home Journal* and a director of the Curtis Publishing Company when Charles Flandrau arrived in France in the mid-1920s, followed by Blair and Grace in 1930. Charles, Blair and Dick were old chums, and, after meeting, Grace and Dick felt instantaneous rapport. He and Alice Lee, his wife, became Grace's close friends and corresponded with her over many years.

Myers was a gifted amateur pianist and composer. His tall, capable wife, who ran a women's dress shop in Paris, was a superb hostess. They gave memorable parties at their rue Visconti apartment. The Flandraus were devoted to both. From their first encounter Dick Myers showed enthusiastic interest in Grace's literary career and took every opportunity to boost it, but he was equally enamored of Charles's writing and often read *Viva Mexico!* aloud to friends.[29] Charles, however, who had reconnected with Dick and his wife in France five years earlier than Blair and Grace, must have felt increasingly sidelined after his brother and sister-in-law's arrival in Europe in 1930.

The Myers circulated with the celebrated colony of expatriate American artists and writers living in Paris after World War I, throughout the 1920s and into the Depression. These included Jerome Hill, Ernest and Pauline Hemingway, Archibald and Ada MacLeish, Nadia Boulanger, Scott and Zelda Fitzgerald, and Gerald and Sarah Murphy. At the Myers's rue Visconti flat Charlie, Grace, and Blair ran into the others. In fall, 1931, Americans in Paris must have been buzzing with the news of Grace's success at *Scribner's*. Henry Miller, an impoverished, little-known American writer then living in Paris, sought her assistance in finding a publisher for his *Tropic of Cancer*.[30]

Charlie also stayed on in Europe that fall, alternating between his house in Bizy and a hotel in Paris. He began dying his hair.[31]

After the family argument at Bizy, whenever he was in Paris, Charles made a point of calling on Grace or telephoning her. He seemed to be in a chastened mood and had temporarily stopped drinking. Grace's letters to Blair in late 1931 revealed sympathy for her brother-in-law. Thinking their quarrel at Bizy had been partly her fault, Grace was attempting to mediate between the brothers. She also felt guilty about staying behind in Paris and spending money.

After lunching with Charlie in Paris one day, Grace wrote Blair: "He was quite sober and very nice, not a bit smug. I think he has learned a lot. . . . Also he has felt very lonely and realized a good many things. He spoke today of his loneliness." She urged Blair to call his brother once in a while when Charlie returned to St. Paul. Grace also mentioned to Blair that it had been ages since she had heard from him.

She explained her perceived need to be by herself for a while: "A lot of things are milling about inside me and doing me a great deal of good. . . . I hope for your sake more than mine . . . And that is why I am staying by myself . . . Why I must be alone a little longer."[32]

Shortly thereafter, in the same vein, Grace wrote:

> Blair, we would not be as happy as we should and shall be unless I really
> get the best of some of the things you know. And I think I understand it

all a little better all the time. Oh, Blair, you are partly to blame. You have spoiled me too, been too little exacting. Talk about monsters—I've been one or was gradually getting to be. . . . [Now I am becoming] more like the me of 20 years ago than you can imagine. It was Bizy that did me in!

Grace admitted she wasn't working but was just spending money. She had ordered three new dresses: "Please don't die of fright. I bought a little more than I expected. Day after tomorrow I go into a retreat absolu to finish my story and get it off. I have been so gay, I haven't worked." She continued, "But oh, how little [difference] a superfluity of rich things to put on your gullet makes! Or a superfluity of anything except love, and loveliness and dignity and charm. And you oh my darling have all these things, and we have them in our life. I do miss you, fearfully, my darling love, but it won't be long now."

Grace repeated her oft-expressed longing for a different lifestyle than she and Blair had: "And when I get home Tudie we must try to live more for ourselves and to ourselves . . . how silly for us to bore and tire ourselves with other people all the time."[33]

Perhaps Dick and Alice Lee Myers, noticing Grace and Blair's frequent separations, made comments to her about her career's demands. In a note from the Pont Royal Grace explained to Alice Lee how important writing was to her: "Writing is my straw in the slow drowning of life—clinging to straws—and I have so few."[34] No doubt the Myers's busy family life, which included three children, many friends, and their friends' children, made Grace feel envious and unfulfilled. Naturally the recognition she attained as a writer gave her compensating status and the raison d'être she desperately sought. Writing Dick Myers before leaving Paris, Grace described the comfort she gained from her friendship with him and Alice Lee:

Give her [Alice Lee] my love and a big hug. Tell her I think of her so often and would give anything if she could just sweep in in her majestic way, bringing that wonderful feeling of reassurance and security and general darlingness she always does. I, always having more or less a broken wing, would like to climb right into one of the children's cribs and be taken care of by Mummy.[35]

Before returning to the United States, Grace again expressed gratitude to Blair for his patience, understanding, and generosity: "I want to know if you're all right, but I'll have to cable soon. Tude, you are so generous—in money—in spirit—in every way. You are so sweet about my staying a little while here, and I know you must be lonely." She wished Blair would offer his brother the olive branch: "Blair, it isn't worth bearing a grudge any longer against Charlie. He's old, he's sad, he is very, very lonely. He'll be awfully glad if you telephone, as if nothing had gone wrong."[36]

Good-hearted Blair, who had already resumed correspondence with Charlie, received this note from his older brother late in November 1931: "As you have taken to dating your letters, you no doubt have given up all hope of ever acquiring an artistic temperament." On the surface, the brothers had returned to their bantering relationship as if nothing had happened.[37]

Charles's spirits revived in fall 1931 with D. Appleton-Century's publication of *Loquacities*, a book of his revamped newspaper essays and other stories including "The Bustle." The coaxing and prodding of James Gray had finally brought results. In 1930 Charles Flandrau signed with his old publisher, D. Appleton-Century, for publication of *Loquacities* (after failing to get it published by Alfred Knopf, Houghton-Mifflin, or Charles Scribner's Sons.) Although the book—which was dedicated to James and Sophie Gray—was a critical success and was simultaneously released in New York and London, it sold only a few thousand copies. A critic writing for the *Saturday Review of Literature* described Flandrau as "an author whose writing is of purest ray serene" but said of his book: "Most of the time the author is saved by an engagingly mordant quirk of wit . . . he is occasionally tiresome and almost never flat; probably the genre can merit no higher praise . . . a curious but unmistakable Harvard Club accent; the faint snobbishness of Mexican and Laorcan turismo . . ." A *London Times* critic called Charles Flandrau at sixty, "a man living in the past."[38]

Years of living among tolerant, sophisticated Europeans gradually allowed Charles the freedom to let his childish eccentricities show, and the person to whom he revealed them most openly was the young St. Paul critic who had become his closest friend, James Gray. His letters to Gray in the late 1920s and early 1930s reveal Flandrau's quirkiness and boyish delight in debunking sacred cows and inflicting "pranks" on the unsuspecting—usually women.

Writing Gray from Stockholm, Sweden, in fall, 1929, Charles—an inveterate animal lover—described "circusing with the birds" on his ship, the *Kungsholm*. Fed by a deck steward, Flandrau wrote, the stow-away birds slept in potted bay trees on the promenade deck at night and played with him by day. "Oh, how we romped and romped!" Charles confided.[39]

To Gray, Flandrau described his enjoyment of a Beethoven concert in Sweden but added: "I still maintain that in certain respects Beethoven was a pig-headed, long-winded old ass."[40] In other correspondence with James Gray, Charles, really letting his hair down, described his boyish delight in tricking a woman friend in Paris:

> Charlotte Kett has just written to thank me for 'the dozens and dozens and dozens of exquisite tulips' sent anonymously to her flat the other afternoon. I immediately replied with a prettily abashed, shy, boyish admission that I had, indeed, been unable to resist sending them, which of course I never did or even dreamed of doing, and when, as is inevitable, she finds who the actual donor was, she will be as mad as <u>hell</u> at having written me a somewhat scented note of thanks. Why does one take a diabolical delight in playing such pranks? I always have.[41]

Gray's responses to Charles took on a similar tone. Their letters shared gossip about St. Paulites as well as their pet peeves among the prominent. In one letter to Charles, Gray confided: "[Thomas Edison] was a mere mechanic and a manipulator of other men's ideas."[42]

In another, Gray expressed disdain for Maude Adams and Otis Skinner, a view he knew Charles shared. Puncturing another sacred cow, James Gray ridiculed Ethel Barrymore, who, he said, was "drunk and doped" on stage. Gray complained too about the religious hysteria in St. Paul over "St. Alice" and said he was "tired of worshipping at her shrine.[43] (In 1930–1931 Alice O'Brien led a successful capital campaign to build the St. Paul Women's City Club and received much praise for it. No doubt, however, underground misogyny flourished among diehard chauvinists.)

While Charles was still at Bizy, Gray sent news and greetings from their crowd in St. Paul, among whom he listed "Clara Mairs, Clem Haupers, Marion Blodgett, Anne Ueland Taylor, Frances Boardman, Gerald Seabury, Harriet Bunn, the Ingersolls, Christopher O'Brien, Louise Foley, Jay Heavener, Badge Fuller, and Walter Lindeke."

A theme of tolerance for—even championing—hard drinking runs throughout the Charles Flandrau–James Gray correspondence, explaining one aspect of their bond. Both were products of the then-prevailing culture that took a winking attitude toward habitual semi-inebriation.

In March 1932, James Gray's flattering profile of Charles Flandrau appeared in *St. Paul Magazine*. Describing his idol, Gray wrote: "[Charles Flandrau was]...one of the finest, most completely mature and civilized natures of our time." Realizing his resuscitation was now underway, Charles thanked his young protégé profusely.[44]

CHAPTER XII

Voice Found

*"You belong with the very first of American writers. I want you to get
that feeling about yourself very strongly in case you haven't it now."
Kyle S. Crichton to Grace Flandrau, January 12, 1932*

GRACE SAILED FOR AMERICA in late fall 1931. After her return to France
with Blair in early winter 1932 they rented rooms for several months in a
boardinghouse in Chesières, Switzerland. Chesières offered inexpensive rates,
seclusion for work, moderate climate for Grace's figure skating lessons, and
nothing more distracting than rummy and backgammon with Blair in the
evenings. Although Perkins and Crichton were asking for a full-length manuscript, progress was slow on Grace's novel. She continued working on short
fiction.

In January 1932 she sent off another long short story, "The Happiest Time,"
to *Scribner's*. In mid-month Kyle Crichton responded enthusiastically:

> We grabbed the story the minute it was off the boat and have written Mr.
> Liveright saying that we want it for the magazine. The price will be the
> same as for "One Way of Love"—$500.00. [Grace briefly contracted with
> agent Horace Liveright in 1932 to sell her short fiction but later broke the
> contract.]
>
> As for the story itself, I think it is magnificent. Whether this is the
> general opinion I don't know, but I am very reserved in saying that I think
> it your best piece of work.
>
> We are so keen about your work here that I am venturing to ask you a
> personal question about your publishing connections. If I am correct,
> it has been some time since you had a book appear, and it may be that
> you are not tied up. If you do have a book in mind and are rather looking
> around, we should be very happy to see it here and I think there would be
> no trouble at all about reaching an arrangement on it.
>
> It seems to me that you have been badly treated in the way of critical
> acclaim, and I feel certain that your next book will bring you everything in
> that line that you may have hitherto hoped for. You belong with the very

first of American writers. I want you to get that feeling about yourself very strongly in case you haven't it now. Please be very frank in writing me as to how things stand with you.[1]

Thrilled by the letter, Grace sent Dick Myers a copy and confided: "I continue to have love letters from Crichton of a chastely literary tone naturally." She began thinking about returning to America.[2]

Early in February Max Perkins followed up Crichton's letter, reinforcing his praise:

> Mr. Crichton has shown me your letter in which you were so very good as to say that you will offer your novel to us. I cannot tell you how much your saying this pleases us. We have always been interested in your writing ever since your first novel. . . . Everything that you say about it leads us to look forward to it eagerly, and as to the matter of adequate critical consideration, I think we can surely say that you will have it.[3]

Two months later Perkins again wrote Grace, asking to see the novel she was working on. Crichton sent word that he didn't think she needed to contract with another agent.[4]

Grace sailed for New York on the Hamburg-American line early in April 1932, planning to divide her time between Manhattan and Farmington. Blair settled in for a long stay by himself at the Hotel Banastron in Menton.

At fifty-seven, Blair was an appealing and outwardly contented gentleman, someone who had settled for his lot in life and had plenty of opportunities to socialize. His description in a letter to Grace of spraying his closet at the Banastron against a colony of moths and brushing his clothes as he unpacked is a touching picture of a tidy and careful man, well trained and unresentful at having to manage his own domestic life. Although Blair might have been vulnerable to romantic adventure, the Hotel Banastron probably offered more intrigue than he was prepared for.

Friends remember Blair Flandrau as an elegant man, as fashionable a dresser as Grace. He made impressive "entrances," often sweeping in with a cape and a broad-brimmed fedora pulled down rakishly over one eye. Long after Blair's death Grace described him to a younger relative who hadn't known him: "When I heard his foot on the floor I saw an eighteenth century French gentleman with lace at his wrists and more panache than any man I ever knew."[5]

The Flandraus liked the Maziroffs, owners of the Banastron, with whom they became acquainted the previous year. The hotel served good continental cuisine and attracted an interesting clientele — retired military officers, dispossessed White Russians, and assorted Europeans and Americans. Some of the latter were escaping expensive divorces at home or were entertaining mistresses in anonymity. (Flandrau friends dubbed the Banastron "the hostelry de luxe and de loose.") Blair thought of writing about the hotel's interesting characters whom he described to Grace in detail in his letters.

On their previous visit to the Banastron the Flandraus had met an attractive young woman named Rema, an employee of the Maziroffs. When Blair returned to the Banastron by himself in spring 1932, Rema immediately endorsed his application for membership at the New Club in Menton where she was, by then, an employee. Rema and Blair spent considerable time together that spring.

Blair described Rema to Grace as "a beautiful girl and so nice." When she introduced him to members of the New Club, Rema said, "I want you to meet my best friend, Mr. Flandrau."[6] Blair and Rema frequently had drinks together at the New Club and took walks into the village of Menton. Sometimes they took the bus to Nice or Monte Carlo for lunch. Soon, as Blair wrote Grace, Rema invited him to go on a driving trip to Central Europe in the company of an elderly English woman, who was also a guest at the Banastron. He decided he wanted to go.[7]

Several weeks later the trip was cancelled, because Rema — a Russian — couldn't get the visas she needed and the Englishwoman suddenly backed out. Evidently the Maziroffs influenced the elderly woman in her decision and also advised Blair not to go. Who knows what intrigue Blair escaped due to his uncanny knack for being looked after?[8]

En route from Paris to Cap d'Antibes, where they were loaned the Gerald Murphy's house, Dick and Alice Lee Myers looked up Blair in Menton. Rema was with him. When Dick wrote Grace about it, she responded:

> I was glad you saw that darling Blair. But, oh, Dickie, I cried about Rema. I was so terribly afraid that was all a smoke screen so you and Alice wouldn't think he was lonely. I won't have that. He must come back here at once if he gets lonely, the dear darling. Everything I know about the innermost depths of feeling and loyalty in the human heart I have learned from Blair. If it hadn't been for him I'd be brittle as glass. Nobody hardly but me and

a few old friends knows the real Blair. They see such an inadequate little surface. But down deep is a well of truth and feeling and wisdom I am not likely to see in any other person in my life.[9]

"The Happiest Time" appeared in the June 1932 issue of *Scribner's*. The story is a strong exposition of the smoldering rage of two grown daughters, Lily and Amy, who are breaking away from a mother who infuriates them. Amy, the younger, is especially angry. (Amy represents Grace, Lily is Lucile, and Mrs. Miller, their mother, is Mary Staples Hodgson). The pages fairly crackle with Amy's contempt for her mother, who has "a certain smile, timid, deprecatory, wistful" and is "gentle and coquettish" in her pathetic efforts to identify with and appease her daughters. Amy is interested in money and society, like her father, who has left his family for an upper class married woman, abandoning his childlike wife, whose relatives have gone downhill and are "hardly more than ordinary farmers" in Amy's resentful words. Writing the story was obviously a vehement catharsis for the author.

After seeing the power of Flandrau's autobiographical fiction in "The Happiest Time," Perkins and Crichton urged her to continue revealing herself more to readers. Vivid as some of them were, Grace's African stories had created distance between author and readers. Although her editors entered "The Happiest Time" in *Scribner's* annual short story contest, however, and it got much attention, Grace's strong piece did not earn the prize. According to a letter she wrote Richard Myers early in July, Kyle Crichton informed Grace that, "the "$5,000 prize would be divided between Wolfe and Hermann. Soskin of the *New York Evening Post* [one of the judges] was determined it [the money] should go undivided to me [Grace], but Burton Roscoe wouldn't agree.... Burton Roscoe is a critic of the type who couldn't possibly like my kind of thing. He adores the hard-boiled babies with loud speakers—and he-mannishness and lots of red blood—But it's nice to have Soskin on our side.[10]

James Gray lauded "The Happiest Time" in private correspondence to Charles Flandrau and praised it in an out-of-town review Grace didn't see. It was Gray's first coverage of her work. When Kyle Crichton informed her of Gray's praise, she wrote the St. Paul critic thanking him profusely.[11] Meanwhile, Gray published another flattering profile of Charles Flandrau in the December 1933 issue of *Golfer and Sportsman*.

Grace's prolonged stay in the United States in spring and summer 1932 yielded favorable results. After she recovered from a spell of rheumatism and migraine complicated by dental problems, Crichton invited her to meet his celebrated boss, Maxwell Perkins. Although they corresponded several times between 1930 and 1932, Grace and Perkins had never met. After the three lunched together in mid-April, Grace described both editors in a letter to Dick Myers from the Lexington Hotel:

> [Crichton] is a big, blond sort of man, intelligent but not brilliant, and very serious. Extremely radical in his politics or perhaps philosophy and quite allied with lots of the critics and especially the *Nations* group.... [12] Perkins is a much younger-looking man than I expected and strange. I don't know if he's a little deaf or has an impediment in his speech or what. There is just something—like a veil over his personality.[13]

Perhaps Perkins, a laconic New Englander, was more impervious than most men to Grace Flandrau's charms. Nevertheless, their encounter further cemented collaboration between her and Charles Scribner's Sons. Crichton's praise and encouragement augmented. Grace transmitted this news to Dick Myers in June from Farmington:

> Have just come back from a thrilling time in New York, ushered in by a visit to my hotel from Crichton. I had sent him the two little shorts ["What Was Truly Mine" and "She Was Old"] I told you I had written and he came bouncing over to say he considered them the finest stories that had come to *Scribner's* since he went there! He says that if I go on doing things like the last two I have only to wait. But he says the critic situation is bad. You see all my things deal with undercurrents in people not so easily seen and there is a mania in letters here as in philosophy for behaviorism, which is at the other pole. He says he fears I'll have to write and write before they will really see and appreciate what I'm driving at.[14]

That summer Grace and Crichton established a strong friendship based on mutual interest in writing, long discussions about communism, and probably much self-disclosure. In correspondence they addressed each other as "Mrs. Flandrau" and "Mr. Crichton." Grace wrote Alice Lee Myers: "Tell Dickie I am becoming Communist due to the influence of Crichton of whom I am very fond. He is a dear. Awfully warm-hearted and genuine and unworldly."[15]

To Crichton she wrote she confided in him because he was "such a dear and so warm-hearted. I love warm people and I hate fishes."[16]

While in New York City, Grace stayed at the Lexington Hotel in midtown Manhattan and often had tea with Crichton at the Plaza or dined with him at the Lexington. Crichton also invited Grace to his home that summer to meet Mrs. Crichton. The kind, open-hearted editor was ten years younger than Grace, who described Crichton's wife as "nice, rather ordinary."[17]

"What Was Truly Mine," "She Was Old," and "Affair of the Senses" quickly followed "The Happiest Time," all published by *Scribner's* in 1932. Although Charles Flandrau privately praised "Affair of the Senses," to his protégé, Gray reviewed none of these stories in his popular *Dispatch* literary column. The first two were powerful vignettes of Grace's feelings about people close to her at various stages of her life. "What Was Truly Mine" described the constancy of a devoted husband toward his sick wife and probably portrays Blair and Grace's relationship. "She Was Old" is the story of an elderly woman's children putting her in a nursing home, very likely a portrait of Mary Hodgson and her female relatives. Grace confided to Crichton that St. Paulites were weeping over it.

In the 1930s *Scribner's* annual short story contest drew a lot of critical attention. Having *Scribner's* editorial staff enter your story in the contest was almost as prestigious as winning. Grace's editors entered both "She Was Old" and "What Was Truly Mine" in annual contests, but neither won. (*The Best Short Stories of 1932* included "She Was Old," and "What Was Truly Mine" appeared in the *Best Short Stories of 1933*.)

Crichton and Grace confessed to being baffled at times by the critics' selections of winners. During the Depression, however, writing about social protest and social reform was in the ascendancy. Grace complained: "Edmund Wilson no longer believes in art for art's sake but only for things about the Peepul and the radical movement. It's all very annoying."[18]

When she visited Thornton Wilder and his sister in New Haven in July 1932 Grace found Wilder discouraged too: "He [Wilder] seems sadder and older than last time [we met]. I think he's disappointed at the critical attitude toward his stuff. And who can blame him? They're fools, the critics, they really are."[19]

But there were signs of recognition too. Theodate Riddle was convinced Grace was on her way to becoming an important American author. After "One Way of Love" appeared in the October 1930 *Scribner's,* Theo wrote:

"You certainly have hit a very high key . . . [it] places you with the Big Boys where you certainly belong." The following month Theodate invited Grace to join the board of the Avon Old Farms School.[20]

In late spring 1932 Theodate made a further gesture of recognition. In mid-May, while he was still in Menton, Blair received word from Grace that the Riddles were making a house on their estate available to her permanently as a haven for writing. The "Gundy" was an eighteenth-century house charmingly restored by Theodate and joined to another historic structure with an enclosed passageway. The other half of the Gundy, a Farmington landmark, served as a teashop for students at Miss Porter's school.

Calmly accepting this news, Blair said he thought Grace would be able to accomplish a lot of work at the Gundy whereas he knew she couldn't do so either in St. Paul or at Hill-Stead.[20] After experiencing Charles's moods and the contention between the Flandrau brothers at Bizy the Riddles no doubt realized that working at home in St. Paul was impractical for Grace. [21]

From Menton Blair notified Grace that his St. Paul brokers had sent bad news about his investments. He also reported that Charles was frantic about the continuing doldrums of the stock market. He worried about his brother's solitude at Bizy and commented, "What a spoiled old man baby he is."[22]

The Flandraus exchanged news of other relatives during their long separation in the spring and summer of 1932. Despite strained finances during the Depression, Blair and Grace decided to send forty-five dollars a month to Lucile Willis after her separation from Ralph Willis. It was just enough, Lucile wrote gratefully, for her to live on. Although she had probably received a modest inheritance from Mary Hodgson's estate, by 1932 Lucile, an alcoholic, was living in extremely reduced circumstances in California. Although the foster sister she had grown up with had become a near stranger, Grace wrote Blair: "We mustn't be too hard on Lucy. She's never had much of a chance of any kind. She would do as much for us if she could."[23]

A happier event eclipsed all other news, good and bad, that summer. Grace arranged a meeting in Manhattan with her birth brother, William Hodson. (William Hodson, the son of Anna Redding Hodson and Edward John Hodgson, never changed the spelling of his name to his birth father's nor did his mother change the spelling of her name to "Hodgson.")

Hodson, who was six years younger than Grace, graduated Phi Beta Kappa from the University of Minnesota in 1913 and later earned a degree from Harvard Law School. After serving as the first director of the Children's

Bureau in Minneapolis and authoring the Children's Code in the Minnesota statutes, William moved to New York in 1923 as director of child welfare legislation for the Russell Sage Foundation.[24]

When Grace met him during the Depression, William Hodson was serving as executive director of the New York Welfare Council and as a member of Mayor Fiorello La Guardia's cabinet. In 1932, Hodson's political friends were urging him to pursue a mayoral candidacy in the approaching fall elections.

William's Minnesota relatives had barely known him in his childhood. Drusilla Hodgson, Grace's first cousin, told her children she remembered seeing William on campus at the University of Minnesota when they were students there about 1912, but she never spoke to him.[25]

Once she became acquainted with her highly regarded and accomplished brother, Grace no longer hid the truth about her own birth. She began admitting quietly that William Hodson's mother was her mother too, for Flandrau relatives and their close friends in St. Paul became aware of the truth about this time.[26]

Blair carefully dated and neatly typed his response to Grace's proud disclosures about William. He wrote:

> My Tudie: Yesterday I got two letters from you and today another one. I love so to get them. One of them was all about seeing your brother William. I am so glad you looked him up and that everything is so satisfactory with him. I think his great success is mainly due to two things, first that he was born with a keen mind and second that, fortunately for him, he had to use it. But I think he is the kind of person who would have used it anyhow, no matter in what situation he had found himself. Rewriting the laws concerning the status of illegitimate children is an amusing note.
>
> I'm glad he has lost all his former bitterness as it is all perfect nonsense [sic] anyway, but I suppose when he was a boy and very young man he couldn't help feeling as he did. To my way of thinking, you and he are about the luckiest two people I know, not to have been born half Steples [sic]. It's a very good thing that he has at last recognized that fact.[27]

Though little is known of the reaction to this news in Minnesota, Grace told Blair that two close friends, society matrons from St. Paul, snubbed her when she ran into them in Manhattan. Blair later confided to Mary Griggs

(Mrs. Theodore) his surprise that Grace hadn't told him the truth about her illegitimacy much earlier.[28]

After hearing much about Rema during the months of their long separation in the spring and summer of 1932, Grace apologized to Blair for her selfishness. She spoke of both spouses' worry about the results of the Depression on their financial future and expressed her determination to keep working. Grace felt guilty about the pain she had inflicted on her husband because of her ambition and the costs of her career.

> My dear, my dear, all I want is to be with you quietly and Keekie don't worry. When we get a little work I'll write hard and you have your income and maybe you could get some sort of job on a salary—I hesitate to suggest that because I don't want you to do anything my dear that would be humiliating or painful to you in the way of taking a bum job—.

Grace continued, speculating about what their life might be like after returning to Minnesota:

> But my darling if we're poor we'll just go off to Hastings [a river town south of St. Paul] or some place to live and be happy together. You are so precious to me—such a rare and wonderful and beautiful person that I only ask for one thing and that is to make up to you in some way for all the stupid, selfish, inconsiderate, self-centered asininity I've inflicted on you.... I have never done my part or been the help to you my love that I should have been. I want you to know right now that from now on I stand by you. I can make money too and I will.... This trip was the last and perhaps as far as money goes, the most gigantic folly of all but it's opened my eyes more than all the rest.[29]

Blair replied, "To me you are absolutely perfect and I wouldn't have you any other [way] than you are for anything in the world. I love you with all old heart and soul and am always worrying about you."[30]

Shortly after hearing from Blair at last Grace communicated with Dick Myers, revealing an adult perspective about Blair and Rema's friendship and double standards concerning Flandrau finances:

> Your letter came with one from dear Blair. I'm so glad he had Rema with

him [when Dick saw them] and anything he does or thinks is all right with me because he's the world's truest and kindest person. If he had a little flick, which I really in my heart don't believe, for her, it's surely coming to him and I hope he enjoys it. The only thing that scares me is money. He has no business to be spending much money foolishly as we are perhaps more broke than he realizes.[31]

When it appeared the worst of the Depression was over by summer's end, 1932, the Flandraus returned to the United States. Grace arrived in St. Paul first, late in July. Anne (Mrs. Edwin) White helped her reopen the house at 548 Portland.[32]

Friends gave Blair and Grace a warm welcome. In early August Grace made a speech entitled "Literature Turns to the Left" at the new Women's City Club in St. Paul. Alice O'Brien told her the audience of 250 was the largest crowd the club attracted since its opening.[33] A newspaper story covering the speech quoted Grace: "In many books today, social conditions become the real hero or heroine. But I don't know one of these more or less propaganda books that I would term a success. To me, the individual with his human emotions is of much more interest than a book painting the world as someone thinks it should be."[34]

Her point of view put Grace squarely at odds with Communist-leaning writers like Kyle Crichton, John Dos Passos, and Meridel Le Sueur.

In an interview with columnist Agnes Kinney, published in an August 1932 edition of the *St. Paul Pioneer Press* shortly after her return from France, Grace waxed eloquent: "Since my return home I have been struck again with the fact that there are more charming and delightful people in St. Paul than anywhere else in the world."

Nothing succeeds like success.

No record of Charles Flandrau's reaction to the news of Grace's illegitimacy exists, but subsequent events indicate that it may have fanned James Gray's determination to revive his idol's career and restore Charles's local literary preeminence. Friends may have begun taking sides at this juncture. As their literary rivalry heated up, surely both Grace and Charles Flandrau must have had critics aplenty.

Alexander Woollcott's article, "Reading and Writing: the Underwriters," appeared in the February 1932 *McCall's*, ostensibly in response to publication of Charles's *Loquacities* in fall 1931. In it Woollcott—a great admirer of

Flandrau's prose—took his old Harvard friend to task for not writing more. Woollcott wrote:

> Indeed, I can think offhand of only three writers of our day about whom I feel (with a kind of grudging admiration, mind you) that they have not written enough—Not enough to satisfy you and their public, their audience, me. I am thinking of the matchless poet, A. E. Housman, Kenneth Grahame (*The Gold Age, Wind in the Willows*) and, just at this minute, of the most exasperating underwriter of them all, Mr. Charles Macomb Flandrau of, among other places, St. Paul, Minnesota, Cambridge, Massachusetts, Mexico, and the Island of Majorca.... Charles Macomb Flandrau is the most civilized and reprehensible loafer in the world of letters.

CHAPTER XIII

A Contest of Wills

"Savage mockery in the wild-shrewd, wild-hard little eyes, irony that
mocked what he praised, the true drunkard's ambivalence that disbelieves
what it believes, hates what it loves, scorns what it desires the most."
Grace Flandrau, Indeed This Flesh, 1934

BY 1932 GRACE'S WRITING ON AFRICA and her connection with *Scribner's*
had solidified her national literary reputation, but, equally important, her
work and Blair's support of it had gained credibility in St. Paul. Now it was
obvious to everybody that Blair's role as business manager of his wife's expand-
ing affairs was essential. And the Depression made it clearer to friends and
relatives that the Flandraus needed Grace's income from writing, something
affluent people can be maddeningly indifferent to when a wife acts as breadwinner.

His brother's management skills impressed Charlie enough to tell friends
that Blair handled all his and Grace's bills and that "he is on to the technique and doesn't mind the labour." Charlie, who depended on his factotum,
Richard Walsh, to manage every aspect of his household, including check-
writing, couldn't have conceived of taking on such a chore.[1]

Although Grace was professionally committed at this stage and knew
Perkins and Crichton were counting on her to produce a new novel, in the
early 1930s she continued to let short fiction absorb most of her energies. From
1930 to 1938 Max Perkins, however, alternating between kid gloves treatment
and stern professional management, persisted in his efforts to coax the full-
length manuscript out of Grace he seemed convinced she had in her. He may
have suspected she badly needed to tell her own story.

When Perkins had asked to see her novel-in-progress the previous winter,
Grace sent this brief description from Switzerland:

> My novel is a character study of a man during the great boom period
> of the Northwest and incidentally of his wife. A study of failure, ambi-
> tion, blindness, hope, love, human misguidedness generally. Although it
> is of the time of my parents, the period is not important. It is first and

last the delineation of a person, a sensitive, naively ambitious and terribly misplaced man of an essentially noble and perhaps even spiritual character, but [who], not knowing himself at all, was somehow utterly defeated by circumstances from realizing any of his possibilities.[2]

This man was Edward John Hodgson. Grace's novel—autobiographical fiction since she would play a part in it too—was to be based on her father's life. She agonized over it.

By January 1, 1933, Grace finished the manuscript but wrote Perkins she was too ill to proofread it. She was laid up in bed and her doctor prescribed recuperation in a warm climate.

The Flandraus departed for Florida, and while Grace recovered slowly at Casa Ybel on Sanibel Island, Max Perkins stayed in touch. He sent her books to read—a well-documented Perkins strategy for stimulating creativity—and occasional notes. He assured her that Scribner's would be glad to wait until she was ready to let them see her novel. Late in January Perkins wrote:

> It seems as though there were an immense amount of hard luck about in the world even apart from the depression; but I am informed by an astrological friend that while this is true, it is to be accounted for by something that Saturn is doing but he is soon going to stop doing. Then everything will be better.[3]

After returning from Florida, the Blair Flandraus declined an invitation to join the Riddles and Charlie again at Bizy, although Grace wrote "I wisht I could be dar."[4] They had good reasons to stay at home. Grace was still polishing her manuscript, and Blair wrote Charlie in Europe: "After what happened . . . the heart of Bizy has gone out of it for me."[5]

Grace wrote John and Theo that, besides working hard, she had acquired a new interest. Through exposure to the problems of adolescents at Avon Old Farms School for Boys, she became interested in juvenile delinquency in St. Paul. She sent this description:

> I have now acquired a little sideline in the way of a group of delinquent boys, the present Ramsey street gang, John. (John Riddle often reminisced about the Ramsey Hill gang known as "the Mickeys.")
> I became interested in them through Juvenile Court and the other night

had them all up here, twenty-two of them, for a turkey dinner. . . . Charlie
Bell came and showed them the African movie. They had such a grand
time! Many of them had never had a piece of turkey in their lives, few of
them had ever been at a party. They saw everything in the house, every
picture, every book. Their interest was extraordinary.

Nothing, I am happy to relate, was stolen although every boy here except
the three very little ones, has been in court. Such intelligent, potentially
decent little human beings. . . . One of them is collecting stamps, John, so
if you go to any foreign places besides France, do send me cards or something with the different stamps. . . .

The thing they loved best was the dogs. The Pomeranian ["Chico"] was a
wonder to them. . . . He is of course very racé [Fr. for highly bred] and has
great style, being a tawny "sable" Pom, with a great feather of a tail and the
most spirited, proud, gallant, little ways. They held him so tenderly and
were delighted too with Cucaracha ["Cuka"] who is an enchanting and
rather comic creature. Most of them are too poor to have even a cur dog.
And every single family is living on relief. The unemployment and poverty
in this part of the country are terrible.

Grace's letter to Riddle included a positive message about a young St. Paulite
at the Avon Old Farms School, someone who was known to be an awkward
teen-ager. She wrote, "Clothilde Irvine told a whole room of people that she
thought the transformation in [. . . .] was simply incredible. . . . And it's all
that school that has done it."

This was welcome news to Theodate. Avon Old Farms School for Boys
depended heavily on her faith and largesse. She needed encouragement.
Because it was a progressive school, Avon Old Farms had a hard time draw-
ing full-tuition-paying students away from traditional schools. Many students
held scholarships.

Grace reported to the Riddles that she had learned to drive so that when
their chauffeur, Allan, "can find a decent job and leaves us, I shall be able to
captain the Buick. Blair doesn't have any confidence in me yet, but I hope
to win him over by degrees." Although they employed a cook, a maid, and a
chauffeur, Blair and Grace borrowed money to buy a car.[6]

Grace's new manuscript about her father arrived at Charles Scribner's
Sons late in April 1933. Perkins notified Grace he would read it immediately.
Within a week, however, Scribner's turned the book down. Perkins criticized

the "rather chronicle-like method in which it is written" and said she hadn't managed the power and truth to be sufficiently effective. When Grace asked for a more detailed criticism, he advised: "Deal with the hero's childhood more. The author should take readers into the mind and emotions of the hero more. Your treatment is too objective. Don't use chronological sequence."[7]

Thanking Perkins for his criticism, Grace said she regretted not sending in the unfinished manuscript eight months earlier, admitting she wasn't satisfied and asking for comments. She lamented:

> That book has been a perfect thorn in the flesh. I got no pleasure from it at all, no aesthetic satisfaction—on the contrary—and the disappointment of not publishing it right away is insignificant compared to that inner disappointment.[8]

She said she was working on other things but felt sure she could make a new book of it.

Grace went east in July to work alone at the Gundy, taking Mary O'Malley with her. She stayed for several months, leaving Blair in the care of their new maid, Delia Newell. Once she began revising the book, she decided to submit it to Harrison Smith, who had left Harcourt, Brace to found his own publishing house. Smith had been a true believer in Flandrau's work ever since *Being Respectable* and *Then I Saw the Congo*.

Grace most likely justified her decision to spend the summer in the East on the basis of needing income. After consulting with Edwin (Ted) White, Blair gave her a full accounting of his holdings in a letter on July 19, 1933. He owned 796 shares of St. Paul Fire and Marine, worth approximately $90,000 on the current [1933] market, and Charlie owned 1,300 shares, worth $145,000. Some of the bonds Blair bought before the Crash for $25,000 were now worth only $14,000. Ted White told him the older bonds were doing fine but not the newer issues; $10,000 of the newer ones would probably default. But, White assured him, the Flandraus were ninety-nine percent better off in terms of losses than almost anybody else he knew of.

Blair said he figured Charlie's income was about the same as his and Grace's, but he feared his brother was slowly selling his holdings to maintain his lifestyle. (Later, Blair began liquidating equity shares to maintain lifestyle, but his remark in 1933 indicates such sales were not yet a habit.) He assured Grace he would talk it all over with Alice O'Brien.[9]

These disclosures imply that Grace's earnings yielded about half of her and Blair's total income in 1933. The financial facts of Blair's letter suggest too that he had lost a significant portion of his inheritance due to the Mexican revolution and perhaps in the auto business. Those losses, however, taught him prudence. Medical care for Grace's uncertain health—health insurance didn't exist in the 1930s—travel and the costs of home ownership at 548 Portland most likely explained the discrepancy between Blair and Charlie's holdings by 1933.

Rosier financial times, however, were ahead. The U.S. economy began its slow recovery from the Great Depression, and within five years St. Paul Fire and Marine stock would almost double in value, allowing both Flandrau brothers to live comfortably off their capital. In the mid-1930s, Charlie's letters to Blair and Grace began referring to Frederick Bigelow, president of St. Paul Fire and Marine, as "our blessed savior" and "our divine redeemer." Under Bigelow's leadership, the value of the shareholders' St. Paul Fire and Marine stock exploded into new fortunes. Instead of paying annual or quarterly dividends, the company's strategy in 1933 was to plow earnings back into growth, in effect building up savings in the value of its stock. Shareholders were rewarded over and over by receiving stock splits and stock dividends instead of cash dividends.[10]

This fortunate result validated Alice O'Brien's consistent advice to the Flandraus never to sell their Fire and Marine stock when others tried to buy it from them. In the 1920s and 1930s a tightly limited number of the company's shares were outstanding, and the value of those original shares ultimately went to the moon. Blair's holdings in West Publishing Company were also destined to soar, and his investment in a relatively new company, Minnesota Mining and Manufacturing, showed promise. In 1933, however, one could only be cautiously optimistic.

Probably social demands and "the pressure of personality" in St. Paul also provoked Grace's decision to work alone at the Gundy in summer 1933. During her absence Blair moved briefly to Charlie's. Then he made a long visit to Theodore and Mary Griggs and their teen-aged daughter, Mary, at Forest Lodge, the Griggs's summer home at Cable, Wisconsin.

Although he assured Grace that a recent medical exam found nothing wrong with him and that he had gained some weight, Blair was suffering uneven health. Early in August he reported that Mary Griggs had invited him to stay at Cable for the rest of the summer: "She says I am family not company. . . . I certainly feel wonderful here. No one drinks at all. Not even one cocktail."[11]

After returning to St. Paul, Blair wrote Grace again, this time with new resolve about his drinking. On August 8 he reported:

> I have got to know Little Mary [the Griggs's daughter] very well, and she is a perfect darling. . . . I had nothing whatever to drink while I was up there and certainly feel a hundred percent better for it. I don't intend to have a drop here [in St. Paul] either. In fact I think I'm off it for good and all. Mary and I had some fine talks.

At the end of his visit he wrote: "Mary [Griggs] has certainly been a godsend to me this summer."[12]

On August 29, 1933, the Flandraus had been married twenty-four years, but when the day arrived Grace was still away. Blair sent a loving anniversary message. Addressing her as "Darling Tudie," he expressed worry about Charlie's excessive drinking. He thought his brother was bored and lonely because his stomach was upset all the time, and he never saw anybody. Women friends like Anita Furness, Helen Bunn, and Badge Fuller complained that Charlie never returned their phone calls. (Privately, Charlie referred to these women friends as "the sexually unemployed.") Sending "All old love to the Queen of them all," Blair signed his letter, as usual, "Keek." He included his characteristic cartoon of himself and Grace—a tall stick figure with arms outstretched toward a tiny stick figure, also with outstretched arms—labeled "hugs."[13]

Crichton and Perkins continued to write Grace at the Gundy, and in August 1933 *Scribner's* published her short essay "A Great Life." The story was another generic Flandrau piece of lightly cynical social satire, this time aimed at the frivolous and semi-inebriated lives led by many society women in the 1930s. Columnist James Gray, who had never before critiqued Grace's *Scribner's* stories in his column, wrote in the *St. Paul Dispatch*:

> The idiom and the intonation in Mrs. Flandrau's sketch are quite perfect. She successfully eludes the temptation to be reproachful about the utter uselessness of this creature who accepts no responsibility, fulfills no function, but devotes her waking hours to staggering daintily from one party to another But there she is in all her delicious and maddening sloth: well-groomed, fastidious, physically alluring, sufficiently intelligent and entirely without reason for being.

Gray's review augmented Flandrau's essay into a sledgehammer. No doubt local resentment exploded. Grace's story may have been pertinent but it was not calculated to win friends in St. Paul whom the description may have fit to a "T." Retaliation would come later.

Early in September 1933 Grace sent *Scribner's* two new African stories and notified Perkins that Harrison Smith and Robert Haas had accepted *Indeed This Flesh* for publication. She took the unorthodox tack of offering to recall the manuscript if Charles Scribner's Sons wanted to reconsider it.[15] Perkins quickly rejected that idea but continued corresponding with Grace. Within a few days he accepted "Giver of the Grape," which he labeled "a fine strong story." He rejected "The Way Out."

After her return to St. Paul that fall Grace's friends told her about a writing course being taught by literary trailblazer Meridel Le Sueur at the downtown Minneapolis YWCA. Several of Flandrau's women friends were enrolled in the course and they obtained a copy of Le Sueur's syllabus for Grace. LeSueur's ground-breaking ideas about writing must have impressed Grace for she filed a copy of the 1930s syllabus in her papers.

Meridel Le Sueur—a novelist, journalist, and poet variously described as a "prairie populist," a "passionate proletarian writer," and an "old style Midwestern radical"—was an ardent Communist and feminist when she befriended the Twin Cities society women who studied writing with her in the early 1930s. Among her students were St. Paulites Maude Moon (Mrs. Charles) Weyerhaeuser, Hilda (Mrs. Pierce, Jr.) Butler, and Alice O'Brien. During this period, despite political and lifestyle differences, Flandrau and Le Sueur formed a brief friendship. Grace could relate well to people from all walks of life, and Le Sueur, a radical with a proletarian background, must have appealed to Grace's rebellious, anti-establishment streak.[16]

Charles, Blair and Grace Flandrau, and Meridel Le Sueur encountered often at gatherings of Twin Cities literati that included Brenda Ueland and other Ueland family members, William J. McNally (the New Richmond writer) and his sister, Stella, the James Grays, writers Joseph Warren Beach and wife, Dagmar, and Richard and Mathilde Elliott. Beach, a poet and professor of English, and Elliott, a professor of French, both taught at the University of Minnesota.

Le Sueur had met and admired Grace from afar in her high school days and was about fifteen years younger. In spite of their age difference, however, during the Depression. Le Sueur's writing career was in the ascendancy, while

Grace was trying to recast herself from short fiction writer to modern novelist. A number of national magazines, including *Scribner's*, regularly published Meridel's stories about class conflict and need for social reform in the 1930s.

In a 1990 interview Le Sueur remembered Flandrau this way: "She [Grace Flandrau] was a double person, who dressed one way for her writing friends and another way for her society friends. . . . In her public personality she exhibited outrageous humour, brilliance, guts. In her private personality she was gentle, modest, frightened, easily hurt."[17] On a postcard to the author agreeing to our interview, Meridel wrote: "Grace Flandrau was a beautiful woman and I loved her. She is a neglected Minnesota writer, but she should have written more. . . . She was wasted in the St. Paul aristocracy of thieves."[18]

Le Sueur spoke frankly about her society students. She declared that she had been fascinated and appalled that many of the wives of "the great looters were like brood mares" and were "poverty-stricken, sex-starved women" completely controlled by husbands who gave them little or no spending money. To pay for their writing classes, these "impoverished" women allowed Le Sueur to use their charge accounts at department stores. "People could never understand such oppression," stated Le Sueur—at ninety-five, still an iconoclast—"if they have never slept with a Puritan." According to Brenda Ueland's diary Le Sueur couldn't believe capitalists had happy marriages and generally disdained affluent people.[19]

Le Sueur insisted that her students open themselves to realism—in feeling and in observation. Her teaching reinforced Perkins's and Crichton's advice to Grace. Meridel's 1933 writing class syllabus stated:

> The era of the concocted or invented story is dead, has been dead for three or four years and I hope forever. The invented story, the O. Henry, de Maupassant story, is too small a frame for the great social implications with which we have to deal in fiction now. Freud, Einstein, the machine, the growth of social consciousness . . . these have killed the old story. . . . The writer of the present and of the future is the one who steps out boldly into this adventure of recreating the very world of man. . . . There are no rules now . . . to which the artist must or even may conform. HE MUST FORGE HIS OWN FORM OF HIS OWN FEELING.

Le Sueur's must have been a profoundly liberating voice to establishment women of the 1930s. In a May 1934 profile, James Gray wrote of Le Sueur:

"[She has] spiritual vitality, a controlled but intense ecstasy is expressed in her face, gesture, intonation. Meridel is brilliantly alive."[20]

Gray's growing admiration for Meridel strongly influenced him toward the political left, a subject about which he and Grace began to have heated arguments.

Le Sueur's message was clear: truth, no matter how harsh, was more acceptable in writing and behavior than pretense. That had been Grace's private credo for years, but she had vacillated between daring to profess it and denying it. No doubt her frankly erotic African stories in *Scribner's*—"Affair of the Senses" and "Giver of the Grape," 1932 and 1934, respectively—were outlets for Grace's repressed sexuality. According to Le Sueur, Grace "had no sex life."

Influenced by American writers of the "lost generation," Grace had already moved toward realism and feeling in her writing but she never moved toward socialism. Her father's brand of Republicanism was conservative populism, and, although Charles E. Flandrau had been a Democrat, there was no radical influence in Grace's early conditioning or in her married life. Nevertheless, the hardship she experienced in youth bred empathy with ordinary people, although aspects of her youthful conditioning had been sophisticated and upper middle class. It is no surprise, therefore, that, although Grace and Meridel, identified briefly as humans and writers, Le Sueur later described Grace as "double" and asserted that Grace and Alice O'Brien "had no social conscience."[21]

The compassionate and frank narrator of *Then I Saw the Congo* and the autobiographical stories in *Scribner's*, 1930 to 1933, spoke in a different voice than that of the glib sophisticate who had written satirical fiction for popular magazines a decade earlier. "One Way of Love," "The Happiest Time," "What Was Truly Mine," "She Was Old" and "A Great Life"—all published in *Scribner's* before Grace obtained a copy of Meridel Le Sueur's syllabus—are based on Flandrau's own life experiences of girlhood, marriage, family life, and travel. They are modern in their realism and light-years removed from the tone of her earlier work.

Le Sueur's milieu and subject matter were proletarian, while Flandrau's were more upper middle class. Their friendship did not withstand this difference. Grace loved elegant living—haute couture, fine food, first class accommodations, refined taste. She never rebelled against her social class; her revolt was against wastrelism and upper class complacency.

In the years between 1932 and 1934, four nationally published collections of prize-winning short stories included Grace's work, all of them previously published in *Scribner's* and *Smart Set*. Frances Boardman's October 26, 1933, *Pioneer Press* column, conceded: "Grace Flandrau is nationally recognized as one of America's leading writers of short stories."

Two months later, however, on December 31, 1933, Boardman's column ranked a number of famous Minnesota authors. She placed Charles M. Flandrau, Scott Fitzgerald, Sinclair Lewis, Margaret Culkin Banning, Tom and Woodward Boyd, Maud Hart Lovelace, Joseph and Dagmar Beach in her first paragraph and placed Grace Flandrau in a second paragraph with Meridel Le Sueur, Gladys Hasty Carroll, and Brenda Ueland.

In 1935, the *St. Paul Dispatch* hired Grace Flandrau as its new guest columnist "on any subject she wanted to write about." She would share space with columnists James Gray, Frances Boardman, and Katherine Gorman (later Mrs. Lawrence Boardman).

Although the decline in market value of most American stocks and bonds and the drop in dividends and interest began to reverse course slowly, a tight squeeze on American incomes persisted throughout 1934. Blair tried his hand again at getting published. Grace asked Meridel to critique his work and Le Sueur's response was favorable. She wrote Grace: "Blair's things are extremely good and interesting... They're really <u>fine</u>... very direct and simple and yet <u>subtle</u>." She advised Blair to "write as nearly as you can like you talk." Apparently, however, none of his work from this period reached publication.[22]

In fall 1933 the Flandraus took a driving trip to Mexico. They spent several months in Taxco in a house rented from Señor Saenz, Mexico's minister of education. En route Grace wrote a long letter to Kyle Crichton giving random details about her life. He was assembling material for a profile on Grace to appear in a future issue of *Collier's*.

In her letter Grace informed Crichton that she was born in St. Paul, attended public school, went to "the oldest and worst school in Paris" and then to finishing school in St. Paul after her return home. She said that she was "still abysmally ignorant but fond of books" and that she had devoured Dickens, Browning, and Shakespeare by the time she was twelve. Noting that she had married very young, Grace confided that in her early married life she had fallen "madly in love with a handsome Mexican and he with me" and that during her marriage she had had three affairs, "only one of which counted."

Flandrau's letter shared other facts with Crichton: "[I can] cook extremely well, keep house if I have to, adore dogs and cats, [am] interested in primitive peoples and history of religions, [am] still ignorant and un-scholarly. [I] no longer like what is called society and particularly abhor meeting 'Lions.'"

Continuing her letter to Crichton, Grace complimented other American writers: "The more you read of Hemingway and Faulkner, the more highly you think of them. Faulkner has that sense of fate . . . one of the things that makes him the fine artist he is." [23]

On a trip from Taxco into Mexico City to pick up mail at Wells Fargo, the Flandraus ran into Minnesotans Kate (Doodie) Skiles and her mother and stepfather, Irene Skiles Siems and Claude H. Siems, at a restaurant in the Zona Rosa. The youthful Grace, forty-eight, and Kate, just nineteen, hit it off immediately. As a result, the Flandraus invited Kate to spend a month with them in Taxco. She accepted and so began a long friendship. (Kate Skiles later married Horace (Bud) Klein, Jr. of St. Paul. Their daughter, Kate—"Minty" or Mrs. George Piper today—became Grace's goddaughter and their son, Blair, is Blair Flandrau's namesake.)

While the Flandraus vacationed in Mexico Lucile Willis paid a visit. Soon, however, Blair and Grace began getting on each other's nerves, and Blair returned to Minnesota alone. His poor health had become an exhausting problem. After his departure, Alice O'Brien and another St. Paul friend, Xandra (Mrs. C. O.) Kalman, joined Grace in Taxco.

The three women visited Mexico City and then traveled to Vera Cruz, Jalapa, and Misantla in search of information about the Santa Margarita ranch and Flandrau belongings left behind in the revolution. Grace learned that, unlike many other properties owned by Americans, the Santa Margarita had remained untouched. Arbuckle's had paid Blair's taxes for nearly twenty years and thereby acquired ownership.

Grace was gloomy. She and Blair had quarreled before his departure for St. Paul, and once again she began apologizing in her letters that, due to her "nerves," she hadn't been herself. Writing him from Mexico she referred to her "horrible depression" and said "the terrible melancholia that began this winter seems to get worse and worse." On her return trip from Vera Cruz to New York via steamer, Grace wrote Blair: "As you have never written me I have no idea what your plans are." [24] Arriving in Farmington, however, Grace found several affectionate letters from him. Blair wrote: "I will be much better about writing from now on, but they will be shorts probably instead of longs.... There was never anyone in all the world as wonderful as you. Don't ever think I don't know it."[25]

When she returned to St. Paul Grace found Blair planning a trip to San Diego with his chauffeur, Allan. Advised by his doctor, Blair sought a month in warm weather for his pleurisy. After he departed, Grace wrote him: "The house seems AWFUL empty without my beloved darling. I miss you so already.... Dear heart, I felt so badly when you drove off with Allan I thought I'd die. I wisht I was dar."[26]

While she awaited release of *Indeed This Flesh*, Grace turned out more short stories. Since Crichton no longer worked at *Scribner's*, Max Perkins assigned short fiction managing editor, Alfred S. Dashiell, to Grace. During their brief relationship, despite an active correspondence, Flandrau never learned to spell Dashiell's name correctly and, as usual, she did not date her letters.

Although Perkins's expectation was that Grace would eventually produce a new novel Charles Scribner's Sons wanted to publish, he and Dashiell probably recognized that, because of her confidence in writing short fiction, they should encourage her in that genre too.

Dashiell accepted Grace's charming, two-part short story "Return to Mexico" for the December 1934 and January 1935 issues of *Scribner's*. And during their abbreviated period of collaboration, Dashiell also agreed to publish two pieces of Grace's critical writing—one a vehement refutation of a new book on Africa and the other her review of Kay Boyle's book *My Next Bride*.[27]

Meanwhile, Harrison Smith and Robert Haas brought out Grace's fourth novel and fifth book, *Indeed This Flesh*, in May 1934. The book is an ambitious, philosophically probing novel, dealing with the universal themes of fate and human suffering. The story was a major departure in subject matter and feeling from Flandrau's earlier mannerist novels about debutantes and dowagers. She told the hero's story with sympathy and revealed cynicism and pessimism about human nature and life in general. Describing the class of men the book's hero belonged to, she wrote this preliminary outline:

> These men [like Will Quane, the book's hero] still believed in the Victorian God of respectability and success, whose first mandate to His chosen was to prosper largely in this unworthy world, to achieve wealth and a social position better than that to which they had been born. They believed in property, in education, in hard work, in duty to their families,

in material advancement, in the sanctity of custom and convention and the sinfulness of flesh. They believed in almost everything but <u>life</u>.[28]

In *Indeed This Flesh* Grace undertook the challenging task of portraying her father ("Will Quane" in the book) as a sympathetic but tragic figure, powerful but flawed in the Greek sense. Quane is brilliant, ambitious, and achieving—proud but also naïve. He rises from humble origins to become a lawyer and mortgage banker of wealth and prominence in St. Paul only to be brought down by a profoundly disappointing marriage, naive business decisions, betrayal in a business deal and scandal contrived by his enemies. His character, crumbling under these stresses, slowly becomes double and he becomes intimate with his pre-teen daughter, Norah (Grace). Readers feel the author's pity and love for her father.

Anna Redding, Grace's birth mother, is "Norah" in the book and Grace is also "Norah," a child who comes with her mother to visit Will and Martha Quane. "Norah," the mother, falls ill and dies, leaving the child "Norah" to grow up in the Quane family. The author's use of the name "Norah" for both mother and daughter is probably Grace's way of explaining to herself her father's abuse. This literary device implies that a deeply frustrated man, who was not able to live with his child's mother, might substitute the child for the mother in an intimate relationship. There can be little doubt that Grace fully intended to imply incest between her father and herself as a child in her auto-biographical/biographical novel. Although *Indeed This Flesh* is presented as fiction, Flandrau's use of accurate place names in her family story (eg., "Red Wing," "St. Paul," and the "Isle of Man") and her substitution of "Castle County" for "Castle Rock" (the actual location of the Hodgson family farm) and "Charollet Pearson" for "Charlotte Hodgson," her real grandmother, indicates the author wanted Minnesota readers to know whom and what she was talking about. No stretch of the imagination is required to recognize too that the author intended to present a long-concealed family story she had strong feelings about. She succeeded in thoroughly shocking St. Paul society and no doubt infuriating her relatives.

Flandrau knowingly describes the circumstances in which deviant behavior such as incest takes root and flourishes. Will Quane disrespects his child-like, unbookish, spendthrift wife, Martha. She embarrasses him socially. His highly intelligent little daughter, Norah, begins to disrespect her too. Will's affection for and pride in Norah—the only family member with whom he can communicate on an equal basis—gradually changes from companionable to intimate. She sits on his lap as he reads to her every night, with her arms wrapped around his neck, "divinely happy and secure," even after "of course, she was too old for that."

One day her father takes her on a drive in the country in "a yellow shining trap with two pale brown horses with bobbed tails and silver harness. No one was invited to go but Norah, not Flossie nor her mother." The book's descriptive passages become more explicit:

> It was at this time he first took her on a railway journey.... In the train her father went into another car to talk with some men and was gone so long she was afraid something had happened to him. But he came back and told her to get into the berth and undress. She was almost asleep when he came and lay down beside her.... After that they took many trips together. They slept in strange exciting hotel bedrooms, with dingy paper on the walls and clattering steam pipes and nothing out of the window but tall gray walls. She was far from home in a strange city.... But she had never felt so safe and wonderful as she did sleeping in a wide squeaky bed with damp new sheets and thin blankets, beside her father.[29]

Eventually Norah outgrows her childish adoration of her father. When she attends a fashionable girls' school in St. Paul and makes friends her own age, her father's unkempt, eccentric appearance embarrasses her.

What was Flandrau's purpose in exposing this damaging story to the world? First of all, the nineteen-thirties was a period in which writing teachers like Meridel Le Sueur and eminent editors like Maxwell Perkins were urging "realism" in fiction and Grace simply followed their advice. Perkins was known to believe that if an author had a compelling story to tell he had better get it out or it would be very bad for him.

And no doubt Grace needed catharsis. She had buried her explosive family story deep within her psyche for decades, since childhood. As writer Zora Neale Hurston once said, "There is no agony like bearing an untold story inside you."

Moreover, Flandrau had been a self-described rebel in her youth, hard for her gentle stepmother to manage, and she became a truth-teller in her writing. She had, if anything, too much courage. At age forty-eight and by 1934 a famous American author, Grace probably thought she could get away with self-revealing frankness just as male Lost Generation writers seemed to. She was wrong.

Mixed reviews of the book, ranging from dislike and disinterest to high praise, appeared in national newspapers. A critic in the May 12, 1934, *New York Post* wrote: "One of the most impressive novels I have read this year and one of the most penetrating novels by a woman about a man that I have ever read . . . the kind of novel I have been hoping she [Flandrau] would write some day."

On May 14, 1934, on the page listing Scott Fitzgerald's *Tender is the Night* among the top ten best-sellers in New York bookstores, the "Books" editor of the New York *Daily Mirror* said of Flandrau's portrayal of Will Quane: "I don't remember a fictional character out of that time and turmoil, in this country at least, so masterfully and so beautifully integrated and objectively absorbed."

One critic called *Indeed This Flesh* "a distinguished novel." Another reviewer compared Flandrau's portrayal of Will Quane to Sinclair Lewis's *Babbitt* and the Salavin novels of Georges Duhamel. He asserted that Flandrau was "more humane, more subtle and more magnanimous than Sinclair Lewis and vastly more intelligent than the pretentious Duhamel."[30] The *New Yorker* called the book "somber but interesting."[31]

The influential critic of the *New York Times*, Harold Strauss, however, panned the novel. The Boston *Evening Transcript's* reviewer said: "[*Indeed This Flesh*] really has no plot. It merely wanders. It has no distinctive style." Bess M. Wilson, writing in the *Minneapolis Journal* of June 10, 1934, praised the execution of the work but wondered whether Quane's story was worth telling. As an unprecedented attempt by an American woman writer to portray and explain a dark side of family life, however, *Indeed This Flesh* was a ground-breaking masterpiece.

Critic James Gray of the *St. Paul Pioneer Press* wrote: "The triumph of Mrs. Flandrau's characterization is that though she has been mercilessly revealing, she remains compassionate, like Quane himself. . . . *Indeed This Flesh* is boldly conceived and expertly executed."[32] Gray's review was his first local coverage of a major Grace Flandrau literary effort.

Despite mostly favorable feed-back, *Indeed This Flesh* was not a popular success. And Grace was stung when Kyle Crichton wrote a bland, curt review and she didn't hesitate to tell him. She felt he had praised her writing in person and betrayed her in print. But Crichton replied in a cordial letter that he liked her short fiction best.[33]

Kay Boyle, a younger writer also working in the Harcourt Brace–Harrison Smith stable, admired Grace's writing and complimented her on her "capture of time, place, and personality" in *Indeed This Flesh*. But she, like Kyle Crichton, said she preferred Grace's short fiction.[34]

Perhaps Grace agreed. Although she outlined plans for new novels, describing their main characters and plots in correspondence with Max Perkins, she again let other work distract her.

Negative criticism of *Indeed This Flesh* boiled down to the perception that, although most readers thought Flandrau had rare insight into human beings and considerable descriptive skill, the book was flawed by its weak structure and inadequately sustained character development and plot. Many found the book too cynical and pessimistic.

Indeed This Flesh yields numerous examples illustrating Flandrau's rare understanding of human personality and mastery of psychological detail. Portraying a habitual drunkard, a colleague of Will Quane's, Grace wrote: "Savage mockery in the wild-shrewd, wild-hard little eyes, irony that mocked what he praised, the true drunkard's ambivalence that disbelieves what it believes, hates what it loves, scorns what it desires the most."[35] Perhaps there has never been a more telling description of the hardened and self-defeating perversity of the confirmed addict.

The following contemporary example affirms Flandrau's insight. In *Rabbit Redux* John Updike describes sexual addict Harold ("Rabbit") Angstrom as "hard-hearted in his helplessness." Updike, like Grace Flandrau, points out that cruelty characterizes late-stage addiction. Kindness to self and others is gone.

In July 1934 Grace initiated discussion with Maxwell Perkins about Charles Scribner's Sons' publishing a collection of her African stories in book form. Perkins rejected the idea, insisting that Grace needed to bring out a new novel before a collection of her old stories. Reminding her that, while *Indeed This Flesh* had "very fine reviews," it had not succeeded commercially, Perkins explained that anthologies of stories were always even more of a gamble commercially than novels. When she persisted, Perkins discussed the idea with Charles Scribner and reported to Grace that his boss agreed with him: the firm would stand by his decision not to publish her African stories as a book. Perkins stuck to his guns for another two years.

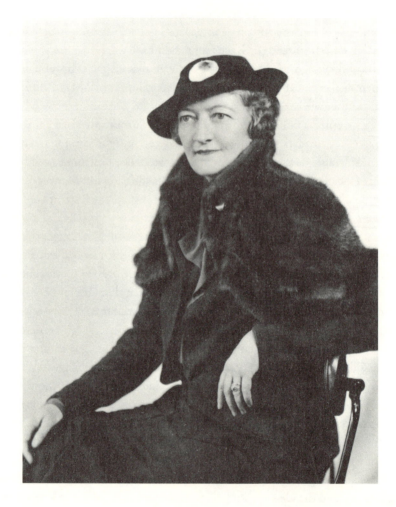

Grace Flandrau, ca. 1936
MINNESOTA HISTORICAL SOCIETY

CHAPTER XIV

The Turning Point

"Why will one not accept the judgment of
people whom they trust, as I trust you?"
Grace Flandrau to Maxwell E. Perkins, 1937

IN DECEMBER 1934, the Twin Cities' leading society and culture magazine, *Golfer and Sportsman*, published Brenda Ueland's profile of Grace Flandrau in the monthly column, "Among Those We Know." Ueland's flair for description and skill at interviewing presented the essential Grace Flandrau at forty-eight. Grace's fourth novel, *Indeed This Flesh*, had just arrived in local bookstores.

The detailed interview wove together many aspects of the author's life. Ueland's coverage subtly alluded to St. Paul's consternation over Grace's exposure, however veiled, of her abuse as a child:

Grace Flandrau has written a remarkable, a great book I think. [I was] lost, absorbed, frightened and illuminated by it. [I am indignant] that few in St. Paul seem to know how good *Indeed This Flesh* is. The book was appreciated in the East. On the jacket you can read the earnest rhapsodies of the most eminent critics. In Minneapolis it has sold well. But in St. Paul no fanfarade, no rataplan of drums. On the contrary her [Flandrau's] best and tenderest friends hover around protectively and wish silently and prayerfully that she would not write such things.

Describing her childhood as "anomalous," Flandrau told Ueland in the interview that her experience at the French school she attended in Paris had affected her life very much. She had felt isolated, lost, alone but not lonely or unhappy:

Children do not repine or know that they are unhappy. But it cut me off from the everyday emotional exchange of family life. It was kind of a sleepwalker existence, and the queer thing is I still have it a good deal. I had to live entirely in myself, mingling with no reality. There I was, a little wisp of a thing, all alone for nearly five years among French people in a fusty old school. And even now I sometimes look at my friends, my husband, and realize that my relation to them is in the same way unreal, uncomprehended.

I did, however, gain a deep affection for France and the French and I learned their language well and still feel more at home in France than any other place. But when I came back to St. Paul as a young girl I felt queer and apart from the other young people. All slang was a closed book, any colloquialism. This feeling of apartness was a misfortune, I think.

Grace spoke frankly about writers and writing in the interview: "As I grow older I have a compulsion that will not let me compromise on the characters I feel and try to cheat on the thing I want to say, even at the expense of popularity, friends, money."

Illustrating her point of view, Grace spoke of a popular and talented American writer:

> I know him and his wife. They have in some ways a beautiful and romantic life but their life is also at times as squalid, quarrelsome, ugly as any life can be. Now when this man writes about his own life (which in a disguised way he mostly does) he throws around these sordid realities a rainbow glaze, a veil, a glamour. About them, in other words, he rather subtly lies. That kind of writing is diametrically opposed to what I believe.

(Later, Grace would deeply regret this thinly disguised public "dig" at Scott Fitzgerald's writing and wrote him an apologetic letter about it, marked "never sent." But in 1934 Charles Flandrau's privately expressed literary opinions, disparaging the works of both Fitzgerald and Lewis, heavily influenced her.)[1]

Among her favorite authors, Grace told Ueland in the interview, were the Russians Fyodor Dostoevsky and Anton Chekhov. "What the great Russian writers want to show, in my opinion, is that nobody is so bad, greedy, malignant but what it tortures himself," she explained. It bothered her, Flandrau said, that American readers couldn't seem to accept any flaws in a book's characters as real or plausible, whereas: "Instead of improving life by sentimentalizing it, I think it infinitely more majestic as it is. I think it more touching to know that human beings may be and often are, at one and the same time, ignoble, false, greedy, cowardly, vile and also noble, tender, aspiring, good."

No doubt Grace was speaking of her brilliant but divided father, Edward J.

Hodgson. No wonder her friends trembled for her. In revealing the dark side of her youth in *Indeed This Flesh,* Flandrau was bravely exposing her vulnerability. Had over-confidence made her drop her guard? Eventually she would pay dearly for her frankness.

The interview concluded with an expression of Flandrau's views on education and raising the young:

> I feel . . . that the present civilization is not right or fertile or beautiful. For one thing, at home, in the schools, in the universities, everywhere, the emphasis has always been placed for the young on getting ahead as individuals. Personal ambition and the acquisitive instinct—that is the principal thing that is taught them, that ever was taught me. The emphasis has been upon Me! Me! even among painters and poets. But look at great people anywhere, in any time, and you will see that the more they cared about something outside themselves, whether it was their fellow human beings or an abstraction like truth, beauty, knowledge, the greater they are. It is the old thing . . . losing your life to find it.

That comment, uttered half a century before Americans labeled the 1980s "the Me Generation," demonstrates Flandrau's prophetic insight as well as her tendency to sound oracular and opinionated to others.

The Ueland interview also reveals that Flandrau at forty-eight had become more self-accepting than she was earlier. Her newfound openness did not go unnoticed. While no record exists of Flandrau family reaction to her self-exposure, probably Charles Flandrau and James Gray, as writers, secretly admired her honesty in *Indeed This Flesh.* After her talk on Mexico at the Women's City Club in October 1934, in a private note James Gray praised Grace's "fundamental wisdom and insight" which he found "in a curious way very moving."[2]

Gray, who had high hopes for his own literary career in the mid-1930s, gave strongly favorable reviews to Grace's subsequent works up through 1937. He produced three new nationally published novels himself 1935–1938. All earned favorable reviews but not lasting national attention or significant commercial success—the fate of most writers.[3]

A close friendship between Grace and Kay Boyle began around 1933 just before publication of *Indeed This Flesh.* Boyle, a Francophile like Grace, had roots in St. Paul. Her grandfather had founded West Publishing Company and had known Judge Flandrau. Intimate involvement in each other's lives, cooperative publishing ventures, and correspondence between Boyle and Flandrau continued over the next quarter-century.[4]

After Grace's two-part story "Return to Mexico" appeared in *Scribner's* in December 1934 and January 1935, Kay Boyle and her then husband, Laurence Vail, asked her to contribute fictional sketches of pre- and post-revolutionary Mexico for an anthology they planned to publish in London. The collection of stories, *365 Days*, would, via the work of many writers, include one vignette for each day of the year. Grace notified *Scribner's* of the request and went to work. Boyle wrote: "I would be pleased beyond words to have things of yours in the book."[5]

Flandrau's nine finished sketches for *365 Days* drew Boyle's praise: "Your work is so calm and certain and I want to read more of it. Your beautiful short things in our book fill me with peace every time I re-read them." After the publication of *365 Days* in London in 1935, Harcourt, Brace and Company brought out an American edition in 1936.[6]

Flandrau's correspondence with Max Perkins about writing in general, and her next novel in particular, continued into the late 1930s. She never hesitated to share her views with him, negative and positive, on other writers published by Charles Scribner's Sons. Her criticism of the 1930s magazine work of Fitzgerald and Sinclair Lewis was outspoken. She observed to Perkins that "Lewis has too many brains and not enough talent while Fitzgerald has too much talent and not enough brains."[7] When St. Paulites wondered why Charles Scribner's Sons published Zelda Fitzgerald's book, *Save Me The Waltz*, Grace passed the query along.[8] She scoffed at Ernest Hemingway's *Green Hills of Africa* to Perkins. (James Gray shared her disdain.)[9]

Everything conspired against Perkins's efforts to get Grace to settle down to work on a new novel. Although she had committed to Boyle and Vail's anthology and continued turning out short fiction for *Scribner's*, in May 1935 Grace also agreed to write a column for the *St. Paul Pioneer Press*. The column, called "My Week," continued intermittently into the 1940s. In "My Week," Grace reviewed books, covered her weekly activities, and wrote opinion pieces about world and local affairs.

Grace continued to seek seclusion away from home for writing. By late summer 1935 she and Mary O'Malley were again in Farmington at the Gundy. Blair was conducting his life from 548 Portland in St. Paul with Delia, their maid, and the dogs, Chico and Cuka. The Flandraus were more than ever leading separate lives, but their habitual frequent correspondence continued. Alfred Dashiell accepted a short story, "Gentlefolk," for the December 1935 issue of *Scribner's*, and Grace was at work on another short piece, "Going to the Lake," for the June 1936 issue.

In February 1936, Max Perkins, reversing his previous stand, notified Grace that Charles Scribner's Sons would agree to bring out a collection of her African stories before expecting a new full-length manuscript. Perhaps he had read her potent Mexican sketches in *365 Days*, just released by Harcourt, Brace and Company. He advised that she would receive a lower royalty per book—ten cents per copy instead of fifteen cents—because of the risky reputation of story collections in the publishing world.[10]

Grace immediately headed to Florida from Farmington to begin work. At first she stayed alone in Miami. She started revising her African material and writing an introduction for the collection with Alfred Dashiell's supervision from New York. Once in Miami, fretting about expenses, Grace shopped for cheaper rooms. Her concern probably reflected renewed feelings of guilt about the costs of her career and her inability, unlike Blair, to curb her taste for luxury. She was, after all, working in Florida at the height of the winter season, despite the fact that she had two other residences, but, prone to bronchitis, she again sought warmth.

From Key West, Grace wrote Blair: "I am going to start work right away and it ought to be a heavenly place for that, with nobody around I ever heard of." At Key West there was "a lovely, divine, clean, grand beach" for swimming and there were also friends from St. Paul. One of them, Sam Shepard, took her out to dinner.[11]

Soon Perkins himself took over Dashiell's assignment, gently urging expedition. Trying to stimulate creativity and encourage enterprise, he again sent Grace books to read—*The Last Puritan*, a biography of Santayana, and *Portrait of an Era*. Grace assured him there would be no interruptions on Key West "in the form of bourgeois dinner parties or communist dialectics" and that she would continue working on her book.[12] To Blair, Grace reported that she was turning down all invitations and that Max Perkins had asked her to deliver a letter from him to Ernest Hemingway:

> But the last thing on earth I would do is look up a celebrity. My god, he [Hemingway] is so hounded by people now, he doesn't know what to do. People here are in a perfect tizzy about him all the time.... They drive

back and forth in front of his house, they ring the doorbell on invented excuses, they become absolutely breathless when his name is mentioned. And I must say, I have a very high regard for his ability. . . . Vital, readable, intensely personal, which always makes good reading.[13]

Blair declined to join her in Florida, saying he was perfectly comfortable at home. The winter of 1936 was particularly cold and he thought Cuka and Chico would freeze in the baggage car if he took them by train to Florida. He also sent social news, sometimes about widows who called or paid attention to him at parties and his bridge lessons at the Minnesota Club. In his customary careful way, Blair also attended to Grace's personal and business affairs at home. He reminded her of department store bills to be paid from her New York bank account and notified her that a *Fortune* editor had wired for information on *The Taming of the Frontier.* He reported that Charlie, who received the inquiry first, remarked to him, "Of course, you're just Grace Flandrau's husband now."[14]

Even Blair's extraordinary patience sometimes wore thin. His response to too many insistent queries from Grace came in a neatly typed letter dated February 17, 1936:

> If I get another letter about the box and the furs I'll go mad. . . . In the first place your furs were in the box—both pieces, the fox and also the little funny you wear about your shoulders. So for heavens sake don't worry about them any more. They are packed away on the third floor and it would take a pretty adventurous artic moth to venture up there. I almost passed away this morning when I opened a letter from you and you asked about them again. I have written and telegraphed about them for the last two weeks.

When Blair made no plans to join her, Grace told him she would come home soon. Learning that he was having tests for high blood pressure, she expressed concern and asked for the results. But in February Blair advised her not to come home:

> Now Tudie, don't bother about me. I'm all right. Just stay down there as long as you want to and if you want to stay in New York for a time do that also. Although of course I miss you awful I think we ought to carry out

the original plan and let you be alone to work for as long a time as you feel necessary. I'll run things here. What you must do is forget everything but your work. Don't think about anything else. All old love to Tudie.[15]

After returning to St. Paul, Grace continued collaborating with Max Perkins on Scribner's edition of her African stories. Editor and author discussed every detail—selection of the book's title, order of the stories, the importance of having a British publisher, the best reviewer (she suggested her old friend, Steven Vincent Benét). Perkins complimented her on the revisions she made to the original stories and the promotion piece she wrote for the book at his request.[16]

Competition for Grace's professional skills increased. In June 1936, KSTP radio offered her a radio show and she immediately accepted the job. Nash coffee and the Soo Line railway sponsored her fifteen-minute spot, "Grace Flandrau Edits," on Mondays, Wednesdays, and Fridays, first at 10:30 A.M. and later at 9:45 P.M. She began by broadcasting vignettes of Northwest history selected from her writing, but her scripts expanded to other topics. Flandrau's warmth, flair for the ironic, and familiarity with vast amounts of information—about travel and literature, history, food, fashion, and theatre—made the show an instant success. She became an overnight radio celebrity. Fans responded with enthusiasm: "Well, at last they have a woman who knows how to talk," wrote Jessie G. (Mrs. Lucius P.) Ordway.[17] John K. Donohue, director of the Ramsey Midgets (the boys' club befriended by Grace) wrote KSTP about the author, saying "She is a swell talker and a good egg."[18]

Grace notified Perkins about her radio show. Though most work for her story collection was complete, final details were still under discussion. One can imagine Perkins's thoughts upon hearing about Flandrau's radio work in addition to her newspaper column. Perhaps she was familiarizing him with the professional demands on her time, hoping to offset her reputation as a social butterfly. Did she realize that accepting KSTP's job offer made her seem less than serious about writing novels? Probably not. Grace often seemed unaware of how her actions appeared to others, but she always managed to live up to professional commitments. For her to produce the expected novel, Perkins was no doubt depending on her pride and her talent. Why was she putting him off? Was her renowned confidence faltering?

Behind Grace's compulsive workaholism—besides habit and the belief that doing work she excelled in was therapeutic—was her conviction that she and

Blair, despite appearances to the contrary, desperately needed her earnings. Later she was proved partially right. In the mid-1930s, as the American stock market slowly recovered, Blair gradually began going through his capital to meet expenses, but he was also content with less materially than Grace. She needed her earnings more than he.

Flandrau's book of short African fiction—*Under the Sun: Stories of Love and Death*—appeared in bookstores throughout the country in October 1936. Favorable, well-placed reviews in both the *New York Times* and the *New York Herald Tribune* pleased both Perkins and Grace.

The collection drew critical praise, nationally and in Minnesota. John Sherman, book critic of the *Minneapolis Star*, wrote: "Mrs. Flandrau has painted a vivid panorama of the White Man's Africa in these 'stories of love and death.'"[19] James Gray extolled the "fine and subtle gifts of Grace Flandrau" in the most favorable review of her work ever published in his column.[20] Brenda Ueland praised the stories in a full-length article in the *Golfer and Sportsman*, saying, "I am in awe of her [Flandrau] for having an eye and brain, a gift and insight that can write so."[21]

But sales of *Under the Sun* were disappointing. A critic in the *Philadelphia Inquirer* may have put his finger on the problem: "Mrs. Flandrau is a sound, conscientious worker, and everything she has to say is interesting. She is slow in working up her effects, but the undertones of her stories are well sustained and never too obtrusive."[22]

The reviewer in the *Greenwich Graphic* put it another way: "Mrs. Flandrau again proves herself a writer of exceptional ability with a fine understanding of the true function of the novelist. She 'neither judges or condemns,' she 'records and interprets,' as the author's introduction to *Under the Sun* explains."[23]

The essential theme of Grace's African fiction (most of it based on firsthand observation) was portrayal of the deterioriation of white colonial character resulting from the exploitation of blacks for profit. That message, told with restraint and subtlety in a variety of stories with minimal plots, may have gone over the heads of many readers or disinterested them. Again, the author's point of view on the subject of race was ahead of its time. Sales continued to lag.

Grace insisted that Scribner's wasn't giving the book enough advertising support, but Perkins assured her they were marketing *Under the Sun* according to its advertising budget, explaining that every other week or so ads would appear in the *Times*, *Tribune*, and *The Saturday Review*. Although she admitted he had been right in the first place about publishing a novel before the

stories, Grace's complaints about lack of advertising continued. She protested
to Perkins that she was hurt and humiliated by what seemed to be Scribner's
lack of interest and reported that the book had been killed in Minnesota. She
was stung when Charles Flandrau and her St. Paul friends asked her: "What
has Scribner's got against your book?" In spite of her disappointment, however—or perhaps because of it—she forced herself back to work on the novel
she had promised Charles Scribner's years earlier.

Tom Wolfe's very successful books *Look Homeward Angel,* 1929, and *Of Time
and the River,* 1935, both autobiographical novels lovingly midwifed by Perkins
and published by Charles Scribner's Sons, strongly impressed Grace. When the
latter book came out in 1935, Grace lauded it to Perkins in a letter he forwarded
to Wolfe. Wolfe told him, Perkins reported, that Flandrau's was the best of the
hundreds of letters he received.[24]

At last Grace seemed ready to mine her own life for a full-length manuscript, but she found the process problematical. She sought Perkins's views:

> I want to ask your opinion and advice about a very important thing. I find
> that one whole section of my book could be conveniently taken out and
> put forward separately. It is almost wholly autobiographical. The point is,
> is it wiser to present it in the first person or in fiction form? As autobiog-
> raphy or as a novel? There are several things, it seems to me, to be said on
> both sides. It deals with my girlhood in France, briefly, and the four years
> we were in Mexico during the beginning of the Mexican revolution.
>
> Do you think people like to read things written in the first person as
> well as if it is presented as fiction? Especially if the events themselves have
> not been of really startling importance? Of course, that was an interest-
> ing and important period in Mexican history. Our life in Mexico City, in
> the diplomatic society of the time, was interesting, and our life on Blair's
> remote coffee plantation even more so. But it is not merely a chronicle
> of outside events. I come into it. Now, if it is written as thinly disguised
> fiction, it gives me much more leeway, I can be franker, I can tell more.
>
> On the other hand, to write it as straight reminiscence would give it a
> certain ease and simplicity. And value too. I could speak by name of the
> various people of prominence we knew in Mexico City, and of the purely
> historic succession of events of which I was a witness. As autobiography I
> could call it a Mexican Memory. As fiction . . . the name of a woman, with
> more to follow in subsequent books. Please write me what you think.

Grace quizzed Perkins further about Wolfe's technique:

> I suppose Wolfe's books are almost pure autobiography, aren't they? Yet, he has used the fiction form. Anyhow, I shall be eager to have your opinion. Especially as to the relative chances of getting it <u>read</u>. Which form, on the whole, would be most apt to sell well? As a memoir it would be necessarily a little less personal, I mean as to the inner events. But there is plenty to tell objectively in that particular period.[25]

Max Perkins replied thoughtfully:

> Although I do not fully understand the problem that confronts you—that is, I do not understand the relations between this narrative about a girl's life in France and the Mexican episode and the complete novel—I am pretty well convinced that the narrative should be in the form of fiction because of the different and deeper quality that that form seems to give. There is also the practical reason, which always intrudes itself upon a publisher, that unless a reminiscent volume has some other features that give it salience aside from that of quality, it is very hard to get attention for it, or a sale.
>
> But in fiction the question of the intrinsic quality counts for far more. I shall think over the question some more, and maybe you will tell me more about it, but I am sure that put in the form of fiction it would be more effective and wiser, unless you have strong reasons on the other side that may develop.[26]

In an outpouring of apology for her past intransigence, Grace asked Perkins for more advice:

> Since writing you I find that the problem almost answered itself. It seems better all round to do it in novel form and I, without thinking at all, found myself writing "she" instead of "I." And I found also that along with facts, just about as much crept in that was fiction.
>
> I wish to God I had done this last winter, instead of fussing with the Congo book. You were right of course, and I shall confess to you that just now it's a little hard for me to keep my spirits up as well as they should be because I feel disturbed and disappointed. Not because the Congo book

isn't a best seller, and not because critics don't lie down and scream with enthusiasm. But because they don't seem to grasp what is in it, along with whatever faults it may have. It seems to me, what is the use? It seems to me as if nothing I wrote could possibly be liked or read or understood except by people who, by some awful malevolence of fate, can't help the book, don't count.

I have a feeling of being doomed, and it is hard to rise above it and work with the gusto that I otherwise would have. Here I am, knowing how at last, with the material at my fingertips, being more interested, more in this [her autobiographical novel] than I ever was in anything, and yet my heart is squeezed with a kind of despair, I am weighed down with a sense of defeat, of a fatal sense. Why will one not accept the judgment of people whom they trust, as I trust you? You published these [African] stories, I know, a little against your will and certainly against your judgment, and now I see that this that I am doing now, should have come first.

Well, never mind. You asked what all this part has to do with the novel I have underway. Well, it's a kind of major operation. I was swamped before, I couldn't write anything until this present thing [Her remorse? Her inde-cision between fiction and "memoir"?] is off my chest, and yet, it got as much in the way of what I was really doing as a grand piano would in the back of a sedan. Once I get it out, the sedan will run again.

Grace continued to describe her work in process:

It [her novel] covers the life of a weird family, and especially a girl, from the time she is a child and goes to Europe to school, through her teens, her marriage and four years of life in Mexico City and on a Mexican planta-tion during the revolution. It will be about half in half, truth and fiction.

In conclusion, she hoped for renewed self-confidence: "Well, if you know of any magic springs, any source of psychic ultraviolet vibrations that will restore hope and faith and the minimum of self-confidence not to say ardor . . . tell me where to find them, no matter how long and dangerous the journey. Faithfully . . . Grace Flandrau."[27]

But, as subsequent events proved, Grace didn't want to fictionalize her personal story; she wanted to write it as memoir. However, reluctant to dispute Perkins's advice again, she abandoned the project. *Under the Sun's* failure, however, taught her an important lesson. Never again would she stray as far from her own and her readers' reality as she had in the African stories.

The commercial failures of *Indeed This Flesh* and *Under the Sun* within two years were humbling shocks to Grace as a writer. Undeniably, in the latter case her ego had forced a sympathetic publishing professional to act against his better judgment. The disappointing results hurt her pride and diminished her literary reputation.

Meanwhile, thanks to the unflagging efforts of James Gray, Charles Flandrau's resuscitation was flourishing. D. Appleton—Century's new edition of his *Sophomores Abroad* (first published in 1901) appeared in national and Twin Cities bookstores in 1935, and the same publisher brought out Charles's classic *Viva Mexico!* again in 1937 (the fourth of five eventual editions). Next, Gray's crowning paeon to Charles Flandrau, "Minnesota Muse," appeared in the *Saturday Review of Literature* on June 12, 1937. In the story Gray mentioned other Minnesota writers but lionized his idol, making him the focus of the story. By 1937 Charles Flandrau's literary reputation again overshadowed his sister-in-law's, mellowing him.

In his new preface for Appleton-Century's 1937 edition of *Viva Mexico!* Charles paid rare compliments in print to both Grace and Blair. Describing the neglected, ill-fed animals of Mexico, Charles referred to the "wistful, yearning, never-fed, stray dogs of which my gifted sister-in-law has elsewhere since written with such poignant beauty." (He didn't name his sister-in-law nor her charming story, "Speaking of Cats and Dogs" in *Harper's*, July 1937.) Of Blair, Charles wrote in the same introduction: "Kindness of heart and perfect manners do not make spectacular entries on the account book, but my brother has always had them."

The late 1930s were years in which Grace might have summoned all her gifts—now more open to criticism and less encumbered by ego—to the realization of her full potential as a novelist. She still had Max Perkins's belief, but Fate had a different plan.

With Blair's deteriorating health, Grace's low spirits, frequent trips to HillStead for Avon board meetings, and the demands of newspaper and radio commitments, Grace couldn't seem to muster the energy (the "libido," as Theodate would have said) to produce the major novel Perkins hoped for. Nevertheless, many drafted segments for her book in "memoir" form turned up in her papers after her death. How long she continued to work on the drafts is unknown as is the reason she never submitted them for publication.[28]

What is certain, however, is that the voluminous, non-fiction drafts about her youth, worked over and over and over again for perfection and clarity of expression, demonstrate Flandrau's urgent need to explain the stark reality of her childhood to the people who seemed the most skeptical about it—her Hodgson relatives and Blair's friends in St. Paul.

After Grace revealed her low morale to Perkins he stopped nudging her about a book. She must have admitted she felt up to short fiction, however, because, anticipating termination of *Scribner's* magazine, Perkins recommended New York literary agent Carl S. Brandt, of Brandt and Brandt, Inc., to her. Subsequently, Brandt became Grace's agent and supportive friend, successfully representing her in the magazine market for the next twenty years. Flandrau's and Perkins's communication all but ceased after 1938.

In accepting radio, public speaking, and newspaper assignments Grace was shoring up her credibility at home and sticking with work that reinforced it quickly. Later, when she called Perkins's attention to her article "Black Potentates of Africa" in *Pictorial Review*, fall 1937, and reported that her talk on Africa at the University of Minnesota's Northrop Auditorium in October 1937 drew more than five thousand people, she revealed her continuing quest for his approval. When she subsequently sought Perkins's advice about doing radio work for Charles Scribner's Sons, Inc., his terse reply went right to the point: "I think radio talks are good if they do not take too much out of you. They ought only to be incidental. Writing must be the main thing for anyone who is really doing it. Ever sincerely yours, ME."[29]

In the late 1930s, Grace's jobs in print and broadcast journalism prevented her from writing even short fiction. The worst drag on her will, however, was the old stress of living with Blair's drinking. It was the same old story. When they were apart—and that was often in the years 1935 through 1937—the Flandraus exchanged devoted, newsy letters, and Blair's friends kept him busy. When they were together their dispositions grated like sandpaper. But others besides Grace worried about Blair's drinking. One was Alice O'Brien.

In winter 1936, Alice wrote Grace that she had seen Blair at a party, and reported, as Grace informed him, "you were so sweet and dignified and sober." But, Grace also wrote him: "You were one of the few people on earth she [Alice] loved enough to have it make her wild with nerves, to see you . . . slowed up, eclipsed." Her letter included a lengthy description of him when he wasn't "sweet and dignified and sober." The frank but fair and loving four-page letter was an eloquent plea to Blair to believe what she said. Her words had the ring of finality.[30]

Alcoholics Anonymous was in its infancy in 1936, but Al-Anon, a support group for families of alcoholics, did not then exist. Nevertheless, Grace contacted Alcoholics Anonymous for help as early as 1936, but Blair's health, morale, and will were by then too frail for recovery.[31]

Grace's zealous pursuit of fame and fortune as a writer throughout her marriage, which must have looked to Flandrau friends like the most callous selfishness on her part, was partly her survival instinct at work. Very likely, after her first bout with nervous exhaustion in 1918, therapists advised her to lead her own life and not get bogged down in futile attempts to change or accommodate to Blair's drinking. At least, Grace behaved that way after she left Purinton Inn at the end of World War I. Perhaps as early as 1918 counselors advised spouses not to behave in what today's therapists label "codependent" ways and not to "enable" another's addiction.

Nevertheless, self-absorbed ambition and moneymaking zeal were neurotic excesses in the personality of the immature Grace Flandrau that her husband enabled and perhaps shouldn't have. Those characteristics and Blair's loneliness during his wife's many absences may have exacerbated his habitual drinking, but he was most likely a chemical dependent in boyhood, long before he met Grace. No one's self-destructive behavior can be blamed on someone else.[32]

Blair was a boyish, charming, and non-threatening man. Because of their own habits, however, some of his friends and his older brother enabled and probably reinforced his excessive drinking. Grace's self-disciplined, independent behavior undoubtedly irritated and threatened not only Blair but some of his associates, male and female. Some were more likely to blame her instead of him or themselves for his overindulgence.

Grace referred to "your girlfriend" when she wrote Blair from Farmington in the summer of 1936.[33] The woman in question was a beautiful married woman, a member of Blair's close circle who was known to drink excessively. Blair and his "girlfriend" apparently had been discussing a driving trip together, but when he backed out, the woman indignantly wrote Grace that Blair was "just an opportunist."[34]

Later that summer Blair sent Grace a loving note: "Good night my own sweet darling. I love you more than you will or ever _can_ know. All my dearest, dearest love to HER. Keek."[35] He wrote this and other letters late in August 1936 from Cable, Wisconsin, where he was again visiting Mary Griggs and family. Blair sometimes mentioned but never complained about his chronic stiff neck. He assured Grace he was fine and healthy and passed on compliments he'd heard about her radio show.

As 1937 began, the Flandraus headed away from Farmington and St. Paul, respectively, in two directions. Grace drove to Mexico City with Mary and Bill Bonilla, a couple the Flandraus had known in Mexico many years earlier. Blair drove to California, chauffeured by Allan. He invited Grace's sister, Lucile Willis, to join him and Allan for a tour of the state.

When he heard about Grace's plans, Blair wrote an uncharacteristically stiff note: "If you wish to go on this Mexican trip I have no objection. However, I think it is a silly thing to do. I thought you wanted to go somewhere where you didn't know anybody and write. This seems to me a waist [*sic*] of time. But if you want to go do so. I will borrow some money and place it in your account. All my dearest love, Blair."[36]

As usual, the spouses stayed in close touch during their travels. Blair's letter dated April 13, 1937, sent from Calexico, informed Grace that: "I haven't felt so well for years." He was sixty-two.

In Santa Barbara, Blair lunched with his half-sister, Sally Cutcheon, a widow, but his thoughts were with Grace. In Mexico City she received Blair's frequent notes, begging her to take good care of herself when she was alone: "Be awful careful. Stay in your room most of the time and dine there always."[37]

In Mexico City Grace spent a whole day at the home of Mexican artist Diego Rivera, listening to the trial of Leon Trotsky on the radio with Rivera's friends. Trotsky had been captured in Mexico and was extradited to Russia for trial. Although Communist philosophy couldn't have been further from her own beliefs, Grace, as usual, found her unerring way into the center of the action in Mexico City.[38]

Blair's health failed rapidly during the summer of 1937. From then on he and Grace were reunited in St. Paul. Within a few months he was bedridden, and Grace was at his bedside almost constantly. He had suffered a series of strokes.

On December 29, 1937, Charlie wrote John Riddle: "Blair is a completely helpless invalid. Grace is wonderfully sensible and resigned about it.... His great depression of spirits is the worst thing she has to contend with." [39] Charles went to see his brother for five or ten minutes daily.

When Grace wrote John and Theodate about Blair's condition on November 11, 1937, she asked John to sign a Power of Attorney giving Mr. Greer, a realtor in Butler, Pennsylvania, the power to sell lots for them to raise money. Blair, Charles, and John had jointly inherited real estate in Butler from Rebecca, and property sales required all their signatures. Grace said that she and Blair were "terribly hard up and any extra funds would help pay medical expenses."[40]

Despite Blair's rapid decline, his older brother preceded him in death. Charles suffered a sudden severe heart attack and died on March 28, 1938. According to his will the Flandrau house was left to Blair. Accommodating her husband's dying wish, Grace moved him into his childhood home at 385 Pleasant, giving up their house on Portland. There, after lingering a few months, Blair died on November 27, 1938.

With his obituary notice in the December 1, 1938, *Dispatch* appeared a story headed "Zest for Living Characterized Blair Flandrau" written by devoted family friend, James Gray, "The meaning of his experience is curiously, brilliantly clear. He was one of those rare creatures born to live exultantly and to pass on to those less blessed with vitality a stirring, vicarious sense of zest."

Milton Griggs wrote Grace about his old companion: "The word 'gentleman' fitted him [Blair] better than almost anyone I ever knew."[41] Many friends, including Maxwell Perkins, sent notes of sympathy.[42]

Grace was the principal beneficiary of both Blair's and Charles's estates in one year, and she became owner of the Flandrau home as well. Through slow erosion of principal, Blair's estate at his death was worth only a little more than twenty percent of Charles's: $57,000 vs. $250,000. Blair had known all along that he would be Charlie's main beneficiary and assumed that, no matter which brother died first, Grace would be provided for.

The two men who had depended on Grace's drive and charisma for nearly thirty years and who had conferred on her their companionship, social position, and financial security were now, quite suddenly, gone. And the gentle, generous husband who had quietly managed her financial and domestic affairs for years was no longer there to lean on. In his place was a great deal of money.

CHAPTER XV

Hanging on to the Past

"There was, from the beginning to the end of life, that place where
friendship, like love, leaves off, and each must go on alone."
Grace Flandrau, "A Night in Wamba," Under the Sun, 1936

GUILT AND DESPAIR overwhelmed Grace after Blair's death. Her devastation
surprised Flandrau friends, who probably expected her to take his death in
stride. William J. McNally, *Minneapolis Tribune* theater critic, playwright and
friend from New Richmond, Wisconsin, pleaded with Grace to pull herself
together. She was one of his favorite St. Paul hostesses. McNally wrote her
shortly after Blair's funeral:

> Even without your letter, I realized . . . the mental state you were in. I
> could see it in your face as you stepped into the car . . . at the graveyard.
> But, Gracie, Gracie, Gracie, you must realize that you are doing neither
> Blair nor yourself nor the world nor your friends any good by letting your
> grief master you to the extent of turning yourself into a living suicide.

But McNally's description of Blair explained Grace's remorse:

> I realize . . . what an irreparable loss you have suffered. . . . No one who
> had been in Blair's company for ten minutes could fail to be aware of his
> exquisite gentleness, his tact, his kindliness, his fineness of fibre, his almost
> fabulous capacity for loyalty and devotion. . . . He was one of those indi-
> viduals who forced you to think twice and wonder when you were about
> to give human nature up as a bad job.[1]

Grace confessed her desolation to Jim and Sophie Gray early in 1939:

> I told Jim that night at the B's so much that was in my heart. I couldn't
> help it. How desperately I feared what was coming—how I prayed and
> prayed that I should not have to drink this cup. All that I had feared is
> worse, worse, worse. So much that was unclear even then is clear now. I

never, never thought I should hate life and want to die. I do. I think of
nothing but him, how no matter where I went, or what I did there was
always waiting, his really divine tenderness, divine kindness, divine generosity. I took it for granted, as my right, as one takes sunshine and fresh
air—and now it's gone and I have nothing. I am nothing. I don't exist
except to yearn for him back, and to realize the silence and the emptiness.
What shall I do? How am I going to go on? And for what? And in such a
world as this—alone?[2]

The shock of sudden solitude intensified. Grace had no children, no relatives
to whom she was close. The loss of Blair and Charlie weakened her connection
to their family and friends. Except for dealings with professional colleagues,
Grace was isolated. Now she had only Mary O'Malley and the dogs, Cuka and
Chico, and the parrots, Albert and Lauro, as her family. She soon learned that
even sympathetic friends tolerate only so much grief. She began a diary.

Flandrau's private journal and her correspondence over the next two decades
document her slow adaptation to widowhood and her attempts to come to
terms with her inner self. Although she produced some of her best short
fiction in the early 1940s and some strong but sparse journalism in the late
1940s and mid-1950s, Grace's recording of her own journey toward whole-
ness became her principal writing effort. During earlier therapy for nervous
exhaustion she must have learned that the process of "looking within," no
matter how painful, would lead to recovery. After Blair's death, as her journal
notes, she forced herself to confront the mask of pretense she had worn for so
long—pretense to herself and to others. To the few she felt affirmed by, the
real Grace Flandrau began to emerge. To those she felt unsafe with, however,
her mask grew more impenetrable than ever.

The diary she began after Blair's death continued into the early 1940s. In it
Grace held imaginary conversations with him and with herself, confessing her
faults, scolding herself, expressing resolve. Her inner self was sometimes "you"
and Blair was sometimes "you." In an early entry she addressed both Blair and
herself: "Blair, Blair, every moment, every day, you are with me. I love you and
miss you and long, long, long for you and you alone." His death, she acknowledged, had awakened her to her self-absorption: "You [Blair] were your dear
mother incarnate and I crucified you. . . . I can hardly endure it. . . . I must
have courage."

Addressing herself, Grace wrote: "You're the most entirely self-centered person in the world, I have never seen or known anyone like you, but your intelligence teaches you to recognize it."[3]

Brenda Ueland—divorced, writing, teaching writing, and living in Minneapolis—tried to console her old friend. Ueland was experiencing loneliness too. She contacted Grace in St. Paul six months after Blair's death:

> I know how you tear at your own breast about Blair, because you were not better to him. But you cannot possibly calculate <u>how</u> good you were to him. I <u>know</u> you were. I not only saw it, and he (unconsciously perhaps) told me about it, but I <u>know</u> it.
>
> And he, in separation, feels no doubt just exactly the same about you—and it is agony for him to see your guilt, because it is not justified at all, he knows—how he did not do half enough for you, thinks of frightful omissions. . . . The more we love people and the better we are to them (especially the closer we are) the more we feel this. I do. I cannot take a train, leaving people I love most in all the world, without feeling what a pinched, meagre, inadequate stinker I have always been to them from the go-off. Which is not true at all, of course.

Ueland continued, remembering Grace's troubled childhood:

> I feel there may be a kind of a love-block in you, a stagnation of it, and it makes you feel sad. You have so much of it in you, but it doesn't pour out freely and continuously enough, to give you happiness. And I think perhaps it is because you had not enough practice in loving people, as a child—those years in the Paris school that you told me about. So much temperament, you had, and you had to be so complete in yourself, such a sealed packet.

Ueland concluded with a description of Flandrau at age fifty-three.

> Much love. I see you every day, as you are: beautiful, graceful (so much incomparable elegance! aesthetic sense! so absolutely necessary and brightening in this world)—perhaps one of the most important things in the world—healthy, slim, hazel-eyed, rosy-petal face, fashionable: your

beautiful voice; the sense of excitement, wit, laughter, affection it spreads around, in one sentence. Your ardent gifted wonderful writing. Your incandescence when you are working. . . . Oh I see hundreds of things. . . . See you soon . . . Brenda.[4]

Ueland's letter precipitated a visit between the two old friends. "Long talk with Brenda," Grace wrote in her diary at the end of June, but her comments about Ueland were critical as well as grateful:

There isn't quite enough innocence . . . Isn't it too self-conscious? Too much a contradiction, above all, too egotistical? The revered Ueland and fibster Ueland, but struggling bravely to amount to something both inwardly and outwardly, I think. Certainly kind, generous, and helpful toward her friends, toward me.[5]

Further correspondence between the two women followed, but Ueland's affectionate letter did not rekindle their friendship. By middle age, widely disparate lifestyles separated them, Grace clinging to the safety of social convention and material advantage and Ueland persisting in her nonconforming adventurism.

Passing years also put distance between Flandrau and Meridel Le Sueur. When Le Sueur called on her after Blair's death, Grace wrote in her diary: "I wish she would leave me alone. We have nothing in common whatsoever."[6] In spite of the solitude facing her, Flandrau maintained her chosen mid-life boundaries. Her changed status would challenge other old friendships

A passage from one of Grace's African stories, "A Night in Wamba" (*Under the Sun*, 1936) revealed acceptance of the fleeting nature of friendship: "There was, from the beginning to the end of life, that place where friendship, like love, leaves off, and each must go on alone."[7]

On July 15, 1939, after returning from downtown, Grace confided in her journal:

Came home to feel such a smashing wave of loneliness . . . my heart nearly stopped beating. It is a golden, cool, hot summer day. I think of last summer, of him, of all I did not do for him, the little tiny things, when he was so sick, even to not staying with him, God Christ, what suffering, what anguish. And now he's gone, gone, gone forever. It is simply incredible that I could not realize, could not sacrifice, could not do everything, everything, everything, oh, god, like staying with him in the afternoons, like giving him everything to make him comfy, and his dear peace of mind about spending—even that I could not do.

She noted that Blair had once tried to tell her how selfish she was, and "all I did was bawl, understanding nothing." Addressing herself, she wrote:

> That is your major wickedness. Never, never to think for other people. And now you must learn it alone, when you are old and tired and defeated. Could I ever kill myself? I doubt it. I am eating the Dead Sea fruit of self-ishness. Now I have myself and myself alone. I have the house, I have the money, I am the loneliest person in all the world. But I cannot change. Too late.

She recognized the fault wasn't all hers: "And he did spoil me, the blessed one. I alienated his love but kept some of it too. He was too loyal to be able to stop loving no matter what." Finally, with resolve: "Discipline yourself, try to be brave, cheerful, helpful. And now, oh, try to lift this great load of pain, try to write a little and forget."

But instead of writing for publication, Grace continued to journal on many subjects—writing, money, the approaching war, art, her troublesome teeth, her friends, her father, her faults. And Grace soon resumed social life; in spite of her outward independence, she was too dependent on attention to withdraw from her usual activities for long and too good an actress not to be able to disguise her feelings. Her diary reveals that she was becoming acutely aware of how she behaved toward others and they toward her. She recognized that not all of her father's influence had been good: "What I started out with, the one great weakness, was fear, moral cowardice, created in me by Father. The vanity, selfishness and greed were all aided and abetted by my bringing up."

Flandrau reminded herself not to be argumentative, not to let her tongue run away with itself, not to tell people off. A compulsive didactic, she had seldom hesitated to speak her mind on issues she felt strongly about, but her blunt outspokenness, however well reasoned, was often inappropriate. Yet, as her diary reveals, she knew the importance of being herself: "You must stop trying to make people like you. You must stop thinking about whether they do." And she cautioned herself not to drink or to drink very little and be honest in her actions: "It's time to make your acts jibe with what [kind of person] you'd like to think yourself."

Always self-conscious about her appearance, Grace grew more so: "Of course, my teeth are my constant despair . . . and that more than anything has contributed to breaking me down and up into small pieces. It seems to kill all my future. Without that I should have remained cocky. Because that hits me where I live, or always have lived, square in the vanity solar plexus."

With the coming of summer 1939, Grace felt somewhat encouraged. Men and women among Blair's cronies called on her, their visits recorded in her diary. "Nice Billy" (recent widower William J. McNally) escorted her to a party at Gerry (Mrs. Horace "Gokey") Thompson's, she wrote, "so I am not so neglected as I often feel." A later entry says: "Reproach nobody, no matter how much you are neglected." Her confidence ebbed and flowed. She recorded occasional snubs and slights.

Grace turned to many sources—poetry, Sanskrit, the Bible—for consolation. In late summer, her diary noted the mounting threat of war in Europe, but grief still so engulfed her she couldn't think about it. She was reading Antoine de Saint-Exupéry and entered his words in her journal: "You have not to be perturbed by great problems, having trouble enough to forget your fate as a man."

In August 1939, Adolf Hitler's Wehrmacht invaded Poland, and on September 3 England and France declared war against Germany. Grace wrote in her journal: "What horror impends no soul can tell. I am thinking of Bizy, of taking care of children. I feel so incredibly desolate that it is like a disease."[8]

Receiving word of Grace's continuing despair, Brenda Ueland wrote again. This time, speaking out of her own melancholy, Ueland advocated surrender of the ego and spiritual awakening. She wrote:

> I have tried to telephone you many times, and you are out. And I feel in a way, that it isn't company you want but help, a letter. I will pray for you. I mean ("pray" sounds ridiculous.), send you power. I did it for quite a while, after I saw you that time. I felt you were better.
>
> You say 'Crucifixion, then resurrection.' But 'resurrection' is too strong a word. There is too much final triumph in it. I say to myself instead 'make a tiny ascension.' If we can make just a little one, then this higher level is never lost, but we stay there, though we think, in slumps, that all our gains have fallen away.

Grace, do you work for your ascension? Do you give it ten minutes a day? Please do this, if you possibly can. Shut your eyes, 'looking inward at quiet' as the mystics say. Or begin (before asking, praying, i.e., shutting your eyes and earnestly asking) by writing down what you want. If you have "lost faith," as you say, then write down: 1. I want faith. I want 'just one person near me to love in the <u>nature</u> way, a young person,' as you say. Then ask, for ten minutes at least, with all your imagination. If you do this, something will happen.

Some sad night if you want company, telephone me. Will come over. Heavens I have frightful melancholy too; it is intermittent anxiety, self-disgust, and often a loneliness that is a bursting chest. But I have learned (I think) to make these times not destructive, but to 'grow' in them . . . per-haps a very little. That is, if I can go through them manfully, without getting drunk, or flying into the comforting herd of talkers, feeders, gossipers, etc. I feel so wonderfully light and even powerful, later.

By an enormous imaginative effort all day long (not often successful), I try to keep my spirit way up there, high, and I say to my dark abdominal self, to my dragons of bile: 'Seethe, dragons. Go ahead and seethe. All you want to. You are not me. My spirit is separate and way up here;' etc. I don't mean that a device like this makes me a bit happier, but I always feel a queer gain afterwards, in courage, in escape from the mean, timid, covet-ous, self-preservative self. The Self is all right. I don't want to be hard on the Self. But it has to go, as one grows up.

Now, as for me and a report. Yes, the war [World War II]. Was terribly depressed. I try to think of it as a volcanic disaster, now, not malevolent. The most depressing thing about war is the malevolence.[9]

Ueland's insightful letter reached Flandrau a decade too soon. In 1939 Grace wanted to recover her old life, her old zest, in the same old way. She existed in a world far removed from Brenda's bohemian life style. In spite of her self-investigation, Grace resisted inner change.

The harsh reality of widowhood increasingly impacted her. The defer-ence always paid her as a married woman was a thing of the past. The long-concealed jealousy of other women surfaced. Naturally there was pent-up resentment at the attention Grace had always received, professionally and socially. Speaking of this deference, Kate Klein confided in a 1993 interview: "People adored Grace Flandrau and always just gravitated toward her."[10] But

Grace's diary recorded a painful episode: "I didn't mention that awful affair yesterday. The coldness of people . . . I shant forget Ruth P. turning her shoulder to me, I don't remember it ever having been done before. Giving me the cold shoulder in very truth, strange, I didn't expect it."[11]

Grace, with survival instinct intact, sought contacts with men but probably didn't understand how threatening that made her appear. A few months after Blair's death she began to entertain a little and described with frankness an intriguing visitor in her journal:

> I made a great effort—Mitropulous [Dmitri Mitropulous, conductor of the Minneapolis Symphony Orchestra (1937-1949) and something of a womanizer by reputation] came for lunch. Knew he didn't like to talk while he ate, so we just masticated and looked out of the window. Afterward he wanted to sleep. I took him out on the lawn, he slept there—a peasant—not used to polite society.[12]

Grace's old boss, Ralph Budd, came to call: "Yesterday Ralph came [and] spent a half an hour. I was glad to see him. I think I like him best still of any living person."[13]

Budd had stayed in touch with Flandrau ever since publication of their railroad pamphlets in the 1920s. He kept trying to engage her in his ideas and repeatedly tried to hire her for other assignments, but she usually declined, giving her radio and newspaper work as excuses.

Occasionally, however, Budd persuaded Grace to edit his speeches and his writing on railroad affairs; their correspondence continued for many years. Sometimes he escorted her and his wife to railroad dinners and other official banquets. Eventually both Budd and Flandrau became members of the Executive Council of the Minnesota Historical Society.

Requests to speak and encouraging letters from Dick Myers, Kay Boyle, and Carl Brandt nudged Grace back to work within a year after Blair's death. When an English teachers' organization in the Twin Cities invited her to speak to them again—many teachers still remembered her talk given two years earlier—Grace's spirits revived. Addressing herself, she wrote in her diary: "Well, that was your role. You should have known it years ago."[14]

Just three weeks after the outbreak of war in Europe, the Minneapolis *Times-Tribune* sought Grace's participation in its radio campaign for American neutrality. On September 21, 1939, she appeared with author Margaret Culkin

Banning and Bernice B. (Mrs. John) Dalrymple on the newspaper's radio program broadcast by eight stations around the state.[15]

In January 1941, Grace was again featured speaker at the Minnesota Historical Society's annual meeting. For the occasion, which celebrated the centennial anniversary of the founding of St. Paul, Grace delivered her famous sketch, "St. Paul—The Personality of a City," later published in *Minnesota History*.[16] Three weeks afterward, on February 9, 1941, she gave the same speech at the Women's City Club in downtown St. Paul. Grace wrote Richard Myers in Manhattan that she was always expected to speak "on state occasions."[17] Whether she liked it or not, hers was the fate of a compulsive ham who had a unique, entertaining approach to dry subjects.

Myers's artistic soul and appreciation for Grace's writing (and her appreciation of his musical talent) fed their enduring friendship. He peppered her from New York with letters urging her to resume writing. A few months after Blair's death Myers wrote from Manhattan: "I feel more sure than ever that your work is at its peak . . . But you must sit down and start your long novel—and write a short story whenever the spirit moves you—but write you <u>must</u>."[17]

In 1940 and 1941, Kay Boyle, divorced from Laurence Vail, was living in Europe with her third husband, Baron Joseph Frankenstein, and their six children. Carl Brandt was Boyle's agent too. As World War II began Boyle sought Grace's assistance in securing passage for Frankenstein, an Austrian Jew, and their children out of Europe to the United States. Grace signed papers, tried but failed to get Joseph a teaching position at Avon School, and sent a $500 letter of credit. Urging Grace back to work, Boyle stated: "You have no right to remain a non-writer."[18]

Although she now had no financial imperative, Grace resumed her former life, the only one she knew: writing for publication, newspaper and radio work, public speaking, social life, trips to Farmington for Avon board meetings, writing long letters to friends, and travel. Resumption of the old modus vivendi meant donning the same old public mask—the always-poised, entertaining, sophisticated literary celebrity Grace Flandrau. In the early 1940s Blair's old friends occasionally got in touch with her. Jack (John G.) and Charlotte Ordway took her out to dinner when Jack's sister, Katherine, visited St. Paul. Louis W. Hill, Jr. and his wife entertained her. She often had tea by the fire at Katherine (Mrs. Roger B.) Shepard's on winter afternoons and sometimes traveled with Mary L. Griggs (Mrs. Theodore).[19] Although she continued to see old friends like the Edwin Whites, the Tom Danielses, and the Kleins, as every new widow or widower knows, things change after a spouse's death. She hid hurt feelings and loneliness. Flandraus' letters at that time refer to her troublesome health.

Between 1940 and 1949 sixteen pieces of Grace's short fiction and journalism appeared in *Harper's, The New Yorker, Good Housekeeping, McCall's, Collier's, Scholastic Magazine, Minnesota History, The Saturday Evening Post, The Yale Review,* and *American Quarterly.* Although her fiction output ceased after 1945, Grace's journalistic skills strengthened.

Her first stories to appear after Blair's death were "To Lose One's Life" in *Good Housekeeping* (1940) and "Nice Man" in *Harper's* (1942). Both explore the issue of marital fidelity versus unfaithfulness; whether to give up your husband to his lover, as in the first story, or to stay with your wife and give up your mistress, as in the second. In "To Lose One's Life" an attractive, wise wife faces and accepts the need to eschew possessiveness and set her husband free. In "Nice Man," an English gentleman, while drinking in the club car on the train, makes the decision not to leave his wife.

Both stories reflected the author's European view of marriage, decidedly not the conventional American one. Instead, Flandrau's premise is that because each person's life is just one brief chance for fulfillment, marital infidelity should be understood and tolerated. Both stories present enlivening metaphors and wisdom about human nature. The style is skillful and is typical of much of the light fiction in popular magazines of the 1940s.

Three *New Yorker* stories in 1942–1943—"Princess," "All the Modern Conveniences," and "What Do You See, Dear Enid?"—present Grace Flandrau at the peak of her skill as a short fiction writer. She drew on her own experience in all three stories, and Houghton Mifflin Company's *The Best American Short Stories of 1943* included "What Do You See, Dear Enid?"

"Princess" describes Marianne, an African girl of royal descent from Madasgascar, the cousin of Grace's classmate, Lucie. Both Lucie and Marianne are upper-class mulatto and black students at the French convent school attended by young Grace Hodgson in turn-of-the-century Paris. Respect and tact characterize the author's sensitive representation of the two young women, both exemplifying the exotic influences encountered abroad by the youthful St. Paulite, 1900 to 1903. The story subtly contrasts the crude manners of Mademoiselle Bouleau, a demoiselle (teaching nun) of common background, with those of the well-brought up blacks, Marianne and Lucie, sophisticated aristocrats: "[Marianne had] the aloofness without condescension of a person not only accustomed to deference but also trained to minimize, politely, that deference." As usual, Flandrau is upending conventional premises.[20]

"What Do You See, Dear Enid?" is a delicious story based on Grace's memory of her adolescent visit with Mary Hodgson and her foster sister, Lucile, to the Isle of Man, Grace's first encounter with her Corrin relatives. Twelve-year-old Grace's distant cousin "Enid" often "had visions" (not unusual among Celts on the Isle of Man) and recounted them nightly to the expectant family circle around the hearth. In the story Grace unforgettably and lovingly described both the Isle of Man—"mist-hung, storm-blown, goblin-haunted, charming"—and the Manx people. She characterized the latter this way: "[Their mixture of] stodgy provincialism and Celtic lunacy were instantly familiar and understandable to me, just as the better fairy tales, which are compounded of this same mixture of magic and homely fact, are familiar and understandable to children." Readers learn that "Mona" is the poetic name for the Isle of Man and "Cutty Sark" is a Celtic goblin.[21]

Another choice story, "All the Modern Conveniences," appeared in the April 1943. *New Yorker*. The sidesplitting essay grew out of Grace's stay with friends in a rented house in Acapulco, Mexico, in 1940. She depicts the confusing mixture of the primitive and the up-to-date encountered by American tourists in Mexico at that time. The plot begins with the Americans' need for repair of a standard household mechanical system and then moves to confusion, disbelief, outrage, and finally, slapstick comedy. The author gives readers an affectionate but exasperated look at the workmen's tendencies to exaggerate, fabricate, goof off, and cover up.

Not all the short fiction Grace produced in the early 1940s was up to the standard of her *New Yorker* stories. In June 1942 Carl Brandt returned twelve unsold stories, asking whether she wanted to redo them. Those he placed were light fiction based on war-related episodes. "A French Woman Too," "Palm Beach Soldier," "Beyond Price," and "White Horse," appearing in *Collier's* and *McCall's* from 1943 to 1945, provided short human-interest stories in wartime settings, brief but revealing epiphanal episodes. Flandrau seems to have decided to unburden her heart with brief messages about her own transforming insights, told in a light way.

The most self-revelatory of the latter stories are "Palm Beach Soldier" (*McCall's*, December 1944) and "White Horse" (*Collier's*, July 1945). Both stories illustrate children's vulnerability to damaging influences and experiences in youth. In "Palm Beach Soldier" the author acknowledged awareness of her father's exaggerated reverence toward people of wealth, which, she believed, had fed her own deep-seated insecurity and tendency toward pretension. In "White Horse" a little girl finds that love for and from an animal can feed the heart when parental love is absent or uncertain.

Grace produced no more fiction after 1945. Drafting notes for a speech or column on what she read and how she worked, she wrote: "I don't like fiction. With certain notable exceptions, I don't like to read it. Except for the occasional great novel, I'm not interested in it. I am interested in what Ring Lardner . . . laughingly nick-named "life." I'm interested in facts, in actualities—the actuality of those bewildering organisms known as human beings. They intrigue and excite me beyond belief. [22]

Those are the words of someone who, having endured misjudgment since childhood due to the gulf between perception and fact, is passionate about truth. Undoubtedly the mature but now unprotected Grace Flandrau recognized how vulnerable she was to harmful speculation and must have admitted to herself that her life had always invited gossip and misunderstanding.

After turning to journalism Grace contributed a bit of literary history about herself and Scott Fitzgerald to James Gray's "Books" column in the St. Paul papers. Scott died in 1940 and, though his literary reputation had been in limbo for years, his reincarnation was under way. By 1945 Grace began to question his growing deification by historians. When the *Nation* published an article comparing Fitzgerald "to Shakespeare, Racine, Voltaire, Goethe, Balzac, Byron, Dostoevsky, Wordsworth, Keats, Shelley, Samuel Butler, Shaw, Proust, Stendahl, Yeats, Gide, Henry James, George Eliot, and Homer," Flandrau spoke up.

In her piece, "Fitzgerald Panegyric Inspires Some Queries," Grace revealed Fitzgerald's own reservations about *The Great Gatsby*, expressed in a private letter he had sent her many years earlier after her negative review of the book. Responding to Flandrau's criticism that Gatsby's character was badly drawn, that he was not a criminal type but a dreamer, Scott wrote: "You [Grace Flandrau] are right about Gatsby being blurred and patchy. I never at any time saw him clear myself for he started out as one man I knew and then changed into myself—an amalgam that was never complete in my mind." Flandrau concluded her column with this comment: "Critics turn authors into their gods and are possessed by them."[23]

Never shrinking from an argument in print or in person, and, disregarding criticism and misunderstanding, Grace still conducted her private, middle aged life according to her own principles, as expressed repeatedly in her writing. She continued cultivating friendships with men—but usually not in St. Paul.

Several bachelors were attentive to Grace during the 1940s. Among them were Twin Cities newspaperman Joe Macgaheran, New York columnist Franklin P. Adams ("What's My Line?" panelist), who lived in Westport, Connecticut, and Edward V. (Ted) Steele, a charming transplanted Englishman born and raised in France. All three men corresponded with her when she wasn't in their vicinity. According to Kate Klein, Grace got a kick out of Macgaheran's wild, Irish sense of humor but decided he was a little rough around the edges.[24]

From Connecticut in 1942, columnist Franklin P. Adams sent two notes concerning a speaking engagement he had in Minnesota and accepting an invitation to "a quiet luncheon" at Grace's in St. Paul. As late as 1944 Adams was still writing Grace, inviting her to join him on a trip to London. Because Adams lived near Farmington, the two may have met frequently in the East or may have visited London together. They had friends in common in the Manhattan publishing world.[25]

Ted (Edward V.) Steele, a recovering alcoholic, was a close friend for many years. He made Grace's acquaintance in the East just before Blair died and visited Grace when he came to St. Paul in 1940 on a fund-raising mission for Alcoholics Anonymous. One communication from Steele is a page torn from the March 1936 *Philosophical Review* with this handwritten note: "In memory of a certain evening in an unforgettable house. T.V.S." The note probably referred to the Gundy house.[26]

After visiting Grace in St. Paul in 1940, Ted Steele wrote her: "In these crumbling days it is so reassuring to find genial, tolerant, graceful people like you. With you I felt my spirits rear up and paw."[27]

Besides knowing how to touch a literary woman's heart and mind, Steele had other appealing qualities. At one time he recorded as a vocalist with John Scott Trotter's band in Hollywood and he recited poetry in French.[28] French idioms sprinkled his letters. Steele had a modest inherited income and took care of his elderly widowed mother in Tucson, where both resided. He was attentive to his mother's aging friends. Grace became acquainted with them after she began wintering in Tucson in the late 1940s.

Flandrau and Steele shared an Old World respect for the elderly—an attribute of genteel manners they agreed was disappearing from the modern world. Ted deplored the way Americans treated older people, such as one mutual friend, a woman named Josephine. Grace, who had a boundless, unsatisfied need for parenting and acceptance, probably projected that longing to older people and they never failed to respond. Steele wrote Grace: "Josephine [has to live in] a world which has become alien and confusing to so many people … and particularly to elderly, aristocratic women with very small incomes; I rather think you and I mean more to her than most of her friends. Her respect and admiration for you are limitless."[29]

Steele pursued and was pursued by other women. Comparing Grace to one of the more zealous, he wrote: "You are virtuous, sensitive and a very finely tuned instrument indeed, you never clutch at anyone (in point of fact, you don't clutch enough)." He also described her in a 1948 letter as "the world's most patient friend."[30]

Whether Flandrau and Ted Steele ever became lovers is unknown, but their friendship spanned more than twenty-five years, 1936 to 1962. Although he lacked Grace's financial resources, Ted traveled too. He repeatedly suggested meeting her in some mutually favored European city. Gaps in their correspondence during the 1940s suggest they did travel together or meet at the Gundy. Steele, however, eventually married someone else, and his wife became as fond of Grace as he.

In Minnesota Grace gradually moved away from the couples in Blair's old crowd, and they from her. She reached out more to both single men and women and to different social groups. She sought friendships with Minnesota writers such as Duluth novelist Margaret Culkin Banning and with members of the English Department of the University of Minnesota. When novelist Robert Penn Warren joined the university faculty in the 1940s Grace invited him to tea.

Although she reviewed his book, *The Illinois*, 1940, favorably in her *Dispatch* column, Grace's friendship with James Gray slowly diminished. After the Flandrau brothers' deaths in 1938, Gray didn't review Grace's work again. But in the 1940s novelists drew critics' attention, not writers of short fiction. Had that master craftsman of short fiction, Anton Chekov (one of Grace's favorites), been a mid-twentieth century writer his stories might have gone unreviewed too.

Although James Gray was a much admired book critic, in the East as well as in Minnesota, after production of four novels, 1925–1938, commercial success and fame as a novelist still eluded him. His fictionalized biography of Charles M. Flandrau and fifth book, *Vagabond Path*, 1941, did little to augment his literary reputation as he had hoped. After that disappointment, Gray grew increasingly cynical. Joseph Warren Beach, a poet, good friend and University of Minnesota professor of English, wrote Gray in 1942: "Nothing has given me more distress of mind during the last six months than the discouragement into which you have fallen over your writing."[31]

Gray, who received an honorary doctorate in literature from Hamline University in the early 1940s, quit his columnist's job at the *Pioneer Press-Dispatch* in 1946 and moved to Burbank, California, where he briefly became a screenwriter for Warner Brothers Studio. In 1948 he returned to join the faculty of the University of Minnesota as a teacher of writing in the English Department. He ceased writing fiction and turned his career increasingly to journalism.Pondering the constancy of James Gray's worshipful feelings toward Charles Flandrau's writing and the obvious ebb and flow of his interest in Grace's works, one grows certain that St. Paulites must have become involved in the Flandraus' contest for recognition as writers presided over and judged by Gray and the St. Paul press for at least thirty years. In the 1940s some of Grace's personal friends among the local literati challenged the columnist's obvious bias. At the request of Mrs. Harold (Margaret) Wood, in 1943 the St. Paul Public Library prepared a list of forty to fifty famous Minnesota authors. The names of Grace Flandrau and Kay Boyle both appear on the list.

Writing meaty letters to a few friends and other writers, sharing her ideas or challenging their views, gradually replaced Grace's diary as her main form of communication. She indulged her passion for facts and thrived on the interchange of ideas with people whom she described as having a "global point of view."[32] Grace's zest for discourse, however, sometimes threatened her friendships.

Flandrau carried on running arguments about politics via letters with James Gray, Kyle Crichton, Kay Boyle, and Theodate Riddle. They were ardent socialists or, at least, communist sympathizers. Boyle, who was blacklisted in the late 1940s for her left-wing views and activities, was finding American publishers less receptive to her work. She turned to teaching and reviewing books.[33]

Grace spoke from the heart about many things other than politics when she wrote Kay Boyle and often made desperately needed financial loans to the younger writer and her family—there were six children by three fathers. Boyle faithfully repaid the loans and wrote Grace eloquently about her gratitude:

"Again, thank you . . . for your incredible humanness and your devotion." Boyle told Flandrau she was a wonderful friend and was too self-effacing.[34]

To Kay, Grace admitted the uncertainty she felt about the quality of her writing, how loneliness was affecting her will to work, and the despair she felt about the war. News in the early 1940s that both the Edwin Whites' son, Gardner, and the Richard Myerses' son, Dicky, had been killed in action deeply saddened her.[35]

Flandrau also corresponded with writers Earnest Seaman, Frederick ("Heinie") Faust, and Isabel Paterson, book critic of the *New York Herald Tribune*. All knew Grace and had appreciated her work in the 1920s and 1930s. All urged her to keep writing.[36]

Grace and Theodate Riddle continued their long conversations via letter. In spite of Theo's enduring admiration for her, Grace didn't hesitate to write frankly about their political differences. She felt Riddle was a "Parlor Bolshevist" with illogical, unrealistic views on advancing humanity while she (Grace) worshipped facts. When she caught Riddle being inconsistent she didn't shrink from exposing it. Theo's letters were just as frank but not as factual.

When Theodate heaped praise on the New Deal and criticized Big Business and its beneficiaries like Alice O'Brien, heiress to a lumber fortune, Grace was incensed: "Because Alice has a fortune derived from lumber—(a fortune which has been tripled by the New Deal methods, which have caused all the little firms in Florida to go out, while enriching the big ones, and in spite of which, or rather, because of which she is against the New Deal)—you imply something very critical about her."

Heatedly reminding Theodate that she herself had inherited a steel fortune, Grace concluded with a stinging rebuke: "I'll remember that you can't differ in politics without running the risk of having it lapse over all too quickly . . . to the impeachment of one's good will and personal intelligence."

Grace and Theo's correspondence covered subjects such as Charles Lindbergh, Walter Winchell, and Wendell Wilkie's criticism of the New Deal's results. Writing Riddle, Flandrau quoted students at the University of Minnesota, farmers, fishermen in Wisconsin, and others to back up her views. For example, in 1940, Grace pointed out, fifty-two percent of the university's students expressed preference for Wilkie in the presidential election.[37]

Political differences may have disaffected Theodate Riddle from her protégée. Grace's diary revealed concern about a growing coolness:

Today it's about Theo and John, not writing, not caring for me. And yet, do you really care about them? No. But you're uneasy, scared if they don't love you. In some ways it's part of your insecurity. It was part of your vanity to be there. And yet you're bitterly unhappy while there. So, why go? Or care if you don't?[38]

John Riddle died in 1941 and Theodate in 1946. Theo's will named Grace beneficiary of a small trust at a New York bank and gave her a life tenancy in the Gundy house in Farmington.

CHAPTER XVI

Valley of Indecision

"They [people] cling to beliefs even when they are proved wrong."
American psychiatrist to Grace Flandrau, 1948

AS THE 1940S UNFOLDED, a new dilemma presented itself: whether Flandrau should continue living in St. Paul or Farmington or both—or somewhere else. Her inability to resolve the issue for many years grew into chronic, debilitating indecision about many things, especially those that cost money, like trips and house repairs. Although Flandrau could now afford practically anything, she didn't seem to believe it. When she repeatedly sought advice from friends, her tortured indecision began to bore and puzzle them.

Richard E. Myers—Grace had no more devoted soul mate than he—tried to coax her to keep the Gundy in Farmington and rent an apartment in uptown Manhattan where he and Alice Lee lived. Sometimes he threatened to burn down the Flandrau house. Myers understood Grace well and identified with what she loved and found difficult about St. Paul. After being her guest on a visit to Minnesota in the early 1940s, Myers wrote:

> All the way home, I thought of you, of your great intelligence. How you can ever keep [it] all working most of the time is a great tribute to your character and is the reason why your friends beam when you come into a room.
>
> Seeing you in St. Paul makes me realize that you must always go there part of the time—for it has a fine feeling of truly American life as it should be lived—and you understand it. My only fear is that you don't receive as much as you give in the matter of human relationships—and those are so vital to your best work. For those you must go afield—and then back to Minnesota. This was evidenced that last night . . . all those dear people lead very conventional lives—undisturbed and for the most part unstimulated. And they will always cling to you for you bring them stimulation.[1]

In spite of her close friendship with both Richard and Alice Lee Myers and their three children, Grace clung to the safety and familiarity of St. Paul. Radio

190

and public appearances in Minnesota, unlike writing for publication, kept her in contact with people, and she couldn't bring herself to abandon old associations in St. Paul. Although she had always been an independent "loner," she wasn't used to unrelieved solitude. Few friends knew that, increasingly, Grace struggled with depression.

Whether she thought of contacting her mother, Anna Hodson, still living in Minneapolis, or communicated with her Hodgson relatives in St. Paul is unknown. There is no record of Grace's reaction to the news that her brother William Hodson died in a plane crash over New Guinea in 1943, although Twin Cities newspapers carried the story. It almost appears that after Blair's death Grace went back into denial about her illegitimacy. Alice O'Brien, Kate and Horace (Bud) Klein, Jr., and their three children, Blair, Minty (Kate), and Allan, now represented Grace's surrogate family in St. Paul.[2]

When he learned of her low spirits from Alice O'Brien, Kent Curtiss wrote Grace that she was probably suffering from what the Greeks called "acedia," a pathological mental and spiritual torpor, or what the French called "le spleen . . . a deep and appalling ennui, a weariness, a despair, an ache, a cloud."[3] Grace replied that, in spite of her despondence and poor health, "one must live with nobility, somehow." During the 1940s Grace was frequently hospitalized with bronchitis in an oxygen tent.[4]

Having sole charge of her business affairs added considerable stress. Previously Grace had depended on Blair and on the Riddle's Hill-Stead staff to manage domestic finances. On her own, such tedious, unfamiliar tasks as bill paying and checkbook balancing, insurance premiums and taxes, intimidated and oppressed her. Now she had to manage two households herself. A portion of the maintenance and operation costs of the eighteenth-century Gundy became Grace's responsibility after Theodate Riddle's death too. Negotiations with Grace for payment of these costs after 1945, according to Hill-Stead Museum staff today, took place in a state of chronic confusion.[5]

The Flandrau mansion at 385 Pleasant was the essence of Victorian St. Paul, but by 1940 a decaying neighborhood surrounded the antique structure. Photos of the imposing, two-story house, with its bays, wings, and twelve chimneys, convey the certainty of astronomical fuel and maintenance bills, drafts, and mice. Overgrown hemlocks and other mature shade trees darkened the front yard—a terraced bank with two flights of steps from the street—discouraging casual access. Iron fencing set off the yard from the sidewalk along Pleasant Avenue. A sunny, upward-sloping back yard, with vegetable and flower gardens, graves of innumerable Flandrau pets, and a well-publicized outdoor "sculpture" collection were invisible from the street.

Flandrau friends remember little of the home's interior except its darkness and its two always-fire-lit libraries, a large one and a smaller, cozier one, off the main entrance hall. Both libraries were filled floor to ceiling with books. In a 1989 interview, St. Paulite Kate Klein remembered having tea with Grace, Eleanor Roosevelt and Blair's sisters, New Yorkers Sally Cutcheon and Patty Selmes, in the little library. Klein said: "Gracie's houses were always hot because she was always cold. . . . She wore sweaters and shawls a great deal."

Klein reminisced: "[Grace] was warm and outgoing and she adored people. One was struck by that immediately. She always gave close friends nicknames; mine was 'Dolly.' She called Alice O'Brien 'Tude' or 'Moon.'" Coomenting on the author's appearance, she wrote: "Grace's eyes were set very far apart. She had tiny feet and wore lovely shoes, was always well dressed. She adored Hattie Carnegie and Mainbocher suits." Klein recalled Grace's outrageous streak and that she relished poking fun at smug people. She described one of Flandrau's fancy parties at which quite a few "stuffed shirts" were present: "A solemn butler passed dinner to the guests on a huge silver tray. When he lifted the cover off the salver, live puppies were lying in it."

Klein also remarked that Grace seemed unpredictable and helter-skelter to her friends. A chaotic homemaker, she was unusually dependent on servants and friends to help her find something, to mail her some forgotten object, or to do favors in her absence or absent-mindedness. When Grace was returning to St. Paul from a vacation, Klein often received a wire a day or so ahead: "Am arriving Thursday. Please meet me with my mink coat."

Once, before leaving on a trip, Grace telephoned Klein and said, "Dolly, I'm going to be away for a couple of weeks. Would you take my parrots?" The parrots remained at the Kleins' home for two years. One of them bit Horace Klein, Jr. (Bud), and during that whole period an incessant parrot chorus of "Nobody's home" and "Blair, Blair, telephone" rang through the house. When Grace finally came to pick up Albert and Lauro before leaving town again she and Klein had to race on foot down Kellogg Boulevard to the depot, hauling fur coats and screaming parrots in cages, to catch the train. Perhaps Grace thought her St. Paul friends expected her to act zany, that they enjoyed having funny stories to tell about her. Entertaining others had always been a major part of her guise.

An increasingly anguished inner self began emerging from the amusing, poised persona Grace had always projected. Perhaps her growing flightiness and forgetfulness and childish dependence on others, was a means of getting attention and staying in touch with people, but her self-centered habits began to create distance. Although Klein at first said she didn't resent Grace's requests, she admitted later that she came to feel imposed upon—and she told Grace as much.[6]

Klein's description of a flibberty-gibbet, disorganized—almost pathetic—woman, however, bears little resemblance to the hard-working journalist laboring in solitude in her study at the Flandrau house in St. Paul or at the Gundy in the 1940s or the sought-after public speaker in the Twin Cities. The celebrity Grace Flandrau was still in touch with editors and other writers, receiving fan mail, and writing an occasional column, story, or book review. But because she had always managed two distinctly different roles—a social one and a professional one—she went on trying. Her double life didn't shore up her credibility with either socialites or professionals.

The wives of some—but not all—of Blair's old friends stayed in touch with Grace, but, increasingly, her closest relationships were with the other single women in his crowd, e.g., Mary (Mrs. Theodore) Griggs, after 1934 a widow, and Alice O'Brien—but Griggs now lived in Manhattan, not in St. Paul, and O'Brien was often at Captiva, Florida. With their children and grandchildren, the St. Paul couples Grace and Blair had known led very different domestic lives from hers. Grace felt the estrangement experienced by any childless widow.

Besides coping with a sense of increasing disconnection, poor health, and new domestic responsibilities, Grace began to worry about her inability to settle down to work. Looking for a challenging assignment after her decision to stick to journalism, Grace contacted Isabel Paterson at the *New York Tribune.* Years earlier, after the success of *Being Respectable,* Paterson asked Grace to consider writing book reviews. Now the long-delayed moment to reopen that subject was at hand. But Paterson declined the offer. In a terse comment implying Grace didn't need to work and questioning her motives, Isabel said, "After all, you were raised a lady, and can't help it now; you'd better eat cake."[7]

Two events in the mid-1940s revived Grace's spirits and improved her health. The first was the discovery of penicillin. The development of penicillin during World War II and its widespread application after 1945 gave relief to millions from chronic influenza, bronchitis, and other upper-respiratory infections. Antibiotics were a salvation to Grace, relieving her concern that fragile health would undermine her ability to handle writing jobs.

Then, after prodding by Kay Boyle and Dick Myers, Grace sought out new writing assignments in postwar Europe. In summer 1947, Grace spent several months in Paris looking into opportunities for bilingual American writers. She renewed friendships with Sylvia Beach and Beach's companion, Adrienne Monnier, and also saw Kay Boyle Frankenstein and family. She participated in a radio program in French for Free France. The next year Grace signed on to write scripts in French for the *Voice of America* and returned to Paris. She was sixty-two. Hard work at a task she believed in in the city she loved best restored Grace's vitality just as it had nearly thirty years earlier.[8]

In Paris, Grace met John Selmes (Jack) Greenway, a young male relative, for the first time. Greenway, who was on vacation from Yale in the summer of 1948, was the son of Charles Eugene Flandrau's only granddaughter, thrice-married Isabella Flandrau Selmes [Ferguson Greenway King]. He was also Blair Flandrau's great nephew. Jack's mother, Isabella, who became the second Democratic Congresswoman from Arizona, and his father, pioneer mining engineer, John Campbell Greenway, were as prominent in Arizona history as the Flandraus were in Minnesota. (John Campbell Greenway, sr. came originally from Minnesota.)

After Greenway's return to college in New Haven and Grace's to Farmington in fall 1948, she invited Jack to the Gundy for lunch. He described the event and the power of Grace's charm in an often-told family anecdote:

> When I returned to Yale after the war I was invited to the Gundy House for lunch with Aunt Grace. I had heard stories about her for years but was in no way prepared for what was to follow. We started off with a delicious luncheon, served by a pretty Swiss maid, Elise, in a gray uniform with skirts that hit the floor. We talked and talked and laughed and laughed—Gracie knew all about everything—and suddenly it was time for tea. Shortly thereafter champagne was served and tiny points of toast with caviar—you know how the story goes—the richer the people, the smaller the canapés. Before I knew it she had instructed the cook that I was staying for dinner.
>
> By this time I had hit my head on the low doorways of the Gundy house so many times [Greenway is at least six feet two inches tall] that I was in a sort of daze and just agreed, and the next thing I knew I had accepted her

invitation to spend the night . . . and that's how I went to Grace Flandrau's for lunch and stayed four days.[9]

Jack and Grace's encounter launched an enduring friendship. Although he was a resident of Arizona and maintained a law practice in Tucson after leaving Yale, Jack assumed the role of son or younger brother to his great-uncle's widow. In Greenway Grace acquired a literary soul mate, a faithful correspondent, and a lawyer.

Greenway was tall, slender, and cultivated with intellectual tastes leaning to history and literature. He spoke French. Like Blair, Greenway was a storyteller, and, having been raised by a beautiful, intelligent, strong-willed mother, he related well to older women. In a 1987 interview he described his attraction to his great aunt: "Grace Flandrau introduced me to the charm of her generation . . . and to the delights of red wine and cheese."[10]

After returning to the United States when the *Voice of America* assignment ended, Grace produced some excellent journalism. Between 1947 and 1950 she received recognition from audiences she had seldom connected with before—the academic and political communities.

In 1948 *The Saturday Evening Post* published Grace's article "Why Don't We Tell Europe Our Story?" The piece exposed the anti-American bias that flourished in postwar Europe and criticized the lack of information disseminated there about American generosity in rebuilding Europe. The *Post* story drew favorable response from Washington, D.C., including letters from Senator Homer Capehart (R-Indiana) and Assistant Secretary of State George V. Allen. Dozens of readers in Europe and the United States sent fan mail. *Reader's Digest* reprinted her story. Alice O'Brien wrote: "I am glad you are working again. You are never quite right without it."[11]

An American psychiatrist, reading Flandrau's story in *Reader's Digest*, wrote her about bias in human nature. Commenting on the difficulty of changing people's minds, he wrote: "They cling to beliefs even if they are proved wrong." That insight into human intransigence undoubtedly consoled Grace when she contemplated long-entrenched bias toward herself.[12]

Although Flandrau's late journalism never gained the broad public attention her fiction had attracted in the two decades between World War I and World War II, those who followed her career did not withhold recognition. In 1947 Grace received an honorary doctorate in literature from Hamline University. That same year she made a speech in Chicago about the impact of Midwestern writers on American letters and attained listing in the 1947 edition of *Who's Who in the Central States*, published in Chicago. In 1947 the Cum Laude Society of the Avon Old Farms School for Boys also made Grace a member "in recognition of meritorious attainments." In 1949 the American Academy of Arts and Sciences elected Flandrau to membership, and she received the Order of Distinguished Americans.

In 1949, Grace's short essay, "Light on Mexico," appeared in the *Yale Review*. It commented on Herbert Cerwin's book *These Are the Mexicans*. In spring 1949 Grace's comprehensive article, "On What it is to be French," appeared in the first issue of *American Quarterly*, the prestigious new review of the University of Minnesota Press. Grace had admirers among the University of Minnesota faculty, among them Richard Elliott, chairman of the French Department.

In September 1950 John T. Flanagan, a former University of Minnesota professor of American literature and a literary scholar, contributed an article called "Thirty Years of Minnesota Fiction" to *Minnesota History*. He wrote:

> Minnesota writers have produced a surprising amount of fiction of sound merit. From 1920 . . . to 1949 probably a hundred novels with Minnesota locales have appeared in the form of detective stories, satires, realistic portrayals of manners, and historical fiction. The successful authors of the period between wars—figures like Grace Flandrau, Darrah Aldrich, Margaret Culkin Banning, Martha Ostenso, James Gray, Maud Hart Lovelace, and William J. McNally—have been reinforced by such recent aspirants to literary fame as Ann Chidester, Mabel Seeley, Norman Katkov, Herbert Krause, and Neil Boardman.

Of F. Scott Fitzgerald, Flanagan wrote: "Serious effort has recently been made to rehabilitate Fitzgerald's fame; still there seems to be small reason for disturbing his position as a clever and bright chronicler of an age which most people are quite willing to let die."

Public recognition highlighted the loneliness of Grace's private life. By the mid-1940s, as she became increasingly detached from Minnesota, Flandrau gave up her newspaper column as well as her radio show. After 1945 she spent more time at the Gundy than she did at the old family manse in St. Paul. Because she did most of her writing for publication in Connecticut, few Minnesotans apparently read her occasionally published new work or knew of the honors she received. By 1950 Grace Flandrau was a forgotten writer in her own hometown.

She felt isolated in Farmington too and began to wonder if the Riddles' friends and neighbors had accepted her only because of them. In winter the inevitable respiratory infections—antibiotics notwithstanding—aggravated her isolation. Both her residences were in northern climates, and Grace realized she should have followed a fixed pattern of annual retreat to just one sunny place in cold weather. She had always traveled on impulse, frequently alone. Now she was much less adventurous.

After meeting his intriguing relative, Jack Greenway began extending annual invitations to her to visit him and other Flandrau relatives in Arizona, and from 1947 on Grace made short visits to Tucson every winter. But pride made her hesitate to accept Jack's hospitality too readily: she had a congenital dread of imposing on people. And Jack's mother, Isabella Greenway King, who was exactly Grace's age, had never encouraged intimacy. "They were very different," Greenway explained. (Isabella died in 1953. Greenway's grandmother, Patty Flandrau Selmes, had died in 1923, and her sister, Sally Flandrau Cutcheon, died in 1947, before Grace began visiting Arizona.)

By the close of the decade, Grace was finding it difficult to make decisions and her anxiety about the future mounted. When she recognized that a gnawing sense of despair was becoming her daily companion, she began fearing for her sanity. She considered seeing a psychiatrist.

In mid-1947 Grace wrote Ted Steele about her illness, sharing her fears. Steele cared enough to give her his full attention. He wrote: "I do think, after all these years of Arizona and the desert in California, that I know something about bronchitis. Also, it's often been said of me that I have uncanny insight into other peoples' difficulties though none whatsoever about my own. Bronchial asthma is one of the aliments with a psychosomatic link, all the allergic things are, but as for straight bronchitis—it's my right as a member of the partially informed laity to doubt it."

Steele made a strong argument against Grace's seeking psychiatry:

I fear a psychiatrist for you, though not for the same reasons as I do for myself. Widows with plenty of money are the psychiatrists' heaven! I don't mean by that that they are all charlatans, far from it, but just take a squint at it from the common-sense viewpoint. They can only accept a limited number of patients, all of whom are charged from five to twenty-five and thirty dollars an hour, according to their incomes. So it's pretty safe to assume that the psychiatrist angles for (and clings to once he has hooked her) the cultivated, intelligent woman of means—who can afford to go on for two or three years of treatment, never boring the doctor nor giving him guilty feelings that she is being impoverished.[13]

But Kay Boyle urged Grace to seek counseling. She recommended California therapist John Becket, who, she felt sure, could "heal" Grace's spirit. Boyle alternately urged, begged, and challenged Grace to resume professional writing and scolded her for not writing. Eventually a heated exchange between the two old friends took place over the telephone. Alarmed, Boyle wrote Grace: "You are in the grip of some very sick destructive thing—for only that could have made you say the cruel, untrue things last night when I called you full of anxious tenderness because I thought you must be very ill and trying to spare me. I wish I could be with you. I <u>know</u> I could help get you back into the sun, out of this terrible miasma."[14]

One can only guess at the cause of Grace's outburst. Likely, after years of playing Lady Bountiful to Boyle's large family, disguising sorrow over her own childlessness and envy, Grace's restraint gave way to anger. The news that Boyle had just received a special award for her writing, initiated by Maxwell E. Perkins, would have been a bitter pill for Flandrau.

There is no evidence that Grace sought psychiatric care at this point in her life although she was no stranger to the profession. In addition to clinical therapy at Purinton Inn (now the Austin Riggs Institute) in 1918 she had received counseling from Carl Jung in Paris in 1927 and, evidently, from a St. Paul doctor—Dr. Gordon Kamman—after Blair's death. Now, however, she couldn't seem to rise above the profound melancholia overtaking her life. Knowing she needed faith, Grace wrote Ted Steele: "I am almost desperately in search of what will feed my heart."[15]

CHAPTER XVII

Confronting the Demons

*"There is, I suppose, in almost everyone, a bird of
prey, fed a little by the blood of another's heart."
Grace Flandrau to Alice M. O'Brien, early 1950s*

DEPRESSION IMMOBILIZED GRACE BY 1950. She had no interest in work,
in seeing people, in traveling. Poor health often confined her to her bedroom.
Paralyzing indecision over how and where to spend the rest of her days and
irrational, obsessive worry about money—the Flandrau estate was worth
$1,150,000 in 1951—continued to fuel her anxiety. Perhaps she learned of
Anna Hodson's death in 1950 in Minneapolis and grieved over never having
known her mother.[1]

Several interrelated issues seemed insoluble. In addition to the age of both
her houses and the cost of their maintenance was the question of where she
really wanted to live. She wondered if anyone besides herself cared where she
lived? Terror and loneliness forced Grace to confront long-repressed conflicts
in her personality—her neurosis, whatever it was—that had made all her relationships difficult and had brought her to immobility and a feeling of stark
isolation.

In her mid-sixties—for the second time—Grace became her own analyst.
Between 1950 and 1955, her worst period of melancholia, she conducted and
recorded a searching self-inquisition, this time not in a private journal but
in correspondence with a few close friends—Ted Steele, Alice O'Brien, Jack
Greenway, Kay Boyle, and Dick Myers. Focusing her curiosity and passion for
truth on herself, Grace created a brutally honest record of her shortcomings
and her journey from neurosis to health. With the compassionate response of
her correspondents, she slowly gained self-acceptance and faith.

Grace knew she was lucky to have friends with whom to share her emotional
burdens—she often apologized to them in her letters—and those she turned
to did not fail her. Understanding her urgent need, they responded with
wisdom and affection. What she heard wasn't always flattering.

The first alarming truth Grace had to face was that work—the antidote to depression that had never failed her—was failing her now. She wrote Ted Steele:

> <u>Not working</u> is the real reason, trouble, basis for all else. BUT—alas, there comes a time, if one leaves it too long, and permits oneself to sink too low in spirits, abuses and neglects and tortures one's real self or soul too long—then work cannot function as a therapeutic agent. It's as if a person were wilting from lack of exercise, but if he leaves it too long, his muscles so deteriorate he can't make them perform their restorative act.
>
> That is not a good simile. This is more like it: writing even a slight essay, reminiscence, article, is not a detached function. It cannot be entirely an act of will. While there is still enough libido, zest, vitality available to carry on after one has willed oneself to the desk, that's fine. But one must not have exhausted one's store of these in futility—because, much as one may <u>will</u> oneself to the typewriter, or, let us say, to the pump handle, it's no good if the well is dry or the water cemented over, or perhaps drained to an inaccessible level.
>
> And yet, if life turned up a sudden trump—say, a great conversion, a breaking through to a new quality of hope and faith and sense of rapture, then I am quite sure that something at least could be salvaged. Such of the water as had not disappeared altogether, but merely receded to a more remote level, would be reached, and would bring the green again to one's fancy and imagination.[2]

Vacillating views about her residences continued to torment her, but now she couldn't make decisions about even the smallest matters. Ted invited her to meet him and his wife in Venice in summer 1950, but Grace confessed she couldn't face the effort to make the trip. She thought she had discovered too late what people need most in their lives and wrote Steele:

> Old [Charles-Augustin] Saint-Beuve said that all we want, in the end, is to understand. But I think he said that in his study, in some old, time-mellowed chateau, filled with associations of a long life.
>
> Living a long established pattern in which [there] is the deep reassurance of <u>habit</u> [is] so essential, I think, to age and to the possibility of peaceful reflectiveness, a settled, peaceful way of life when one has made up the accounts, closed the books, given oneself final surcease from uncertainties,

indecisions and change. I think the factor which fills the hospitals of the USA with nervous breakdowns is the everlasting pulling up of roots.[3]

At the urging of Jack Greenway, about 1950 Grace began renting a series of houses in Tucson in winter. Each was close to the Arizona Inn, the charming, historic, adobe-style hotel owned and managed by Greenway and his mother, Isabella Greenway King. This new residential option, however, only added to Grace's confusion about where to develop one permanent "strategic base" for her old age. Writing Steele again, Grace revealed dread of oncoming old age:

[I am undergoing] at first faintly, faintly, then with accelerating pace and scope, what I think is the real change of life.... In the earlier stages one forgets it often and for long periods. But steadily and with long strides it advances upon one. That is the realization that what happens to all human beings happens to you.

And if you have lived your life blindly, wastefully, narcissistically and with the stupidity possible only to clever people, then the final, crashing realization that one is no longer and never again will be a young, or youngish person, that the vague something one promised oneself to be or to accomplish, one has <u>not</u> become or in all likelihood ever will accomplish—that what is left is to reap what one has sewn, is simply Man's Fate, The Way of All Flesh et al . . . then the going is really bad, at least for a time. At least and until and <u>if</u> one can stretch out one's hand to the final gifts and be worthy of receiving them—courage and resignation.

In the meantime, it is an appallingly alienating state of mind. It separates one from one's friends, not to speak of one's mere acquaintances; it makes one fit only for the very thing one dreads most—aloneness.[4]

Kay Boyle continued to show concern. Their correspondence in August 1950 reveals that Grace, heeding Boyle's advice, got in touch with West Coast therapist John Becket. Becket gave Boyle his assessment: "She [Grace] feels separated from everything. Perhaps has cut herself off without wanting to."[5]

A year later, still discussing Grace's illness, Boyle responded to Grace's admission that she was "dying from the lack of being useful." Boyle advised her to read Dostoevsky's letters to his wife. "You must love and serve," wrote Boyle.[6]

Boyle's letters to Grace, which continued into the late 1950s, deal with Kay's career, her family's need for money, her blacklisting by publishers, and concern that her left-wing views as well as her morals were being investigated. She persisted in urging Grace to write. In one particularly outspoken letter, Boyle admonished: "I know that the melancholy—which is nothing more than self-love—is consumingly present, to be defeated anew every day."[7]

Grace's understanding grew that all her life she had suffered from a bifurcated personality, one side of which had never been allowed to develop—the personal, real self. She said as much to Alice O'Brien in the early 1950s:

> Darling Moon: I'm going to try to set down something of what's going on in my poor head, because when I'm with you I get simply tongue-tied. Because then, it's not the immediate problems or impasses that keep surging up, but the whole of what I have at last come to see—the blind, shallow, lost, misguided way I have lived my life.
>
> And worse yet, the many and complicated reasons, beginning when I was a little, spoiled girl, going through all the vagueness and insecurity of my growing up, my total lack of education or family training or example or anything—and to make you see, which I have a feeling you do not believe, that <u>I was not that way by nature</u>; the very fact that I have always been so scared and puzzled and rebellious but ignorantly rebellious, striking out at random and with no idea what to do to find, to express and to live, <u>ME</u>, that would give a chance to develop and produce an unknown entity <u>who existed</u>—that other, the real, the total human being I instinctively knew and definitely believe in, who never had a chance; who never came, so to speak, out of the crysallis.
>
> It's that which I always want [to tell you], at the risk, oh, god don't I know, of, in Blair's elegant phrase, "boring you pea~less." Also, I know I've said it to you too many times. So that you know it but only in that not very real intellectual way I know it.

pee·less

The retarded development of her real self as opposed to her public self, Grace now saw, had resulted in "separation from others." She wrote O'Brien: "I have connected with nothing and nobody in any practical everyday sense." Her confession to Alice continued:

> It's only when I am near you that I feel really safe, or let us say, approximately safe. That I have more confidence in the person I was, that is, the <u>best</u> person, because <u>long</u> before then, the other half had got lost or rather,

still remained a feeble shoot two inches high instead of a grown up plant. My whole life has been a blind effort to see it and find it and make it a part of me.

The endless struggle between her two selves, Grace went on, was "the real conflict. Between the longing, the awful <u>need</u> of a perpetual personal god or mother, and the strange wonderful need of a human being to find his or her <u>own</u> strength and reality and soul—even if it seems horribly hopeless, if it comes maybe too late to be effectuated . . . This necessary, useless, painful but somehow reassuring struggle goes on."

Grace admitted that her problems had always stemmed from her difficulty with relationships, but she believed her judgment of each person, apart from herself, had generally been right. She also recognized that she had had a delayed adolescence, manifested in her inability to come to grips with reality and her continuous escape into fantasy. Now, at last, she wrote, she had fully realized her aloneness.

When Grace's self-analysis returned to her current question—what house or houses she should live in and where—she confessed that she had long avoided admitting she was growing old and had put off planning for it. She remembered Alice warning her she must plan for the future right after Blair's death, when she still resided at 385 Pleasant. Grace wrote: "You might as well have talked sanscrit, as it was not possible for me to believe I was getting older, or ever would."

Charlie's will specifying that the Flandrau home be demolished when no family member wished to occupy it further complicated her decision. To raze the residence meant destroying much of the property's value. And the house was so old now that it needed extensive renovation to be livable. Grace viewed either option as a major capital loss. The Gundy house—a house she didn't even own—also badly needed repair and remodeling. The aged kitchen required considerable overhaul just so Mary O'Malley could use it, and a new bathroom downstairs was imperative.

Grace's turmoil continued, unresolved, over many months. She wrote O'Brien again about the unending circle of interdependent, put-off decisions: "As I told you, any new move, any new undertaking, any <u>plan</u> about houses simply throws me in a kind of mental tailspin at the mere thought. It is no longer a question of . . . self-discipline—there was a time for that, God knows, and it was never applied. Now, for the moment, it has gone past."

Grace was convinced that she had taken many wrong turns in her life. She continued her letter in an almost desperate tone:

> The frustration, emptiness, melancholia which have been accumulating for years are at the moment at a strictly pathological point. Included in all this is the terrible realization that I, who so desperately need roots, have pulled them up everywhere. Never made any definite arrangements in Tucson, have spent relatively little time here [in Farmington] in the past years, and have with a queer unwillingness severed myself from Minnesota over a long period of time.

She thought her loss of joy in life began when she and Blair left 548 Portland Avenue just before his death. She felt she had made so many mistakes since then she could no longer trust her own judgment:

> As I told you the other day, the sudden realization of my bad judgment terrifies me. How can I believe in whatever decision I do make . . . ? And the time now is short. I must take the right turnings soon, or I shall be too discouraged to act at all. What is the right way to plan for the next 10 to 15 years? How to find some way of dignity and moderate contentment and enrichment inside, to say nothing of perhaps, still, even a little productivity?[8]

O'Brien's patience ran out. She wrote Grace:

> Why does it [your indecision] have to go on until it kills you? Here's what I think. It's folly to do Farmington and Tucson. I certainly would drop Farmington just where it is. I would rent a Tucson house for the winter and buy a Tucson or St. Paul house next spring. There are many reasons for living in Tucson, but, as always, I feel there are many more for living in St. Paul. I can't feel that you will ever feel 'at home' any place else.[9]

Grace admitted to O'Brien that a growing realization of unfriendliness toward her in St. Paul was causing her to doubt the wisdom of maintaining a residence there:

> But lately, and it has really existed perhaps for longer than I realize . . . and

it has had a lot to do with my hesitancy in coming back to St. Paul—I have had a growing feeling that somebody, or some small group . . . is not friendly. . . . I have a feeling of malice—a genuine malice and hostility, directed against me!!! an active enmity . . . it's a little like going to sleep (even if it was for 67 years) in what you thought was a garden of pansies and buttercups, and waking up in a jungle with teeth and fangs showing through the foliage.[10]

Jack Greenway affirmed in a 1991 interview (twenty years after Grace's death) that Grace's loss of status and credibility in St. Paul probably began in the 1930s as awareness of her illegitimacy spread. Other younger associates, Kate Klein, Meridel Le Sueur, and James Gray, years after Flandrau's death, described her fall from grace or gave reasons for it. Klein declared: "We all thought of her [Flandrau] as kind of a joke" and "she wasn't a good writer."[11]

Klein, however, whom author interviewed several times between 1985 and 1992, admitted she hadn't read much of her late friend's work. She changed her mind about Grace's writing, however, after reading *Memoirs of Grace Flandrau*, a recently published example of the author's fully developed prose style, drafted for but never submitted to Charles Scribner's Sons in the late 1930s. About her previous misperception Klein said: "I'm sorry, Georgie."[11]

The late Meridel Le Sueur commented to the author in 1993: "She [Grace] came from a common background, you know. She didn't belong with all those high society people up on Summit Avenue." Le Sueur, however, also admitted that Flandrau refused to receive her when Meridel contacted her in Tucson in the 1950s and added this illuminating comment: "She [Grace] had a young one in Arizona, you know."[12] Le Sueur's remark, which referred to Jack Greenway without knowing him or understanding his relationship to Grace and Blair, reveals profound misjudgment and the unbridgeable distance between two uncopasetic women who no longer had anything in common.

When interviewed by Charles M. Flandrau's biographer in 1979, eight years after her death, the late James Gray described Grace as "morally tawdry."[13] Whether he was expressing Charles Flandrau's views posthumously as well as his own is unknown. In author's opinion, however, given Grace's enduring friendships in middle age with women like Katherine K. Shepard (Mrs. Roger B.), Anne White (Mrs. Edwin), Mary L. Griggs (Mrs. Theodore), Frances Daniels (Mrs. Thomas L.), Alice O'Brien, Jerusha (Juty) Pillsbury (Mrs. John S.), Bernice Dalrymple (Mrs. John), and Corrinne Roosevelt Alsop (Mrs.

Joseph)—highly regarded women of St. Paul, Minneapolis, Manhattan, and Farmington—it is hard to accept Gray's description of the mature Grace Flandrau as anything but distortion due to personal prejudice.

The words "morally tawdry" sound like the idiom of Charles Flandrau and probably pertain to Grace's immature affair in Mexico about which the whole family knew, as she recorded in an unpublished story.[14] One can assume that as a sophisticated product of the Jazz Age the youthful Grace Flandrau had been liberated and "experienced," and we know that by her own admission she had "three affairs" in the course of her marriage. That record, however, doesn't begin to duplicate the behavior of the young Edna St. Vincent Millay, Brenda Ueland or Meridel Le Seuer in the same era.

What posterity really wants to know is: was Grace Flandrau a significant writer? Apparently, literary scholars in Minnesota, who were her contemporaries, thought she was. It also appears, however, that literary rivals generalized from the particular—i.e. Grace's hints of incest in *Indeed This Flesh*, her illegitimacy, and her youthful affair in Mexico—to discredit not only her moral reputation but to diminish her literary achievement. If their bias went that far it was just as silly as asserting that Johannes Brahms couldn't have been a good composer because his mother was a prostitute and he was born in a brothel.

Nevertheless, it also appears that the good will of a wider circle of her St. Paul acquaintances toward Grace gradually eroded as she aged and her literary accomplishments were forgotten. Long-concealed resentment against the high-living flapper who once satirized St. Paulites in her novels undoubtedly reared its head. Like Zelda Fitzgerald, Flandrau had seemed to be the antithesis of conventional, maternal womanhood, not a propitious image in the conservative Midwest. Compounding that stigma, general awareness of Grace's "anomalous" childhood broadened, providing the climate in which harsh assessments take root and flourish. To her discreditors it also seemed increasingly unforgivable that Grace inherited the entire Flandrau fortune, the St. Paul house, and life tenancy in a house in Connecticut as well. To some that unexpected windfall apparently was reason enough for put-down.

In the 1950s Alice O'Brien continued urging her old friend to return to St. Paul, but one too-hasty decision by Grace complicated things further. In 1952 she first rented and then suddenly purchased a stately white stucco home at 470 Summit Avenue, planning to move into it permanently.[15] Then, hesitant to leave Farmington, she lost interest. And she still hadn't come to a decision about the empty Flandrau house. Grace's catharsis–via–letter continued. She wrote O'Brien:

> Although so totally alone, I nevertheless dread, now, seeing people, espe-
> cially people I've not seen for some time. I dread seeing anybody in St.
> Paul but you. I dread having anyone say how she's changed, how badly she
> looks and seems. [By the early 1950s Grace had gained an uncharacteristic
> and unbecoming amount of weight.] Nor have I anything of interest to
> give or receive while this paramount question of where to live and how
> and for what reason is so hideously uppermost.

Grace confessed that she had finally become aware of her vulnerability. She admitted to O'Brien that she had:

> . . . a fear I never felt before, of people. A fear that one is so vulnerable,
> so far from safe. That any moment someone can turn and tear your very
> heart out for a whim, a misunderstanding, a delight in cruelty or what
> have you.
>
> It is of course the exact reverse of what I felt before . . . that the attitude
> toward me [in St. Paul] was primarily one of unawareness or else a very
> mild good will. I didn't think everybody was filled with sweetness and
> light, or that there might not be someone here and there who actively
> disliked me and whom I had given a reason to do so. But of ill will per se,
> or of being misjudged, of being criticized for all the wrong reasons, instead
> of the right ones . . . well, all that has been so new to me and come so late,
> I haven't dealt with it very well.

Flandrau's admission of feeling victimized evidently provoked a stern retort from O'Brien, but the letter or letters in which she scolded Grace no longer exist. Flandrau's shocked response, however, reveals that O'Brien must have leveled with her, evidently telling her that, for one thing, she faced criticism in St. Paul because people viewed her as a hyper-materialistic snob—or words to that effect. Grace replied heatedly:

> I have had only one criterion for people (aside from the trivial, escap-
> ist relationships)—and that was the extent, well, to use a big, inadequate
> word—[of their] "cosmic" understanding. Which of course, includes the

aesthetic, whether in poetry or what have you, in the arts. Aside from that I had no standard and not much interest. That was the yardstick.

Interestingly too, it can be several things—intellectual, aesthetic, or, as in the case of Martha Breasted [Jack Greenway's sister] ... purely of the heart. A kind of saint-like loving-kindness. Not sappy, not lacking in discrimination, but with a gift of love that transcended everything else.

You can imagine then, Alice, what I felt when you, YOU could believe that I, that I—was only interested in the size of a Cadillac and the price of [St. Paul] Fire and Marine! You could never have thought that up on your own. You, like many artists, are suggestible.

Well, all this is complicated and neither here nor there. There is NO clear answer to human beings, nobody is the kind of person I have found it so easy to transform them into, a kind of benevolent super being, a kind of angel. ... Universal Mother or Deity to whom nothing need be shown or demonstrated, who would just go on believing, caring ... No matter how you persisted in showing him or her or them only your weakness, [you were] sure they would see what lay beneath. ... There is, I suppose, in almost everyone, a bird of prey, fed a little by the blood of another's heart.[16]

Clearly, Grace Flandrau was experiencing the archetypal wounds of "affliction" suffered by other ambitious, achieving women who have "fallen from grace," e.g., Sylvia Plath and Simone Weil, as described and quoted in Patricia Hampl's penetrating essay, "The Smile of Accomplishment," in *I Could Tell You Stories*.[17] It is the special agony of such "afflicted" women that the causes of their pain are often unrecognized and denied by others. Thus the outcasts must not only bear their suffering alone but, if their complaints continue, they are apt to be labeled "emotionally disturbed." That was Grace Flandrau's fate in St. Paul.[18] Hampl writes: "Social degradation is such an essential component of affliction because in a curious way it virtually ostracizes the victim while paradoxically casting her into a glaring public light. When the social degradation is caused by sexual humiliation, the pain is heightened." [Nothing is said about *imagined* sexual transgression.]

Simone Weil's phrase, "Affliction is essentially a destruction of personality, a lapse into anonymity," describes Flandrau's fate as her once-lustrous literary reputation evaporated within a decade. Another Simone Weil quote succinctly characterizes Flandrau's life story and explains her decision to retreat from

Minnesota: "Affliction is a pulverization of the soul by the mechanical brutality of circumstances."[19]

To illustrate the hazards of ambition for women, Sylvia Plath is quoted: "Being born a woman is my tragedy." Hampl adds: "That is, a tragedy for her ambition."[20]

Brenda Ueland and Kay Boyle are further examples of ambitious women who suffered rejection and misunderstanding. Ueland's and Boyle's words of sympathy and advice to Flandrau in earlier chapters of this biography reveal their understanding (and Grace's) that she needed to forget the self and to serve. In 1939 Ueland wrote to Grace: "I don't want to be hard on the self. But it has to go, as one grows up."[21]

Half a century later, Patricia Hampl echoed Ueland's advice. Labeling the egotistical self "the autobiographical self," Hampl writes: "[P]ain is a fact, and the autobiographical self is firm about pain: It is bad. Or at least, it is too bad. The autobiographical self, after all is no fool: It knows who must do the dying."[22]

Grace closed her letter to Alice with an admission of her dependence on O'Brien's friendship and her fear that she might have lost even that.

> Oh, Alice, as I re-read this, I horribly ask myself, is this too an illusion like all the rest? Is this the last stubborn fantasy I must give up? Am I wrong to feel that there is an altogether different dimension in which some few friends sometimes can meet? Do I mistake you? Am I still not awake? Does the full stature of reality still elude me? Am I simply a trial and an object of incomprehensible confusion even to you? Is that the objective reality out in the objective world? And is that the real one?[23]

O'Brien sent her old friend a comforting response. She couldn't have failed to remember how their African journey in 1927 had boosted Grace's morale. After her scolding, O'Brien proposed that they visit France together.

The O'Brien-Flandrau journey to France in the summer of 1953 allowed Alice to return to Verdun, where she had served as a Red Cross nurse in World War I, and Grace to revisit her old haunts in Paris. Thomond (Tomy) and Terence (Terry) O'Brien, Alice's eighteen-year-old twin nephews, chauffeured the two women in a Packard touring car purchased by their aunt and shipped to France. Judy O'Brien Wilcox, Alice's niece, and her husband, Richard, newlyweds in their twenties, joined the excursion.

No one could have understood better than O'Brien how the companionship of young people would nourish the heart of an aging widow who had neither children nor grandchildren. That summer's journey, described by Thomond O'Brien as "a hilarious adventure from start to finish," was just the tonic Grace needed. According to Thomond, Grace had everyone—her companions, waiters, maids, gendarmes, maître d's, concièrges—in stitches all day long:

> Grace had this act—half real, half concocted—of being helpless, and she was terrified by the French traffic. From the moment our Packard rolled onto French soil, Grace was constantly warning us that "the French have never learned to drive" and that they were "tous assassins." [Fr."All assas- sins."] After a few days of Terry's and my maneuvering through whirling, swerving masses of bicycles, motor carts, pedestrians and cars we heard Grace muttering in the back seat, "Nous sommes tous assassins." ("We are all assassins.") She kept telling us that if we had an accident she would refuse to be taken by ambulance to a French hospital, because too many times she had seen the doors of speeding French ambulances fly open and bodies come flying out.

Like many Flandrau friends, Thomond remembered that, because Grace was frequently chilly, she always wore a scarf or boa or fur thrown around her shoulders. Then, after dramatically throwing off scarf, boa, or fur in some restaurant or theater, she inevitably left it behind. "There was non-stop excite- ment, comedy, and confusion wherever we went, but we adored her."[24]

Many Flandrau friends recall Grace's special chemistry with the young. Among them was the late art collector, David Daniels, of New York City (son of the late Tom and Frances Daniels of St. Paul): "She [Grace] used to take me to the St. Paul Hotel on Sunday nights for chicken sandwiches if my parents were out of town. I adored her." Other interviewees made the same observa- tion, among them Saranne Neumann, stepsister of Jack Greenway.[25]

Alice O'Brien reaffirmed her affection for Grace in a note after their return from France. "Every time we are able to spend a nice time together we deepen and strengthen that extraordinary bond between us."[26]

Grace responded with a tribute to the power of love and friendship. Although still undecided about her future, she could at least discuss her persisting dilemmas with her old sense of humor:

Oh, Tude, your lovely letter came yesterday and was a burst of light and warmth in my very heart of hearts. I sit here still agonizing over the house situation in Minnesota, believe it or not. It's abject, it's shocking, it's everything you like, but there it is. I can think of nothing, do nothing, till I settle that at least. It is now two o'clock in the afternoon, and the minute I end this, I shall go to the telephone, send a wire saying: "Tear it [the Flandrau house] down. This is final." or; "Roof and repair and paint and wait till spring for me." And I don't know yet which it will be.

Here in Farmington I feel indifferent and detached. Have seen a few old friends . . . The sink is clogged and the bathroom won't work, and Mary's (Mary O'Malley's) feelings about LIFE are mixed.

About their friendship Grace wrote:

I clung all day yesterday and last night, digging in with all my ten fingers and winding my two legs around the <u>reality</u> of it—of your letter, of you. Oh, Alice, I've loved you in so many ways and never quite so well, so widely, so deeply, with so much understanding and thought and vision as now, or ever could if I hadn't been so down, so far down in the black depths.

My god, there may be something in it all, in what we pretend to believe and think we believe and maybe don't actually believe until this does happen, namely that pain is not all lost and that thus 'comes wisdom to us by the awful Grace of God.' And the Grace of God is surely in friendship—in love—because they are one, and it's a benediction and a glow and it's manna to the hungry and the poor as I so terribly feel myself to be—except for that.

I've written you dozens of letters in my mind, but what I really meant to do and didn't was send you . . . a little volume of the Portuguese Sonnets because they say it all and for all <u>kinds</u> of love which are all one. "How do I love you, let me count the ways."

Of course . . . some of them are specifically love of a woman for a man, but it's only superficial really, and what doesn't show above the surface, all the base and volume of it, is that wonderful and mysterious grace of tenderness and affection and dear love for a dear friend once or twice in a whole life it is one's great good fortune and blessing to feel and to receive. It's a grace you have known how to bestow more than any person I ever knew . . . I wish I could do this other <u>kind</u> of giving . . . write about it, I mean, in a way that would make it real to people, so they would open their hearts to it, be ready for it if it came. I have the feeling the chance of it doesn't come very often to many people in this day and age, or this country maybe.

Blair could give it, you know, way down below the physical differences between men and women, down where people are just people, just two human beings . . . he could give that grace of tenderness and truth. Like you, Alice.[27]

CHAPTER XVIII

Catharsis

"Do take care, dearest Aunt-o, because you are the somewhat casual
custodian of so much that others find so precious in you."
John S. Greenway to Grace Flandrau

AFTER SHE RETURNED TO FARMINGTON and solitude Grace resumed the
former pattern of her life. Although her depression continued, the journey to
France had demonstrated she could still enjoy life. She never again sank as far
into immobilizing despondency as she had in the late 1940s and early 1950s.

Besides O'Brien's reaffirmed friendship, Grace now had growing intimacy
with Blair's kin in Tucson to look forward to every winter. Greenway and two
generations of Flandrau relatives in Arizona corresponded with her when she
was alone in Farmington. Sometimes they visited her in Connecticut too.
Grace's recovery was underway but there were terrifying setbacks.[1]

By 1954, although she had been renting houses in Tucson every winter
for four years, Grace still hadn't made up her mind about her St. Paul and
Farmington homes. Her indecision became almost pathological when she
grew interested in buying a Tucson residence too.

Whenever Grace showed curiosity about Tucson real estate Greenway and
his family made arrangements for showing her properties. After she became
enthusiastic about a Tucson house, however, a young First Trust Company
officer in St. Paul, familiar with her affairs, advised her she couldn't afford it.
He had concluded her judgment about such matters couldn't be trusted. He
also discovered that Grace knew little about her financial affairs, that she didn't
know her tax bracket, and that she was unaware of a First Trust Company
checking account as well as a First National Bank checking account.[1]

The trust officer's opinion drastically undermined Flandrau's self-confidence. Now guilt was added to angst about houses and locales. She was morti-
fied that she had uselessly enlisted Jack's and his sister Martha's help in seeking
a home in Arizona. Grace wrote Greenway:

Jack, it was this blackness which rises up and says, how can you make
a life anywhere that matters a damn, it's too late, too late.... Due to my

own frivolity, no, confusion, blindness, timidities, super-sensitiveness, god knows what, infantilism is a more comprehensive term, I have NEVER known how to live life, but always . . . run away, escaped, hidden or tried to, my <u>real</u> feelings, my need to do for others and to care and be cared for and so on.

It is as painful and boring to me to talk about it as it is for you to hear it. I'm not asking you to understand, because I don't understand myself. But, feel so the ultimate difficulty, Jack, dear, is not the indecisiveness, it is the downright Godawful melancholia that is pouring over me and scaring me to death. It has got much worse in the last few weeks. . . . A kind of what's the use . . . or why should I live another minute . . . and not only why should I but <u>How</u> <u>can</u> <u>I</u>?

When Flandrau wrote that letter, she had just come to Tucson from St. Paul. She evidently had gone to Minnesota to make a decision about the Flandrau house. During her stay alone at the Lowry Hotel, fear engulfed her. Again she was unable to reach a decision. Grace confessed to Jack that her confusion in St. Paul had made her dread coming to Tucson where she would be shown more housing options:

As the days passed . . . I began to realize that I ought not to risk coming here [Tucson], bringing such a thing even to a small degree into yours and Martha's lives. Hanging such an albatross . . . about your blessed necks. I knew I had gone beyond the place where I could really participate in things with normal people. That the effort would be too great and also too unsuccessful. . . . I felt deeply—and now I'm afraid I was right—that I had nothing left. . . . I had just about enough force left to creep into the cottage [Gundy] and pull up the drawbridge and rest from every effort.

Then she confessed the heart of her pain:

Oh, Jack . . . I see how mad and awful it is and I am helpless. And back of it all is something so simple—just sadness . . . but a sadness so great that it paralyses the will . . . a terrible homesickness for the kind of normal giving and receiving of affection I had never had since I was twelve, a home in the deep sense, for the kind of normal give and take of friendships and love [that] my life, mixed up as it was with older and stronger people, even my life with Blair, hadn't provided. . . . What makes it impossible to act is that to act . . . one must feel that it is what one longs for, the ultimate and profound thing one must have in order to go on.[2]

Grace finally admitted what she hungered for, risked asking for it, and used sound judgment in addressing the person from whom she might receive life-giving help. Jack Greenway's empathetic response to Grace's longing for reconnection to family life undoubtedly provided the safety net she needed. Apparently she hadn't been ready to count on Blair's family for support until she showed them her worst side—how frightened, sad, isolated, needy she felt at times—and found she would still be accepted with open arms. In spite of the age difference of forty years, Jack's interest in Grace as a friend and in her welfare nourished her fragile spirit and undoubtedly extended her life.

With Greenway, Grace could let down her hair about her difficult childhood, her illegitimacy, her estrangement from her relatives, Blair's and Charlie's struggle with alcoholism, and her sense of being misunderstood and criticized in St. Paul "for all the wrong reasons." Jack came to understand that Grace's neurotic concern about money stemmed from the time of her father's bankruptcy in 1893, when his insistence on repaying all his customers had thrown him and his dependents into poverty.[3]

And Jack understood Grace's tendency toward morbid self-recrimination. Once when she sent him an anguished letter, apologizing for transgressions or impositions, real or imagined, Greenway replied: "You do suffer for everybody, expiating sins of complacency for us all. To feel painfully that you are always wrong and forgive everybody without any worldly reason—which you do—makes you one of the few altogether plausible humans in an otherwise implausible world."[4]

Grace responded: "I can think of nothing in the universe, which you are less—than complacent. And I am always right. I am never wrong about people, [despite] the fact that I am always wrong in relationships—I mean in contacts—in the connection with me, a little wrong—you know, hesitant, evasive, shy and so on."[5]

To Jack's inquiries about why she never remarried, Grace replied:

After Blair's death I could of course have married again. But in spite of this sudden deprivation of a person who had been in his quiet, tender . . . way a tower of strength and an unceasingly indulgent friend . . . I could not even consider a new relationship of that kind—not even a totally platonic one. Of course, besides those other qualities I have mentioned, he was so exquisitely a gentleman in the rarest and best meaning of the term. . . . So that a close companionship with anyone less endowed with sensibilities and delicacies and utter amenity and—oddly too, his own very definite panache—(all these make up the meaning of the word "virtue" to me) was unthinkable.

Grace began to understand that her own super sensitivity and habitual hypercriticism of people contributed to her aloneness. She told Jack:

> The thought even of the mildest intimacy with any but the most unusually congenial person is strangely repellent to me. In a much broader sense it even includes my horror of hospitals, of the constant presence of trained nurses. . . . And in spite of the terrifying and new experience of loneliness I can't tell you how often the sense of my door closing behind me, leaving me alone, without the boredom or irritation or inadequacy of unwanted contact, of being safe for a time even from as simple and beneficent [contact] as that of my true Mary O'Malley—or with the many acquaintances with whom no fruitful intimacy is possible or desirable, relieves and . . . restores me. It explains too how little adventurous I am in making new friends. I cannot recall in all my life any instance where the normal, friendly advance was not made by the other.[6]

In Greenway, Grace found her literary soulmate. They often exchanged favorite passages of books and poetry shedding light on two issues that absorbed Grace now: the quality of real friendship and the meaning and purpose of life. From Farmington she wrote Jack:

> Well, you'd be surprised if you knew how often I carry on conversations with you as I somewhat morosely tromp around this old dilapidated cottage. Conversations which would, of course, bore you to death, because the only things that seem to be of real interest to me are the ones to which there isn't any answer. Human nature; human destiny; the why of both.
> Just the same, bored or not, it would interest me to know what, if anything, you think or surmise or wonder at . . . or find most incomprehensible about it all. And what, if any, conclusions you have arrived at. Or

whether, mercifully, you are too young, too able to cope with and carry on activities in the objective world, to bother much.

I would also like to know what poets you like and why. I have been undergoing a kind of return to [Alfred Edward] Housman. I always liked him, certain things, but one never likes more than a few things . . . of any poet. But of his I revel in a few. There is number XXXII of the "Shropshire Lad."

> Could man be drunk forever
> With liquor, love or fights,
> Lief should I rouse at morning
> And lief lie down of nights.
> But men at whiles are sober
> And think by fits and starts,
> And if they think they fasten
> Their hands upon their hearts.

It's funny, in view of the fact that the human dilemma has always seemed to me of impassioning interest, that what people, my friends, anybody, actually <u>does</u>, doesn't interest me much. Only <u>why</u> they do it. And even not that so much as what they think—not especially what they think about what they do, but what they think, period. What their <u>ideas</u> are—provided they are the kind of people whose ideas are the kind of ideas which are worth hearing about.

I am sending you [André] Malraux's *Voice of Silence*. Don't let anybody else give it to you. He and Saint Exupéry represent a way-to-be, an elegance of being I think we rather lack in this country. A kind of blend of intellect, spirit and spirituality . . . a great panache in living. Certainly [Charles A.] Lindbergh has had that.[7]

In her letters to Greenway, Grace often referred to passages from Saint Exupéry, describing the poet's view of the qualities of true friendship. Saying she thought the way people picked each other apart was awful, stupid and destructive, Grace, translating from the French, paraphrased two sentences: "True brothers should have a common aim, one outside themselves, in order to breathe, for experience shows us that to love is not to look <u>at</u> each other but to look together in the same direction. . . . A true friend is he who doesn't judge, for he cannot refuse one part of his friend; he accepts the whole."

Grace worried about Jack's health, his drinking, and the state of his liver, just as she had worried about Blair's. When "Aunto" (Jack's nickname for Grace) worried excessively about his health, Greenway countered with worries about hers. Hearing she was again confined to her bed in Farmington under doctors' care, he wrote: "Do take care, dearest Aunt-o, because you are the somewhat casual custodian of so much that others find so precious in you."[8]

Communication about favorite writers inevitably led to discussions about Grace's writing. During her worst depression Carl Brandt had advised Grace her writing reflected her low spirits too clearly and that she should wait for better days before submitting more. When Grace notified him she felt better and wanted to work again Brandt immediately went into action.

Shortly, New York editor Francis Steegmuller proposed that Grace put together a reminiscence of Charles M. Flandrau for an anthology of his best work. Grace, who had preserved all Charlie's whimsical letters about his travels, had often discussed with Brandt the idea of publishing them. Notifying the University of Minnesota Press, she began working on the anthology.[9]

Eventually, deciding Charlie's subtle essay style was too out of date for modern readers, Grace abandoned the project. Brandt, however, soon found her another challenging assignment, one that brought her out of retirement and nourished her recovery.

In 1954 *Holiday* magazine hired Grace to write a story on Minnesota for its series on the various states. The publisher "didn't want a regulation thing [about] history, industry, economics," Grace wrote Jack from St. Paul, "but a personal, reminiscent, purely impressionistic job. It sounds like an amusing way to go about it, but it means coming right back [to Minnesota] and making a rather extensive tour of the state. I would buy a car here [St. Paul] and get a man to drive me."[10]

Attacking the *Holiday* assignment with her old "libido," Grace toured the state in summer 1954, sometimes traveling by train but mostly chauffeured by Blair Klein, age seventeen, the son of Kate and Horace (Bud) Klein, Jr. Flandrau bought a new green Packard for their junkets. Young Blair remembered being surprised and impressed that Grace didn't want to sit up in front with him, that she always sat in the back seat, writing. He also noted that Grace, who invariably wore an elegant suit and hat and carried a fur on her arm, usually had one or two martinis before dinner and that she retired early to work in her hotel room each night. Because she disdained restaurant peppershakers, she carried her own silver pepper grinder in her purse.[11]

Grace's prose was at its descriptive best in the *Holiday* story, published in August 1955. Three paragraphs summed up the Twin Cities' distinctly different personalities and topography:

> Seventy miles south, also on the Mississippi, we come to Minnesota's urban phenomenon—the Siamese but not identical twin cities of Minneapolis and St. Paul.
>
> St. Paul, which had a few years' start, grew steeply up and down her hills and bluffs along the Mississippi. Minneapolis was born on the high, level plateau across the river with all the vast, empty West as her front yard. At her back were the falls, which stopped navigation, a geographic circumstance that made St. Paul a great transportation center but gave the power of the river to Minneapolis.
>
> The nucleus of population in both cities came from the eastern seaboard. But soon Germans in large numbers settled in St. Paul, as did the gifted, generous, always intensely human and therefore incalculable Irish, while an influx of able, hard-working, hard-headed, forward-looking Swedes made Minneapolis one of the largest Swedish cities in the world.

Response to the *Holiday* article from Minnesota was enthusiastic. Among those who wrote fan letters were Charlotte (Mrs. John Gilman) Ordway, Frances Densmore (a scholar of Indian culture), and Harold Stassen, former Minnesota governor.

Grace wrote Alice O'Brien: "Speaking of Minnesota, nothing has so pleased me as the most wonderful letter from Doodie [Kate S.] Klein about the Minnesota piece! I was so surprised. And of course pleased because she is both hypercritical and extremely honest." Shortly thereafter, Kate Klein brought her college-aged daughter, Kate ("Minty"), to visit Grace, her godmother, at the Arizona Inn.[12]

That year, after publication of the Minnesota story, would have been the obvious time for Grace to return to St. Paul permanently. But she continued waffling between her old hometown and Farmington. A new complication arose. Grace wrote Greenway:

> I don't dare even touch on the house situation, because now a fourth alternative has turned up. The [Frederick K.] Weyerhaeusers have offered me a rare bit of land next to them, with the most superb view of the

valley—land almost impossible now to get, with the suggestion that I build a new house for myself on it. But we won't go into all that. A tiresome and grotesque impasse.[13]

Grace now realized that her incapacity to make decisions about "a strategic base" stemmed from her lifelong flight from intimacy. (All interviewees remarked on Grace's customary silence about personal matters, the walling-off of her real self from others.) She began to feel that all her relationships in Farmington were superficial. In a 1954 letter to O'Brien, she admitted that all her life she had relied totally on such friendships.

[Those superficial friends] had got something... from my excitability, high spirits—no, vivacity is a better word, because there was in that easily aroused vivacity something enlivening, while it lasted, which was while I was stimulated by the fun of talking and eating and being with pleasant people.... Well, I see under and beyond all that. I who have relied so entirely on people no longer get anything from that kind of frivolous contact.... I am terrified, saddened, shocked by the silence and emptiness around the real me, around my heart. I'm not asking for pity or trying to make that sound mournful. I am stating a stark and dreadful truth.

Her confession continued: "The nearest thing to companionship I now get is from poetry.... And it's funny, how you are always with me then. As, indeed, Blair was in the old days on Portland when we read poetry together so often in the evenings.[14]

Grace did have friends in Farmington who cared about her and wanted to see her. By the 1950s she had been first a visitor and then a resident of the lovely old Connecticut town every year for over thirty years. Although she had made acquaintances through the Riddles at first, some had become her own friends. Also, after Theodate's death, Grace served as her personal representative on the Avon Old Farms School board. The other board members counted on her judgment and personal knowledge of Riddle's wishes in running the school.[15]

Among Farmington residents close to Flandrau in the 1950s were Wilmarth Sheldon ("Lefty") Lewis and his wife. Lewis, a former Yale football star, lawyer, and literary scholar, was probably responsible for Grace's work appearing in the *Yale Review*. Lewis possessed an impressive Horace Walpole collection.[16]

Corinne Roosevelt Alsop, wife of columnist Joseph Alsop, and her daughter, Corinne Alsop Robinson, were other Farmington friends. Lefty Lewis and his wife and the Alsops, as well as the John Parsons—he was the Avon school's lawyer—were frequent dinner guests of Grace's and vice versa. Still, being a dinner guest is not being an intimate. Grace described the difference in a letter to Jack Greenway from Farmington in the middle 1950s:

> Well, I'm off to N.Y. tomorrow, I don't know just why. And when I get there I'll think it would be less empty in Farmington, and when I get here I'll think, I must go down to N.Y. and have a change. And a great many things are becoming clear to me, or real to me, that were merely academically known, and hence not known at all. That what is outside is of very little significance compared to what is, or is not, inside.
>
> I had a very gay and charming party last night, only the very few I love, the two darling Lewises, Swans, Parsons—they seemed to have a delightful time. It was the kind of thing, which a year ago would have left me with a great feeling of pleasure and satisfaction, but now? Oh, no. Only the feeling, yes, this is pleasant . . . they were friendly and gay—especially Annie Burr's charming and really beautiful young sister-in-law, Janet Auchincloss—and civilized and nice. [Janet Auchincloss was the mother of Jacquelyn Kennedy Onassis] BUT SO WHAT? It is a frightful thing to mistake the peripheral for the—whatever the opposite is. To mistake the side dishes for the main course, let us say, or the paint on the outside of the house for the hearth, for the love and the warmth and the depth of feeling.[17]

By 1954 or 1955 Grace's depression was lifting. She began making repairs on the Gundy. The board of trustees of the Avon Old Farms School, which, under the terms of Theodate's will, owned the cottage and would handle its sale after Grace's death, gave her permission to make any repairs and interior remodeling she chose . . . at her own expense, Grace ruefully wrote Jack: "I am now having the kitchen modernized, cleaned up and so on, plumbers, sink experts, painters, carpenters—presumably a beginning here, for doing all the rest. And why? Answer me that?"[18]

Well-intended but conflicting views about her future from close friends augmented Grace's confusion. When Greenway notified his brother-in-law, Charles A. Breasted, of Grace's desperate indecision over where she ought to live, Breasted wrote Grace from his hospital bed in New York City. Greenway undoubtedly was aware of Grace's dependence on male attention. Breasted's letter and its advice would have buoyed any woman's spirits:

> Dearest Grace: . . . I think incessantly about your situation and the steps which to this adoring observer seem indicated. I'm persuaded that your execution of the HOLIDAY article broke the insidious 'log jam' which for so long held you a prisoner of indecision. Now you are again the Grace I first knew, and it delights and relieves me beyond words. Only two major 'humps' remain to be conquered: you must delete Gundy Cottage from your future plans; and you must tell your Bank to proceed at once with the razing of 385 Pleasant Avenue. Once you've surmounted these two, I'm sure you won't find it difficult to turn the Summit Avenue house into a congenial 'base' for your hard-won freedom to do a thousand interesting things. And don't forget that we're all going to celebrate this victory together in Tucson.[19]

But another cherished adviser, Dick Myers, had a contradictory view. Grace listened, not only because of their long friendship, but because she respected male advice. Except for Alice O'Brien, Kay Boyle, and Theodate Riddle, Grace rarely turned to women for advice. When she continued bemoaning her quandary, Myers wrote:

> You belittle yourself so flagrantly that I must tell you that you are none of the things you say you are. True, you can't make decisions, except through a struggle—but if I were you, I'd struggle and make them. And once made you'll find you are happier even if they are wrong. And you can always change afterwards. You must sell the house in St. Paul [the Summit Avenue house], more from an economic standpoint than anything else—saves taxes—make the Gundy more habitable and modern for comfort.[20]

Although she continued to struggle with competing views, after 1955 Grace took steps toward reconnecting with the people and places she had known the longest. She wrote Jack Greenway from Farmington: "I feel more at home on what is surely the ugliest, most down-at-the-heels intersection in any city in the world, say—7th and Wabasha in St. Paul, Minn.—than beautiful Main Street here."[21]

When Alice O'Brien wrote: "I still think St. Paul is the place for you," Grace replied: "I am writing Mr. Ahl now to tear down the old house. Haven't been able to before . . . Have decided to open that thing on Summit, but keeping in mind building some place in St. Paul where there is a view."[22] But she also made minor improvements and repairs to the Gundy.

Demolition of the Flandrau house took place in 1955, and for a while Grace seemed convinced she should develop another permanent residence in Minnesota. But again she hesitated, giving up her plan to reside in the elegant house at 470 Summit Avenue and selling it instead.[23]

The sudden necessity of helping Lucile and Ralph Willis most likely stalled Grace's further investment in St. Paul real estate. When she visited the Willises in California just after the demolition of 385 Pleasant, Grace found them both in poor health. Shortly thereafter Ralph died, leaving Lucile almost indigent. Grace established a trust for her sister at First Trust Company in St. Paul, and for the remainder of her life Lucile Willis lived in a nursing home under supervised care. Making repairs on the Gundy and simultaneously providing for Lucy probably made Grace reluctant to outlay further funds in the same year. Again she postponed a decision.[24]

After 1955 Grace's attention focused increasingly on Tucson. Having rented homes there for five years, she began putting down roots. Besides the friends made through Blair's relatives, Ted and Louisa Steele, and Betty Foster Vytlacil, her old St. Paul friend of many years, resided there. Jack Greenway, Martha and Chuck Breasted, and their stepsister, Saranne Neumann and her husband, grew close to Grace. They and their children became the children and grandchildren she never had. Each winter they made a big fuss over her arrival in Tucson. Grace described one such welcome in a letter to John Parsons and his wife in Farmington:

> The family, winding up to one of their outbursts, met me at the station with a <u>band</u> and placards of welcome, and it was all most amusing and gay and startled the transcontinental passengers out of their minds. Martha, Chuck, Jack Greenway, the beautiful Mrs. Russell Davenport (Marcia Gluck) and other friends all bearing placards mounted on poles and reading "Welcome to Grace," "Welcome to Aunto," "Welcome to Mrs. Flandrau" and the payoff—Mme. Davenport bearing a placard reading "Welcome to Mary O'Malley." What with the singing and playing of the Mexicans, Mary's banshee screech when she read her name on the sign, and all the rest, it was really very gay and ga ga and uninhibited and fun.[25]

Each time Grace returned to Farmington, however, gloom and inertia descended. She wrote Martha Breasted from the Gundy in the late 1950s, quoting Robert Louis Stevenson to describe what age and illness can do to the human spirit:

> It's that dreadful loss of ganas—zest—response. Oh, Martha, he [Robert Louis Stevenson] describes this state of mind perfectly. It is how he feels when sick and disillusioned, when he always seems to be in the company of somebody who is not moved by the beauty of a fair scene, not up to the measure of an occasion—and then realizes that dull stranger is himself. He cannot recognize that this "phlegmatic and unimpressionable being with whom he goes burthened is the same he knew heretofore so quick and delicate and alive."[26]

Grace continued fretting about money and then admitting money had nothing to do with her indecision. Her regret mounted over not having purchased a Tucson house she had wanted. And her thoughts kept going back to the trust officer in St. Paul who had discouraged her from buying it. He and she, she explained to Martha and Jack, had both been aware that she had practically thrown away three houses in St. Paul:

> The first, Blair's and my adorable Cass Gilbert house, *practically* given away. The old house worse than given away, and finally the third place [470 Summit Avenue]—an extraordinarily nice house built at a cost of $75,000, bought by me for thirty, and after five years sold for less than twenty as well as all the upkeep. It seemed to me . . . that in giving up that place [in Tucson] I gave up my last chance to find a home and to be happy. And it has seemed so ever since. It seems . . . Jack and Martha, that I have so destroyed myself and my life that I have nothing left with which to go forward—no vitality or hope or confidence in myself . . . that I have missed the one chance in Tucson and made everybody angry and bored and that I can't pull myself out of this despair.[27]

But help was in sight. Charles Curley, president of First Trust Company, invited Grace into his office for a private visit on her next visit to St. Paul. Curley told her that the young trust officer she had spoken to earlier had no idea of the effect he was having upon her, that if she had spoken to <u>him</u>

[Curley], he would have insisted that she buy the house in Tucson, not only for a home but as a good investment. That conversation was worth all the money, real and imagined, Grace believed she had thrown away on past real estate decisions.[28]

Another serendipitous event occurred almost simultaneously. A Philip Wylie article in *Partisan Review* deeply impressed her, bringing peace of mind. Writing Wylie, Grace referred to his "Grand Inquisitor" piece, built around a dialogue in Dostoevsky's *Brothers Karamazov*. She said she had been moved by Dostoevsky's "surrender to faith and love."[29]

Writing Alice O'Brien about it, Grace said she believed that such a surrender of the ego could help her dispel "that cloud of pessimism and fear that shadowed the house and all my childhood."[30] She now understood that fear and pessimism—though disguised by her seemingly frivolous nature—had dominated her personality for so long that she had been unable to believe in the future. Alice responded, again urging Grace to move back to Minnesota. She wrote: "Maybe the cloud around you will break this time. Why not give it another try before Farmington? . . . I still think St. Paul is the place for you."[31]

But Grace's life took another direction. Taking deliberate steps, she worked her way toward establishing her "strategic base" in Tucson. Describing what she wanted and why, she wrote Charles Breasted:

> [I long] for a place to which the family and only the family could, when and if any or all of them felt like it . . . drop in any time of the day or night, and find an adequate larder . . . If I never so long as I live give another dinner party or organize a formal social activity it will be the one bright spot . . . and the only thing that can gladden and enrich them [her last years] would be the privilege of exercising, giving effortless love, or affection. That, and books, of course, and ideas—talk—which I love so much. Just enough food for the heart, so that the mind will not, as mine has lately, lie down in emptiness and fatigue and malnutrition and an overwhelming sense of "a quoi bon-ism" [what's the use of it all?].[32]

In 1960 Grace purchased a handsome, two-story, white Spanish colonial home on spacious wooded grounds at 2318 East Elm Street in Tucson. The house, less than a block from the Arizona Inn, cost $96,000. She spent every winter there for the next decade.

$\mathcal{A}$ $\mathcal{H}$ome for the $\mathcal{H}$eart

"I did not <u>live</u> my life."
Grace H. Flandrau to Eleanor Jerusha (Mrs. John S.) Pillsbury, 1950s

DURING HER DECADE OF SELF-ANALYSIS Grace learned that taking risks and making changes in the way she handled relationships were essential. Gradually discarding her celebrity writer persona, she became a more centered, accepting version of her old self. She appeared to have renewed confidence she could handle her emotions or at least not be incapacitated by them.

Although she gave up writing for publication after 1955, Flandrau continued long conversations with friends and literary associates—even with celebrities she didn't know—via letters. She also carried on extensive correspondence with St. Paul lawyers and trust officials regarding her burgeoning fortune. Her papers evidence significant financial generosity to people and charitable causes. She became increasingly involved in the causes and treatment of juvenile delinquency but was too frail for active participation.[1]

Flandrau came to view her forty-year career as a professional writer with skepticism and regret. She felt her ambition had distanced her from people and prevented development of lasting relationships. In the years that remained to her, Grace concentrated on friendship. Blair's family and their friends and others she met in Tucson were barely aware of her past literary celebrity. Jack Greenway said of his great-aunt at our first interview in 1987: "Her charm was in her private life."[2]

Nevertheless, the aging author continued to thrive on lively interchange of ideas. Young and old who knew her in the last decade of her life remember that she relished stimulating conversation with informed participants. As in her previous life, Grace never doubted the value of expressing her ideas.

Patty Ferguson Doar, present manager of the Arizona Inn—a great-great grandchild of Charles Eugene Flandrau and Jack Greenway's niece—was a Bryn Mawr student when she corresponded with "Aunt Grace" in the 1950s. Grace, who was then in her late seventies, was old enough to be Patty's grandmother. Jack, understanding "Aunt-o's" affinity for the young and her need for stimulating conversation encouraged the friendship.

Via letters, Doar and Flandrau held spirited exchanges on the pros and cons of feminism, Patty taking the pro side and Grace the con. Grace's mature viewpoint must have differed considerably from her thoughts on feminism when she and Brenda Ueland had corresponded forty years earlier. Grace wrote Patty:

> I would deplore anything which tended to make women try to resemble, emulate or pattern themselves on men. . . . I think the pair of opposites is far more exciting and productive—not biologically, which would always obtain—but emotionally and therefore aesthetically.
>
> In other words, what was really in my mind was not the inferiority of women to men, but the profound and important difference. A difference which I can't help feeling has been the source of humanity's most . . . divine productions and perceptions . . . my belief being that the state of being in love—'romantic love'—is one of the great insights or sources of aesthetic creativeness; any reconciling of this to changing *moeurs* [Fr. moral customs] is extremely difficult.

Grace went on:

> While women are the equals and sometimes superiors of men in the inter-pretive arts (acting, dancing and so on), they seldom are in the infinitely different and more important creative arts—because theirs is another creativeness—and a very great and proud one.
>
> The greatest project women can have is to seek to become great in their own way. I realize perfectly that I am dealing with the maddest of impon-derables, and yet I dare to suggest it includes giving, loving, mothering in the best sense—something bigger in the way of selflessness and dedication to the proper development of others—namely the young—than anything that is properly demanded of the male, whose roles are less personal . . . to be an inspirer of men, a guide and creator of the rising generation in the way of the heart, the intuit . . . the understanding . . . is as special a creative role as the kind of ultimate artistic . . . creativeness [of] Aeschylus, Socrates, Shakespeare, Beethoven, Leonardo, Giotto et al.[3]

Two other relatives-by-marriage in Arizona, Martha Breasted and Saranne Neumann, described Grace's last years in Tucson in recent interviews.

Breasted said of Blair's widow: "She was terribly good company, more fun to be with than anyone I know, extremely bright and very quick. As relatives, we all really loved her although she wasn't blood kin." In a subsequent interview, Breasted was more candid. Speaking of Grace's hot temper, she said, "Boy, she was colossal." Like all women, whether related to Blair Flandrau or not, Martha Breasted—like her mother, Isabella, and her grandmother, Patty Selmes—had adored him. She remembered him as "a darling." On the sensitive issue of Grace's troubled childhood, Breasted only offered: "The family never got it straight."[4]

Saranne Neumann, a step-sister of Jack and Martha, said: "One of the most lovable things about Mrs. Flandrau was her dependence—some of her charm was in her dependence on friends. She'd ask them what to do, what to wear. . . . She telephoned me every morning and asked, 'What shall we do today?'" Describing Grace as "a cozy person," Neumann, whose home in Tucson was directly across Elm street from Grace's, gave this picture of her life in Arizona: "We'd ask "Aunto" to baby-sit our youngsters in the evening every once in a while. They loved going to her house, because, instead of making them do their homework, she'd serve them sherry and play backgammon with them."

In her seventies, Flandrau began taking long walks in good weather, a remedy some doctor must have advised for osteoporosis and the blues. In Tucson, Grace's daily habit was to have a long, conversational lunch at the Pioneer Hotel with friends and then walk home, a distance of four miles. She regained strength and lost weight.[5]

In summer 1962, the Minnesota Historical Society invited Grace, at seventy-six, to return to Minnesota to give an address on Charles Eugene Flandrau, Jack Greenway's great-grandfather and Grace's late father-in-law. The occasion was the society's annual meeting as well as the centennial of the battle of New Ulm in the Dakota Conflict of 1862. The event also featured dedication of a statue in New Ulm honoring Charles E. Flandrau for his role in defending the frontier town in the famous uprising.

C. E. Flandrau, appointed United States Indian agent for the Mdewankanton Sioux in the 1860s, had been at his home in Traverse des Sioux in August 1862 when the Indians' outrage at U.S. government mistreatment erupted along the Minnesota River Valley. Hearing of the dangerous situation, Flandrau quickly recruited a militia of volunteers from the area to turn back the Sioux's raid on the town of New Ulm. Although some historians have disputed the scope of Flandrau's role, most have granted major credit for the victory to him.

To prepare for her speech, Grace did extensive research in Minnesota. When she arrived in the state the Twin Cities press awaited her. A story appearing in "Today's Personality" in the *Minneapolis Journal* that summer, described Flandrau this way: "She is regarded by many discriminating Twin City folk as the most interesting woman conversationalist in the region." The once-famous author's comments may have surprised them. In the published interview, Grace deplored the pitfalls of excessive ambition, particularly in women. The paper quoted her: "[Mrs. Flandrau] distrusts ambition as mere vanity, a painful straight-jacket which may, especially in women, inhibit the flowering of the personality as a whole."

When reporters quizzed her about the famous Flandrau parrots, Grace said Albert was named for the King of Belgium because she and Blair had plucked him from a tree in the Belgian Congo in 1927 when King Albert was on the throne; they hadn't been sure whether the parrot was male or female, so sometimes they called the bird "Albertine." Lauro, Charlie's par-rot, was "a misanthrope who hated the human race."[6]

St. Paul newspapers also interviewed and photographed Grace for a story in the August 16, 1962, *St. Paul Pioneer Press*. In spite of the obvious age of the subject, her alert gaze directed squarely at the photographer projects the unflappable poise that had always been Grace Flandrau's public posture. With her perky, tan straw boater and again slender, the author still projected unsinkable élan.

To gather information about her late father-in-law, Grace sought help from the elderly granddaughters of the state's first territorial governor, Alexander Ramsey. Ramsey, who was in the statehouse when the starving Indians went on the warpath in 1862, had given Charles E. Flandrau an emergency commission in the state militia. Although they were members of rival political parties, Ramsey and Flandrau were friends throughout the second half of the nineteenth century. Three generations of their families had been intimates. The simultaneous deaths in 1903 of Governor Alexander Ramsey, territorial justice Charles E. Flandrau, and Edward J. Hodgson (Grace's prominent father) had punctuated the end of the state's youth.

While completing her research Grace stayed at the historic St. Paul Hotel on Rice Park. She invited Ramsey's maiden granddaughters, Anita (Anna E.)

and Laura Furness, to dine with her and described their visit in detail to Jack Greenway and Martha Breasted:

> [Anita and Laura were] those two unbelievably entrancing sisters [with] snow white hair en pompadour in semi-evening dress and pearls (artificial) and similar diamond brooches (real), made out of some of 'Mama's [accent on the last syllable] jewels.' Very proper, they had insisted on being 'announced' to Grace by the hotel clerk and were incensed when he told them 'Oh, just go on up.' Anita and Laura, Grace said, had a marvelous, very real sophistication which makes you see why their cousin T. S. Eliot is so devoted to them.'

The two "entrancing sisters" spent a fruitful evening with Grace reminiscing about Charles E. Flandrau ("such a darling man, so charming, so kind, so good-looking, Isabella looked very much like him.") and other members of the Flandrau family. During the evening they shared anecdotes about Flandrau-Selmes and Ramsey-Furness family members with Grace, including Anita's rumored infatuation with the young Charles Macomb Flandrau.[7]

Although she had never known her father-in-law, Charles E. Flandrau, for her speech to the members of the Minnesota Historical Society Grace created a sensitive portrait of a real man. The speech could only have been the result of hours of discussions with those who had listened to stories about him for generations.

Jack Greenway escorted Grace to New Ulm for the society's annual meeting on August 18, 1962. On the eve of her appearance she received a wire from Ted Steele and his family: "Wish we could all five be in the front row for your speech tonight. Much love darling and wow them." Grace was seventy-six and the speech in New Ulm was her last public appearance in the state.[8]

Ted Steele died in 1962. Alice O'Brien died the same year. O'Brien's obituary story said: "The death of Miss Alice O'Brien Friday November 11, 1962, removed from the St. Paul scene its leading woman philanthropist, world traveler and art connoisseur." A woman friend of O'Brien's wrote Grace a letter of condolence: "My husband, Virgil, said: 'Grace is the only friend of Alice's I'd like to see again.'"[9]

Although she abandoned plans to live in Minnesota, Flandrau continued returning to St. Paul regularly. Attendance at meetings of the Executive Council of the Minnesota Historical Society was often the purpose of her visits. Grace had served as a council member since 1949. She also attended stockholders' meetings of St. Paul Fire & Marine Insurance Company (now Travelers). After Alice O'Brien's death, on trips to St. Paul Grace stayed at the St. Paul Hotel.

On these visits, Grace also conferred with officers of the First Trust Company and Francis D. Butler, her attorney at the St. Paul law firm Doherty, Rumble, and Butler. Butler wrote on January 31, 1962, that the revocable trust at First Trust, of which Flandrau was beneficiary, was worth approximately $4,435,000 in bonds, real estate and leaseholds, and miscellaneous stocks. By far the biggest holding—$2,600,000—was in St. Paul Fire and Marine stock. The letter confirmed the wisdom of First Trust's investment strategy: buy municipal bonds with any excess income and don't sell Fire and Marine stock. As the 1960s unfolded, the size of the Flandrau holdings in St. Paul Fire and Marine stock became legendary. Rumors circulated in the Twin Cities that St. Paul Fire & Marine couldn't hold a stockholders' meeting without Grace Flandrau's attendance or proxy.

After a stay in St. Paul in 1963, Grace stopped at the Mayo Clinic in Rochester, Minnesota, for a physical. B. L. Riggs, Flandrau's examining physician, reported that her major physical problems were depression, occasional colitis, bronchitis, back pain, and osteoporosis, probably a fairly typical list for a woman of seventy-nine years.[10]

Craig Reynolds, the California attorney who had been overseeing Lucile Willis's care for several years, corresponded with Flandrau steadily. Toward the end of the 1960s, Reynolds advised Grace that Lucy had taken a fall requiring surgery and that she was no longer ambulatory. Willis was, however, Reynolds wrote, getting along all right, was being allowed two cans of beer a day, and was content.

Flandrau's response was philosophical: "I have an idea Lucile will outlive all of us. She seems to have been born with the blessed inability to worry about anything." She commented on the differences between Lucy and herself, then turned to her own state of mind: "I used to wonder what <u>could</u> be meant by the term melancholia. Now I know. Well, if the Hindus are right, <u>Karma</u> includes all experiences, and until you have them all you don't qualify for Paradise." Quoting Emily Dickinson, Grace added:

> The heart asks pleasure first,
> And then excuse from pain,

And then those little anodynes
That deaden suffering,
And then to go to sleep.
And then, if it should be
The will of the Inquisitor,
The privilege to die.[11]

She concluded: "I find the last line particularly elegant." Lucile Hodgson Willis died in January 1969 in California.

Ann Wooden Rush, a childhood friend of both Jack Greenway and Patty Doar, befriended Grace during her last years in Tucson. Rush, who was a Wellesley graduate and a writer, often lunched with Flandrau at her Spanish colonial home on Elm Street. They had long talks about cooking and books. While Grace was a witty, worldly, and delightful companion, Rush remembered that she never talked about anything personal and never spoke of her family. There was a sadness in her face, Rush remembered.[12]

Tucsonans remember that Grace continued to wine and dine friends and visitors in spite of protesting she didn't enjoy entertaining. Elegant cuisine and impressive guests characterized her parties. Grace continued to mingle stuffy people with bohemian, offbeat types, and her racy wit both charmed and startled her invitees. One distinguished elderly guest was Lawrence Gould. Gould, who had known his hostess when he was president of Carleton College in Northfield, Minnesota, in the 1940s, was a professor of geosciences in the 1960s at the University of Arizona, living in Tucson.

The reliable, devoted Mary O'Malley and Frederick Smith, chauffeur, continued to serve as Grace's domestic support system in Tucson. Smith drove Flandrau's car each winter from Farmington to Tucson and back in the spring, accompanied by O'Malley. Although Grace previously owned unostentatious cars, in her old age she enjoyed the luxury of being transported in a chauffeur-driven Rolls Royce.

Jack Greenway accompanied Grace on journeys by train across country each year, from Connecticut to Arizona and back, assisting with transportation of parrots, furs, books, and luggage. Entering her eighties, Grace's mind began to fail, and she became too confused to travel at all. When Greenway's involvement in her care became even more essential Grace appointed him her legal guardian as well as executor of the Flandrau estate.[13]

Although Grace led a more solitary life in Connecticut than in Arizona, some living residents of Farmington and Hartford as late as 1990 held strong memories of her. One of them, John Parsons, interviewed in his nineties, was a trustee of the Avon Old Farms School and served as attorney for the Hill-Stead Museum. (The Riddle estate, Hill-Stead, became a house museum after Theodate Riddle's death in 1941.)

Parsons and his wife, Katrine, were Flandrau's friends for many years. Recollecting that Grace was "very, very humorous," Parsons said he "loved to talk with her about books."[14] Parsons also respected Flandrau's astute business judgment. He remembered that, when the issue became a crisis, he and Grace both voted to close the Hill-Stead Museum, which had become a financial drain on the resources left in Theodate's will. Grace knew, Parsons said, that Riddle would have wanted the Avon Old Farms School, above all, to survive.[15] (After Flandrau's death in 1971, sale of the Gundy house provided an endowment for development of Hill-Stead as a magnificent residential museum.)

In Connecticut, Grace gradually became an isolated elderly woman with a diminishing circle of friends, and after retirement from the Avon board, she lost contact with community life in Farmington. In the late 1960s, in her eighties, Grace became increasingly confused and frail. Ingeborg Carlson, who worked as Grace's maid for the last nineteen years of her life in Farmington and was with her when she died, remembered the beautiful dinner parties given by the accomplished hostess until the last years of her life. She described Flandrau as a "perfect lady until she got sick. She was very patient with those who worked for her and very down to earth." Carlson, the consummate lady's maid and a model of refinement herself, remembered that her mistress had the "most beautiful feet and legs" and that "she knew it."

According to Carlson, her employer never drank to excess with guests in the house and was always beautifully dressed. But she also recalled that, as Grace became more isolated and addled, she occasionally drank too many cocktails and became quarrelsome with Mary O'Malley. Carlson began to monitor Flandrau's drinks carefully and to spend nights at the Gundy house. She said visits from Greenway, Breasted, and Neumann meant a lot to Grace and those looking after her.[16]

Greenway supervised Grace's care from Arizona by staying in touch with her staff of four. In addition to Mary O'Malley, Ingeborg Carlson, and Fred Smith, a secretary, Elizabeth McCarthy, took care of Grace and her personal and business affairs in Farmington. When Jack's sudden arrival in Farmington befuddled Grace and she wondered whether they were in Farmington or

Tucson, he would reply, "Well, we're having fun, aren't we, Gracie? So it doesn't matter."

Greenway recalled that Grace's childhood panic about money gradually reasserted itself and she lost touch with the fact that she was a wealthy woman. Worrying incessantly about running out of money, she insisted on cutting household expenditures to the bone. She ordered Mary to curtail purchases from the grocery store. "About one chicken a week," remembered Greenway with a chuckle, "was all she would allow."[17]

If they thought a movie would be a good outing for Grace, Greenway and McCarthy invented schemes to fool her into thinking the theater owner had donated tickets for her and the two or three other household staff members to accompany her on such chauffeur-driven expeditions.

Grace died in Farmington on December 27, 1971, at the age of 85. Her funeral took place on a bitterly cold winter day, with burial next to Blair in the Flandrau plot in Oakland Cemetery in St. Paul. One untoward incident marred the solemnity of the occasion. As he led the funeral procession into the cemetery a policeman on a motorcycle spun out of control on the icy road, causing him to dive unceremoniously, unhurt, into a snowbank. Grace would have laughed uproariously.

Epilogue

GRACE FLANDRAU DIED IN 1971 leaving an estate worth $8,000,000. Within two years, while it was probated and bequests were made, its value grew to almost $10,000,000. Ninety-five percent of the money went to charities. Jack Greenway was closely involved in the distribution of bequests from the Flandrau estate.

Under the terms of her will Grace left more than three million dollars in honor of Blair to the National Council on Crime and Delinquency to establish its headquarters in Tucson, and she left an unrestricted gift of $800,000 in stock to the University of Arizona in Tucson. With that sum and the interest it earned, the University built the Grace Hodgson Flandrau Planetarium on its campus. The gift honors Edward Hodgson, Grace's father, a zealous student of astronomy.

Flandrau's will specified several other large bequests. Harvard University received $3,200,000 to establish a Flandrau Fund honoring Charles Macomb Flandrau to encourage good writing and good English usage. Her will also specified a $1,000,000 bequest to the University of Hartford in Connecticut, the largest donation in the school's history. The Saint Paul Foundation received $3,200,000. The Minnesota Historical Society received $100,000 to establish a research fund for perpetuation of the name of Charles Eugene Flandrau in state history. Hamline University received a bequest of $50,000.00.

Flandrau's will specified a number of personal bequests. Mary O'Malley received $50,000, but died shortly after Grace Flandrau's death. The family of Elizabeth McCarthy received $10,000 as did the Avon Old Farms School. Four humane societies received $5,000 each.

Jack Greenway inherited Grace Flandrau's house in Tucson and her Rolls Royce. Bequests of jewelry, furniture, art, Albert (the parrot), and other personal belongings went to Flandrau relatives.

Notes

THE FLANDRAU FAMILY PAPERS (hereafter FFP), MS 1018, constitute a 9,000-document collection of more than forty-five linear feet in the custody of the Arizona Historical Society in Tucson. The collection includes microfilm copies of family correspondence of Judge Charles Eugene Flandrau (Minnesota pioneer, Indian agent, jurist, and lawyer) as well as original correspondence of his second wife, Rebecca Blair McClure Riddle Flandrau, his four children — Martha Flandrau Selmes and Sally Flandrau Cutcheon, Charles Macomb Flandrau, and William Blair McClure Flandrau, husband of Grace Flandrau — and his stepson, John Wallace Riddle.

The Flandrau Family Papers (FFP) also include the papers of Grace Corrin Hodgson Flandrau — the largest segment — and the papers of her father, Edward John Hodgson, St. Paul lawyer, businessman and much-published writer. Copies of many references used in this biography are now in the archives of Hamline University, St. Paul.

The original papers of Judge Charles Eugene Flandrau, Grace Flandrau's father-in-law, are housed at the Minnesota Historical Society, St. Paul. Copies of a number of Charles Macomb Flandrau's papers also reside in the Charles Eugene Flandrau collection at the Minnesota Historical Society (hereafter MHS) in St. Paul.

The letters between Martha Flandrau Selmes and Charles Macomb Flandrau are now in the family collection at Dinsmore Farm, Boone County, Kentucky, the ancestral home of Isabella Dinsmore Flandrau, first wife of Charles E. Flandrau. Copies of this correspondence exist in the Charles M. Flandrau Papers at MHS.

Grace Flandrau, who became custodian of the Flandrau Family Papers after the deaths of Charles M. Flandrau and William Blair Flandrau in 1938, decided to leave the FFP to her husband's great-nephew, the late John S. (Jack) Greenway, her heir and great-grandson of Charles Eugene Flandrau. (Please see Preface to this biography.) According to the late Jack Greenway, Grace Flandrau left a bequest of $100,000 to the Minnesota Historical Society to "keep the Flandrau name alive in Minnesota history."

GHF – Grace Corrin Hodgson Flandrau. Her letters were typically undated, so the
   following notes provide only an estimated date.
WBF – William Blair McClure Flandrau, always called "Blair."

CMF – Charles Macomb Flandrau, "Charlie."
RBF – Rebecca Blair McClure Flandrau
CEF – Charles Eugene Flandrau
MFS – Martha (Patty) Selmes
EJH – Edward John Hodgson
MHS – Martha Staples Hodgson
KSC – Kyle S. Crichton
MEP – Maxwell E. Perkins
TPR – Theodate Pope Riddle
JWR – John Wallace Riddle
REM – Richard E. Myers
ALM – Alice Lee Myers
JSG – John Selmes Greenway

AUTHOR'S PREFACE

1. Brylawski, Fulton. "Works of Grace Hodgson Flandrau," copyright list, 1949–1955, file 90, box 18, Flandrau Family Papers, Arizona Historical Society, Tucson (hereafter FFP). Expanded and updated by author. See Appendix B.

2. See, for example, *Who's Who Among Minnesota Women*, 1924, and *Who's Who of American Women* (1958–59, 1966–67, 1968-69); see also Publication Credits of Grace Flandrau.

3. Grace Flandrau to Alice M. O'Brien (hereafter (AOM), [undated] 1950s, file 26, box 14, FFP.

4. When the Charles E. Flandrau house at 385 Pleasant Ave., St. Paul, was razed in 1955, Grace Flandrau and her heir, John S. Greenway, moved the family papers first to her second home (the Gundy House) in Farmington, CT, and later deposited them in a vault at the Minnesota Historical Society in 1962. At Grace's death in 1971 Greenway ordered the papers brought to Tucson, Arizona, where they remained in their original cartons on the porch of his residence at the Arizona Inn for nearly eight years. In 1979 Greenway returned the Flandrau papers to the Minnesota Historical Society, where they were placed in new cartons and again stored in a vault. In 1983 Greenway ordered the return of the papers to Arizona to establish the Flandrau Family Papers collection at the Arizona Historical Society in Tucson. Record based on phone calls, MHS records and correspondence with MHS staff members Lucile Kane, November 12, 1998, and James Fogarty, November 16, 1998, and January 6, 2004.

5. "Charlie was really terrible." John S. Greenway (hereafter JSG) to author, Aug. 26, 1993.

6. Georgia Ray, "In Search of the Real Grace Flandrau," *Minnesota History*, summer 1999, 308–309, notes 8, 13.

7. Grace Flandrau, "Child Memories," "Memories of a French Convent," and "Mexican Memory". Typed drafts possibly intended for an autobiographical novel, file 139, box 22, FFP; drafts now published as *Memoirs of Grace Flandrau* (St. Paul: Knochaloe Beg Press, 2003) ed., Georgia Ray (hereafter *Memoirs*).

8. Author Files I, C0101, Archives of Charles Scribner's Sons, Dept. of Rare Books and Special Collections, Princeton University (hereafter Scribner's archives), files I and II, box 50.

1. Maxwell E. Perkins (hereafter MEP) to Grace Flandrau (hereafter GHF), April 19, 1935, file I, box 50, Scribner's archives.
2. *Minneapolis Journal*, October 28, 1937; GHF to MEP, undated letter, [November 1937?], file II, box 50, Scribner's archives.
3. 4. Correspondence from publishers and critics to Grace Flandrau about her works, file 91, box 19, FFP; also reviews, file 101, box 20, FFP. See Grace Flandrau's articles, "What Africa is Not," in *Contemporary Review*, December 1930, and "Black Potentates of Equitorial Africa," *Travel*, September 1929. Four foreign language editions ... Grace Flandrau to Blair Flandrau, undated letter from France [1930-1932], file 12, box 13, FFP.
5. GHF to Kyle S. Crichton (hereafter KSC), undated [1934?], file 30, box 14, FFP.
6. GHF to MEP, undated letter, [November 1937?] file II, box 50, Scribner's archives.
7. MEP to GHF, November 8, 1937, file II, box 50, Scribner's archives.
8. Ibid., July 2, 1930, file 91, box 18, FFP.
9. Ibid., February 2, 1932, file I, box 50, Scribner's archives.
10. KSC to GHF, January 12, 1932, file I, box 50, Scribner's archives.
11. GHF to MEP, June 25, 1935; MEP to GHF, July 17, 1935, file I, Box 50, Scribner's archives; GHF to MEP, undated, [October 1936?], file II, Scribner's archives.
12. MEP to GHF, May 8, 1933, file 91, box 18, FFP.
13. Ibid., October 2, 1936, FFP; GHF to MEP, undated [October, 1936?], file II, box 50, Scribner's archives.
14. GHF to MEP, undated [October 1936?]; MEP to GHF, October 13, 1936, file II, box 50, Scribner's archives.
15. MEP to GHF, November 8, 1937, file II, box 50, Scribner's archives.
16. *Memoirs of Grace Flandrau* (see Preface #7).
17. GHF, "Notes and Diaries," file 471, box 50, FFP.
18. GHF awards include an honorary doctorate in literature from Hamline University, St. Paul, 1947, and membership in the American Academy of Arts and Sciences, 1949.
19. Olivia Irvine Dodge to author, St. Paul, December 19, 1995.
20. Kate Skiles Klein to author, St. Paul, June 23, 1993.
21. Brenda Ueland (hereafter BU), diary entries, November 2, 1934, November 13, 1934, March 9, 1935, Brenda Ueland Papers, microfilm edition, roll 1, MHS.
22. Kate Skiles Klein to author, St. Paul, December 19, 1995.
23. Records of the Saint Paul Foundation, St. Paul, Minn.
24. For understanding of Grace Flandrau's archetypal downfall, please see Patricia Hampl's essay, "The Smile of Accomplishment," in *I Could Tell You Stories*, W. W. Norton and Company, New York, 1999.
25. Meridel Le Sueur (hereafter MLS) to author, Hudson, Wisconsin, July 16, 1990.

26. GHF to Alice M. O'Brien (hereafter AOM), undated [early 1950s], file 53, box 16, FFP.

27. Thomas Boyd to GHF, file 76, box 18, FFP.

28. Michael Fedo, "A Literary Life," *View from the Loft* (November, 1999) 5, 17.

29. Louis Auchincloss, *Love without Wings*, (Boston: Houghton Mifflin Company, 1991), 184.

30. Mary Griggs Burke to author, Cable, Wisconsin, September 4, 1994.

31. Constance Shepard Otis to author, St. Paul, 1994.

32. Barbara White Bemis to author, St. Paul, February 26, 2002.

33. "My own strange fate . . . "GHF to Sylvia Beach, August 8, 1955, box 196, Sylvia Beach Papers, CO108, Manuscripts Division, Firestone Library, Princeton University.

34. " . . . distrusts ambition as mere vanity," GHF interview quoted in "Today's Personality," undated clipping [August, 1962], *Minneapolis Tribune*, Minneapolis History Collection, Minneapolis Public Library.

CHAPTER II

1. Martha Ferguson Breasted to author, February 14, 1990, Tucson, Arizona.

2. Obituary of William Hodson, *Minneapolis Tribune*, January 21, 1943.

3. *History of the Hamline University of Minnesota when located at Red Wing . . . from 1854–1869* (St. Paul: Alumni Association, 1907), 172; Theodore Christianson, *Minnesota, the Land of Sky-tinted Waters–A History of the State and Its People* (Chicago: American Historical Society, 1935), 4:185.

4. Death certificate, Anna Redding Hodson, July 25, 1950, #3102, Hennepin County records; Minneapolis City Directory (1901) lists Anna Hodson as "widow of William" at 749 Quincy.

5. Mary Griggs Burke to author, September 4, 1994, Cable, Wisconsin.

6. Jane (Mrs. James) McKay, quoting her late mother, Mrs. James Gray (ex-St. Paulite Betty Bishop Reeves Gray, a St. Paul neighbor of the Edward J. Hodgson family) to author, telephone interview with author, August, 2001.

7. GHF, *Indeed This Flesh* (New York: H. Smith and R. Haas, 1934); fictional character "Norah" is based on Anna Redding Hodson.

8. Obituary, *Minneapolis Tribune*, January 21, 1943, names Anna Redding Hodson as William Hodson's mother and describes William Hodson as the " . . . Dean of all social welfare workers produced by Minneapolis;" Blair Flandrau (hereafter WBF) to GHF, May 8, 1932, file 27, box 59, FFP (confirming William Hodson is Grace's brother).

9. *Indeed This Flesh*, 45–47.

10. Mary Staples Hodgson (hereafter MSH) to Edward John Hodgson (hereafter EJH) from Paris, 1900–1903, file 6, box 63; files 210, 211, box 26, FFP.

11. See note 4.

12. EJH to his nephew, John Edward Hodgson, June 25, 1903; Edward R. Hodgson, *Hodgson-Clague-Corrin* (Sacramento, 1971), 70.

13. St. Paul Chamber of Commerce Minutes for October 1903, Minnesota Historical Society Collections.

14. Albert Willis to MSH, file 6, box 63, FFP.

15. Rebecca Blair Flandrau (hereafter RBF) to John Wallace Riddle (hereafter JWR), August 23, 1909, file 21, FFP.

16. Although they married in 1909, WBF did not learn the truth of his wife's parentage until after she met her brother, William Hodson, in 1932 (see note 8).

17. Muriel E. Nelson (great-niece of EJH), to author, October 24, 1992; Corrin H. Hodgson, great-nephew of Edward Hodgson, telephone interview with author, December 12, 1992.

18. William Hodson became the first director of Minnesota's State Children's Bureau, author of Minnesota's Children's Code, director of child welfare legislation for the Russell Sage Foundation, NY, president of the National Conference of Social Workers, and director of New York City's welfare system under Fiorello La Guardia; undated clipping, author's possession.

19. GHF, *Indeed This Flesh* (New York: Harrison Smith & Robert Haas, 1934); also, GHF to MEP, January 21, 1932, Scribner's archives.

20. Kate S. Klein to author, St. Paul, June 23, 1993.

21. GHF to Kyle S. Crichton (hereafter KSC), fall, 1933, file 30, box 14, FFP.

22. *Memoirs of Grace Flandrau*, "Child Memories," 3.

23. Obituary of William Hodson, *Minneapolis Tribune*, January 21, 1943.

24. GHF to KSC, January 21, 1932, file 1, Box 50, Scribner's archive.

25. *History of the Hamline University*, 175.

26. *Memoirs of Grace Flandrau*, "Child Memories," 4.

27. Thomas C. Hodgson to Drusilla Hodgson, July 4, 1899, GHF Papers, Hamline University (hereafter, Hamline).

28. GHF, *Indeed This Flesh*, 256–261. There can be little doubt that GHF intended to imply incest between her father and herself as a child in her biographical/autobiographical novel, *Indeed This Flesh*. Although the book is presented as fiction, the use of accurate place names (e.g., "Red Wing," "St. Paul," "The Isle of Man") and slimly disguised names for actual persons in her family story, (e.g., "Carlotta Pearson" for "Charlotte Hodgson," Grace's grandmother) indicates Flandrau was disclosing a long-concealed family story she urgently needed to tell. Illustrative episodes are subtly implied. The circumstances in which deviant behavior such as incest takes root and flourishes are knowingly described; the author's mature feelings of love, understanding, and pity for her disgraced father are clear.

29. Georgia Ray, "In Search of the Real Grace Flandrau," *Minnesota History*, summer 1999, 308, note 6 (hereafter *In Search*).

30. Theodore Christianson, *Minnesota, the Land of Sky-Tinted Waters—A History of the State and Its People* (Chicago: American Historical Society, 1935), 4:185.

31. Corrin H.Hodgson to author, November 11, 1998, author's possession.

32. Edward R. Hodgson, Hodgson-Clague-Corrin (Sacramento, 1971), 70; Thomas Hodgson-Charollet (Charlotte) Corrin genealogical chart, author's possession.

33. *History of the Hamline University*, 172.

34. Christianson, 4: 185.

35. GHF, *Indeed This Flesh*, 32.

36. *History of the Hamline University*, 172.

37. Claude Francis and Fernande Gontier, *Creating Colette* (South Royalton, Vermont: Steerforth Press, 1998) 1, 12-13.

38. 1870 Minnesota Census, Red Wing, Goodhue County; Grace Flandrau, *Indeed This Flesh* (see note 29).

39. GHF, *Indeed this Flesh,* (see note 29).

40. Nora Brechner interview with Corrin H. Hodgson, transcribed to Georgia Ray, 1992, author's possession.

41. *St. Paul City Directory,* 1876–1903.

42. Edward R. Hodgson, Hodgson-Clague-Corrin (Sacramento: 1971), 70.

43. EJH obituary, *St. Paul Dispatch*, September 22, 1903.

44. EJH to editors Files 28, 29, box 66, file 3, box 63, essays and manuscripts, files 10-16, box 64, file 19, box 65, FFP.

45. *Catalogue of Hamline University for the Year 1880-81,* 14.

46. David Craine, *Manannan's Isle* (Glasgow: The Manx Museum and National Trust: 1955, printed and bound by Robert Maclehose and Company, Ltd., University Press).

11; H.S. Cuan, *The Isle of Man* (North Pomfret, VT: 1977).

47. *Memoirs,* ("Child Memories") 11.

48. St. Paul City Directory lists Charlotte L. Hodgson (widow of Thomas) living at 518 Dayton, residence of Edward J. Hodgson, 1886–1901.

49. GHF, *Indeed This Flesh,* 245.

50. Ibid, 207.

51. Ernest R. Sandeen, *St. Paul's Historic Summit Avenue* (St. Paul: New Directions Publishing Corporation, 1978) 7-9.

52. Ibid, 99, 101.

53. *History of the Hamline University,* 172.

54. Edward J. Hodgson obituary, *St. Paul Dispatch*, December 22, 1903.

55. Security Trust letterhead, 1890s, Edward J. Hodgson papers, file 2, box 63, FFP.

56. JSG to author, Tucson, Ariz., February 7, 9, 1990.

57. *Memoirs,* "Child Memories," 3.

CHAPTER III

1. *Memoirs,* "Child Memories", 12.

2. Mary Staples Hodgson (hereafter MSH) to EJH, April 30, 1900, file 6, box 63, FFP.

3. GHF to EJH, note enclosed in MSH letter to EJH, August 3, 1900, file 6, box 63, FFP.
   4. *Memoirs,* "Memories of a French School," 73.

5. GHF letters and postcards to Drusilla Hodgson, from Europe, 1900–1901, GHF papers, Hamline University, St. Paul, Minn. (hereafter, Hamline).

6. See note 4.

7. Claude Francis and Fernande Gontier, *Creating Colette* (South Royalton, Vermont: Steerforth Press, 1998), I, 12.

8. *Memoirs,* "Child Memories," 9.

9. Brenda Ueland, "Among Those We Know," *Golfer and Sportsman*, 26.

10. *Memoirs,* "Mexican Memory," 96.

11. *Memoirs,* "Child Memories," 9.

12. William Blair Flandrau's (hereafter WBF) unpublished account of his purchase of the Santa Margarita Ranch, 1904, file 1, box 58, FFP; also, GHF papers, Hamline.

13. *Memoirs*, "Child Memories," 12.

14. CMF to MFS, August 22, 1909 (L.P. Haeg, "Little Corners of Great Places," MHS Collections (hereafter "Little Corners.").

15. Theodore Roosevelt to WBF, August 4, 1906, file 56, box 61, FFP.

16. RBF to JWR, August 23, 1909, file 21, box 57, FFP.

17. Will of EJH, Ramsey County #12637, September 30, 1903.

18. *Memoirs,* "Child Memories," 18.

19. Corrin H. Hodgson, telephone interview with author, December 12, 1992.

CHAPTER IV

1. *Memoirs,* "Child Memories," 11.

2. WBF to CMF, October 26, 1904, file 11, box 58, FFP.

3. WBF to JWR, January 23, 1910, file 48, box 60, FFP.

4. CMF to MFS, September10, 1909, FFP.

5. Ibid., January 13, 1913, January 25, 1915, CMF letters, MHS collections.

6. Paul Revere Reynolds to GHF, November 9, 1917, file 91, box 18, FFP.

7. GHF to WBF, November 14, 1914, file 6, box 12, FFP.

8. WBF to GHF, February 19, 1912, file 13, box 58, FFP.

9. WBF to GHF, July 23, 1918, file 15, box 58.

10. GHF to WBF, undated letter, file 6, box 12, FFP.

11. CMF to MFS, December 27, 1911, Charles M. Flandrau letters, MHS collections.

12. GHF, profile of Charles E. Flandrau, speech delivered at MHS annual meeting, New Ulm, Minn., August, 1962, file 354, box 36, FFP.

13. CMF re WBF, page xvii, introduction to second edition of Viva Mexico! (New York: D. Appleton's, 1908).

14. CMF to JWR, September 1, 1910, July 13, 1911, file 64, box 5, FFP.

15. RBF to JWR, 1883, file 21, box 57, FFP.

16. Biographical sketches of Theodate Pope Riddle and John Wallace Riddle, 1990's, by Hill-Stead Museum staff, Farmington, CT, author's possession.

17. JSG interview with author, Tucson, Arizona, February 1987.

18. Letters between WBF and CMF, 1893–1897, files 3–12, box 58, FFP; letters.

19. CEF to WBF, 1900–1903, files 3–5, Microfilm reel 11, FFP.

20. Greenleaf Clark, "The Life and Influence of Judge Flandrau," *Minnesota Historical Collections*, 10:771-782 (part 2).

21. William H. Lightner, "Judge Flandrau as a Citizen and Jurist," *Minnesota Historical Society Collections*, 10:819–828 (part 2).

22. (see note 12).

23. "Little Corners of Great Places," chapter three; D.P. Skrief, "Viva Flandrau!" *Twin Cities,* February 1986, 32.

24. CEF to CMF, July 15, 1996, file 2, box 1 (microfilm reel 11), FFP.

25. RBF to JWR, file 21, box 57, FFP.

26. RBF to WBF, August 21, 1900, file 16, box 57, FFP.

27. MFS to WBF, 9/19/1900, file 11, box 77, FFP.

28. Will of Charles Eugene Flandrau, #12604, Ramsey County records, St. Paul, Minn..

29. D.P. Skrief, "Viva Flandrau!" *Twin Cities*, February 1986, 34.

30. WBF, autobiographical sketch, file 1, box 58, FFP. GF Papers, Hamline.

31. WBF to GHF, letters from the Santa Margarita ranch, MX, 1912–1916, file 13, box 58, FFP.

32. GHF, biographical sketch of WBF for Harvard class of 1900, box 58, FFP.

33. WBF wrote three articles about U. S. intervention in Mexico, *The Bellman*, May 30, 1914; June 6, 1914; January 16, 1915.

34. WBF to GHF, December 13, 1916, file 13, box 58, FFP.

CHAPTER V

1. CMF to MFS, September 12, 1916, CMF papers, MHS.

2. Ibid., October 10, 1916.

3. Ibid., November 1, 1916.

4. Ibid., February 19, 1917.

5. WBF to GHF, February 5, 1917, file 14, Box 58, FFP.

6. Ibid., February 15, 1917, file 14, Box 58, FFP.

7. Fan Mail, Reviews, "Cousin Julia," 1917–1918, File 77, Box 18, FFP; "Edith" [Wharton] to GHF, 1917, File 69, Box 17, FFP.

8. Ibid.

9. Preface, 1937 edition of *Viva Mexico!* D. Appleton-Century Co., Inc. N.Y., xvii

10. CMF to MFS, May 19, 1917, CMF papers, MHS

11. WBF to GHF, December 11 and 18, 1917, File 14, Box 58, FFP.

12. Ibid., Aug. 2, 1917, File 14, Box 58, FFP; CMF to GHF, May 28, 1917 and March 2, 1918, CMF papers, MHS of Dinsmore Farm, KY..

13. WBF to GHF, December 1, 1917, File 14, Box 58, FFP.

14. Ibid., November 17, 1917, File 14, Box 58, FFP and CMG to TPR, May 17, 1921, CMF papers, MHS or Dinsmore Farm.

15. Mark Hewitt, *Antiques*, October 1988, 848.

16. Character sketches of Theodate Pope Riddle and John Wallace Riddle by Hill-Stead Museum archivists, Sandra Wheeler and Polly P. Huntington, July 20, 1999.

17. GHF's sketch of Theodate Pope Riddle in *Reader's Digest*, "The Most Unforgettable Character I Ever Met," undated, File 221a, Box 27, FFP.

18. WBF to GHF, March 4, 1919, File 16, Box 58, FFP.

19. Ibid., December 1, 1917 and December 5, 1917, File 14, Box 58, FFP.

20. Ibid., August 18, 1918 and November 12, 1918, File 15, Box 58, FFP.

21. Ibid., June 23, 1918, File 15, Box 58, FFP.

22. *Town Topics*, NYC, June 13, 1918, File 77, Box 18, FFP.

23. GHF to WBF, October 24 and October 30, 1918, File 7, Box 12, FFP.

24. Ibid.,Letters from Paris January 1919–April, 1919, File 8, Box 12, FFP.

25. Betty Boyd Caroli, *The Roosevelt Women*, pp 168–169, 172.

26. *Who's Who in American Art*, Minnesota Historical Society Collections, re: Jaccaci.

27. WBF to GHF, January 8, 1919, File 16, Box 58, FFP

28. GHF to WBF, February 13, 1918, File 8, Box 12, FFP.

29. Ibid. February 2, 1919, File 8, Box 12, FFP.

30. WBF to GHF, Ibid. November 4, 1918, File 15, and January 21, 1919, File 16, Box 58, FFP.

31. Ibid., January 21, 1919, File 16, Box 58, FFP.

32. Ibid., April 18, 1919.

33. Ibid., April 22, 1919, File 16, Box 58, FFP.

34. Ibid., May 14, 1919, and May 6, 1919, File 16, Box 58, FFP.

35. GHF to WBF, April 10, 1919, and April 23, 1919, File 16, Box 12, FFP.

CHAPTER VI

1. GHF's correspondence with publishers and critics, File 91, Box 18, FFP.

2. Theodore Peterson, *Magazines in the Twentieth Century* (Urbana, University of Illinois Press, 1964), 143–148.

3. Metro Pictures to "Mr. G. H. Flandrau," November 25, 1919, File 91, Box 18, FFP.

4. "Dukes and Diamonds," *Saturday Evening Post*, November 22, 1919; "Let That Pass," *Saturday Evening Post*, April 17, 1920; "Terry Sees Red," *Harper's Monthly,* December 1920.

5. CMF to MFS, December 8, 1919, File 25.C.11, Box 2, Charles Flandrau letters, MHS.

6. WBF to GHF, December 28, 1919, File 16, Box 58, FFP.

7. GHF to Betty Foster Vytlacil (hereafter, BFV), January 29, 1920, File 47, Box 15, FFP.

8. GHF to Paul Revere Reynolds, File 91, Publishers and Critics, Box 18, FFP.

9. GHF to W. J. Holt, autobiographical letter, File 1, Box 12, FFP.

10. Haeg, Lawrence P., *In Gatsby's Shadow*, biography of CMF, (Iowa City:University of Iowa Press, 2004), 174.

11. Hampl, Patricia, *The St. Paul Stories of F. Scott Fitzgerald*, (St. Paul: Minnesota Historical Society Press, 2004), Introduction, XIV.

12. Paul Revere Reynolds to GHF, File 91, "Publishers and Critics", Box 18, FFP.

13. GHF to BFV, December 27, 1920, File 21, Box 13, FFP.

14. Ibid., December 29, 1920, File 21, Box 13, FFP.

15. TPR to WBF and GHF, September 14, 1920 and April 19, 1921, microfilm reel 40, File 2, Box 76, FFP.

16. MSH to GHF, February 18, 1920, File 36, Box 14, FFP.

17. CMF to MFS, February 23, May 17, and June 7, 1921, Charles Flandrau letters, 25.c.11, Box 2, MHS.

18. GHF to BFV, April 26, 1921, File 21, Box 13, and "publishers and critics," File 91, Box 18, FFP.

CHAPTER VII

1. CMF to MFS, September 29, 1915, Charles Flandrau letters, FFP, MHS

2. MSH to GHF, 1917–1929, File 36, Box 14, FFP.

3. WBF to GHF, File 18, Box 58, FFP.

4. Ibid., April 15, 1921, File 18, Box 58, FFP.

5. Ibid., March 28, 1921–January 30, 1922, Files 18 and 19, Box 58, FFP.

6. GHF to BFV, April 1921, File 21, Box 13, FFP.

7. Brenda Ueland to GHF, File 91, Box 16, FFP.

8. GHF to Kyle S. Crichton, December 15, 1934, File 30, Box 14, FFP.

9. TPR to GHF, April 19, 1921, File 2, Box 76, FFP.

10. WBF to GHF, January 8, 1919, File 16, Box 68, FFP.

11. CMF to MFS, May 17, 1921, Charles Flandrau letters, MHS.

12. CMF to MFS, June 7, 1921, Charles Flandrau letters, MHS.

13. GHF to BFV, undated letter, 1921, File 21, Box 13, FFP.

14. Brenda Ueland to GHF, File 59, Box 16, FFP.

15. CMF to GHF, June 8, 1925, File 7, Box 2, FFP.

16. GHF, Notes, File 471, Box 50, FFP.

CHAPTER VIII

1. WBF to GHF, December 26, 1921, File 18, Box 58, FFP.

2. Ibid., January 9, 1922, File 19, Box 58, FFP.

3. Ibid., January 13, 1922, File 19, Box 58, FFP.

4. GHF to WBF, undated letter, February 1922, File 9, Box 12, FFP.

5. WBF to GHF, January 30, 1922, File 19, Box 58, FFP.

6. Harrison Smith to GHF, January 27, 1922, File 91, Box 18, FFP.

7. Harold Paget to GHF, February 2, 1922, File 91, Box 18, FFP.

8. WBF to GHF, January 13, 1922, File 19, Box 58, FFP.

9. Ibid., January 30, 1922, File 19, Box 58, FFP.

10. Ibid., February 1, 1922, File 19, Box 58, FFP.

11. GHF to WBF, undated letter, 1923, File 10, Box 12, FFP.

12. WBF to GHF, January 30, 1922, File 19, Box 58, FFP.

13. GHF to WBF, undated letter, 1922, File 10, Box 12, FFP.

14. GHF to BFV, undated letter, 1922, File 21, Box 13, FFP.

15. Harold Paget to GHF, October 24, 1922, File 91, Box 18, FFP.

16. Carl Hovey to GHF, December 12, 1922, File 91, Box 18, FFP.

17. Ibid., December 18, 1922, File 91, Box 18, FFP.

18. Alfred Harcourt to GHF, November 22, 1922, File 91, Box 18, FFP.

19. Donald Brace to GHF, December 6, 1922, File 91, Box 18, FFP.

20. GHF to BFV, January 25, 1923, File 21, Box 13; File 76, Box 18, FFP.

21. GHF to KSC, December 15, 1934, File 30, Box 14, FFP.

22. Comments by F. Scott Fitzgerald in the *Literary Digest International*, Isabel Paterson in the *New York Herald Tribune*, and the other named critics are among dozens of favorable reviews of *Being Respectable* in File 76, Box 18, FFP.

23. Tom Boyd, "In a Corner with the Bookworm," *St. Paul Daily News*, Sun. January 28, 1923.

24. Tom Boyd to GHF, File 76, Box 18, FFP.

25. Frances Boardman, *St. Paul Pioneer Press*, Sunday, January 21, 1923.

26. CMF to GHF from Majorca, February 17, 1923 File 5, Box 2, FFP.

27. Scott Fitzgerald to GHF, undated letter, 1923, File 69, Box 17, FFP.

28. GHF to WBF, undated letter, winter, 1923, File 9, Box 12, FFP.

29. WBF to GHF, January 3, 1923, File 20, Box 59, FFP.

30. Ibid., January 30, 1923, File 20, Box 58, FFP.

31. GHF to BFV, undated letter, 1923, File 21, Box 13, FFP.

32. GHF to WBF, undated, 1924, File 10, Box 12, FFP.

33. *The Porcupine*, "Bookshop Trivia," File 76, Box 18, FFP.

34. GHF to WBF, undated letter, winter, 1923, File 9, Box 12, FFP.

35. Ibid.

36. Ibid.

37. Ibid.

38. WBF to GHF, January 3, 1923, File 20, Box 59, FFP.

39. Ibid., January 4, 1923, File 20, Box 59, FFP.

40. Ibid., February 14, 1923, File 20, Box 59, FFP.

41. Ibid., January 29, 1923, File 20, Box 59, FFP.

42. GHF to WBF, undated letter, winter, 1923, File 9, Box 12, FFP.

43. WBF to GHF, February 14, 1923, File 20, Box 59, FFP.

44. Ibid.

45. Ibid., February 20, 1923, File 20, Box 59, FFP.

46. Ibid., February 11, 1923, File 20, 1923, FFP.

47. GHF to WBF, undated letter, winter, 1923, File 9, Box 12, FFP.

48. WBF to GHF, March 1, 1923, File 20, FFP.

49. GHF to WBF, undated letter, March, 1923, File 9, Box 12, FFP.

50. Donald Brace to GHF, March 22, 1923, File 91, Box 18, FFP.

CHAPTER IX

1. John W. Riddle to GHF, March 13, 1923, File 23, Box 68, FFP.

2. Meridel Le Sueur to author, July 16, 1990.

3. GHF to BFV, March 24, 1924, File 47, Box 15, FFP.

4. GHF to WBF, undated twenty-one page letter, winter 1923, File 9, Box 12, FFP.

5. WBF to GHF, September 26, 1923, File 20, FFP

6. GHF to BFV, undated letters, fall - spring, 1923–1924, File 47, Box 15, FFP.

7. Ibid.

8. Ibid.

9. Ibid.

10. Ibid.

11. Ibid.

12. Ibid., December 29, 1923, File 47, Box 15, FFP.

13. Ibid., May 9, 1924, File 47, Box 15, FFP.

14. GHF to WBF, undated letters, winter 1924, File 10, Box 12, FFP.

15. GHF to BFV, March 24, 1924, File 47, Box 15, FFP.

16. Ibid., May 9, 1924, File 47, Box 15, FFP.

17. GHF to BFV, May 20, 1924, File 47, Box 15, FFP.

18. Ibid.

19. GHF to BFV, fall, 1923, File 47, Box 15, FFP.

20. Fan Mail/ Reviews, File 76, Box 17, FFP.

21. GHF to WBF, summer 1924, File 10, Box 12, FFP; Ralph Budd to GHF, summer 1924, File 70, Box 24, FFP.

22. GHF to WBF, summer 1924, File 10, Box 12, FFP.

23. Ibid.

24. WBF to GHF, June 2, 1924, File 21, Box 59, FFP.

25. GHF to Dorothy (Doria) Noyes, summer, 1924, File 30, Box 14, FFP.

26. Ralph Budd to GHF, fall, 1924, File 70, Box 24, FFP.

27. GHF to WBF, undated, summer 1924, File 10, Box 12, FFP.

28. GHF to BFV, undated, summer 1924, File 21, Box 13, FFP.

29. Theodate P. Riddle to GHF, spring 1924, File 23, Box 68, FFP.

30. *Minneapolis Journal*, March 4, 1923, Fan Mail/Reviews, File 76, Box 18, FFP.

31. Fan Mail/Reviews, File 78, Box 18, FFP.

32. Alice M. O'Brien to GHF, 1924, File 26, Box 14, FFP.

33. Grace Flandrau interview, *Golfer and Sportsman*, December 1934.

34. WBF to GHF, November 17, 1924, File 21, Box 59, FFP.

35. GHF to BFV, fall, 1924, File 21, Box 13, FFP.

36. GHF to BFV, late December, 1924, File 21, Box 13, FFP.

37. GHF to BFV, January 15, 1925, File 22, Box 13, FFP.

38. Nurse (for GHF) to BFV, three letters: January 29, February 3, February 10, 1925, file 21, Box 13, FFP.

39. GHF to BFV, February 25, 1925, File 22, Box 13, FFP.

40. WBF to GHF, March 12, 1925, File 22, Box 59, FFP.

41. Brenda Ueland interview of Grace Flandrau, *Golfer and Sportsman*, December 1934.

42. Ibid.

43. Kate S. Klein, interview with author, June 23, 1993.

CHAPTER X

1. CMF to WBF, February 3, 1925, File 51, Box 5, FFP.

2. CMF to GHF, January 6, 1926, File 8, Box 2, FFP.

3. L. P. Haeg, "Little Corners of Great Places," unpublished manuscript, MHS, 259.

4. CMF to GHF, August 16, 1918, "Little Corners of Great Places," by L. P. Haeg, MHS, 258.

5. CMF to James Gray, October 17, 1927, File 69, Box 5, FFP; CMF to GHF, Dec.29, 1933, File 14, Box 2, FFP.

6. James Gray, *The Penciled Frown* (New York: Scribner's, 1925).

7. Duncan Aikman to GHF, February 25, 1925, File 91, Box 18, FFP.

8. Kate S. Klein, January 23, 1993.

9. CMF to WBF, 1926, File 52, Box 5.

10. WBF to GHF, December 31, 1926, File 23, Box 59, FFP.

11. Alice M. O'Brien to GHF, undated letter, 1929, File 53, Box 16, FFP.

12. CMF to GHF, June 11, 1927, File 9, Box 2, FFP.

13. CMF to WBF, undated letters, 1927, File 53, Box 5, FFP.

14. June 28, 1927, unsigned copy of letter to GHF from Charles Scribner's Sons, Scribner's archives.

15. John S. Greenway interview with author, February 1987. Arizona Inn, Tucson, Arizona.

16. *Then I Saw the Congo* (New York: Harcourt, Brace and Company, 1929), 5.

17. Ibid., 38.

18. Ibid., 9.

19. British review, January 29, 1930, File 81, Box 18, FFP.

20. *St. Paul Dispatch*, October 9, 1936.

21. John G. Ordway to GHF, September 23, 1929, File 81, Box 18, FFP.

22. Alice M. O'Brien to GHF, undated letter, winter 1929-1930, File 26, Box 14, FFP.

23. Michels, Eileen, *Women of Minnesota*, Chapter 8, "Alice O'Brien, Volunteer and Philanthropist," 146.

CHAPTER XI

1. CMF to GHF, letters from Majorca, Spain, 1923–1925, files 5, 6, and 7, box 2, FFP.

2. CMF to REM, 1929, file 71a, box 5, FFP.

3. James Gray to CMF, January 13, 1930, James Gray and Family Papers, MHS, hereafter, Gray Papers.

4. William Rose Benét to GHF, file 69, box 17, FFP.

5. CMF to James Gray, file 69, box 5, FFP.

6. Ibid.

7. GHF to MEP, May 27, 1930, Scribner's archives.

8. MEP to GHF, June 6, 1930, Scribner's archives.

9. GHF to MEP, June 1930, file 91, box 18, FFP.

10. MEP to GHF, July 2, 1930, Scribner's archives.

11. Kyle S. Crichton to GHF, July 9, 1930, file 91, box 18, FFP.

12. MEP to GHF, July 11, 1930, file 91, box 18, FFP.

13. Kyle S. Crichton to GHF, July 17, 1930, July 17, 1930, FFP.

14. Ibid., July 22, 1930, file 91, box 18, FFP.

15. Ibid., September 23, 1930, Scribner's archives.

16. Grace Flandrau, "One Way of Love," *Scribner's* (October 1930), 19.

17. CMF to GHF, September 20, 1930, file 11, box 2, FFP.

18. Kyle S. Crichton to GHF, October 23, 1930, file 91, box 18, FFP.

19. CMF to GHF, September 20, 1930, file 11, box 2, FFP.

20. James Gray to CMF, undated [fall, 1930?], Gray Papers, MHS.

21. GHF to Theodate Pope Riddle, October 8, 1930, Hill-Stead Museum Archives.

22. CMF to REM, file 71a, box 5, FFP.

23. GHF to WBF, undated letter, fall 1931, file 11, box 13, FFP.

24. WBF to GHF, April 17, 1932, file 27, box 59, FFP.

25. Ibid., January 10, 1931, file 26, box 59, FFP.

26. CMF to WBF, January 31, 1931, file 57, box 5, FFP.

27. GHF and WBF letters, 1930–1932, FFP; GHF and WBF to Richard E. and Alice Lee Myers, 1931–1932, mss. 27, series I, file 49, box 4, Richard W. and Alice Lee Herrick Myers Papers, Beineke Rare Books Library, Yale University (hereafter, Myers papers).

28. GHF to WBF, undated, fall 1931, file 11, box 13, FFP.

29. See note 27.

30. *A Literate Passion: letters of Anais Nin and Henry Miller, 1932–1953*, edited by Gunther Stuhlmann (New York: Harcourt Brace Jovanovich, 1987), 48.

31. CMF to GHF, January 6, 1923, file 5, box 2, FFP.

32. GHF to WBF, undated, fall 1931, file 11, box 13, FFP.

33. Ibid., November, 1931, file 11, box 13, FFP.

34. GHF to Alice Lee Myers, November 18, 1931, file 50, box 4, Myers Papers.

35. GHF to REM, Aug. 25, 1932, file 49, box 4, Myers Papers.

36. GHF to WBF, November 31, file 11, box 13, FFP.

37. CMF to WBF, undated letter, November 1931, file 57, box 5, FFP.

38. *London Times*, December 10, 1931.

39. CMF to JG, October 10, 1929, file 69, box 5, FFP.

40. Ibid., October 10, 1929, file 69, box 5, FFP.

41. Ibid., February 21, 1929, file 69, box 5, FFP.

42. JG to CMF, October 1, 1931, box 3, Gray Papers.

43. Ibid., September 14, 1931, box 3, Gray Papers.

44. CMF to JG, March 17, 1932, file 69, box 5, FFP.

CHAPTER XII

1. KSC to GHF, January 12, 1932, Scribner's archives.

2. GHF to REM, February 24, 1932, file 50, box 4, Myers papers.

3. MEP to GHF, February 2, 1932, Scribner's archive.

4. Ibid., Mar. 21, 1932, file 91, box 18, FFP.

5. JSG, interview with author, February 1987.

6. WBF to GHF, April, 1932, file 27, box 50, FFP.

7. Ibid., May 27, 1932, file 27, box 50, 1932.

8. Ibid., June 6, 1932, file 27, box 50, FFP.

9. GHF to REM, summer, 1932, file 51, box 16, FFP.

10. Ibid., July 5, 1932, file 50, box 4, Myers papers.

11. James Gray to CMF, June 7, 1932, box 3, Gray papers; GHF to James Gray, 1932, file 2, Box 3, Gray papers.

12. Kyle S. Crichton was an ardent Communist sympathizer in the 1930s when he was associate editor for *Scribner's* and *Collier's* and also wrote reviews for *Life*. In that era, under the pseudonym "Robert Forsythe," he wrote articles for *The New Masses* and *The Daily Worker*, a collection later published as *Redder Than the Rose*. Crichton's son, Andrew Crichton, believes his father was never a card-carrying Communist.

13. GHF to REM, April 19, 1932, file 50, box 4, Myers papers.

14. Ibid., undated letter, 1932, file 51, box 16, FFP.

15. GHF to ALM, June 4, 1932, file 50, box 4, Myers papers.

16. GHF to KSC, undated letters, (summer?), 1932, Scribner's archive.

17. GHF letters to REM, July 18, 1932, file 50, box 16, Myers papers.

18. Ibid.

19. Ibid.

20. Theodate P. Riddle to GHF, November 9, 1930, file 2, box 76, FFP.

21. WBF to GHF, May 13, 1932, file 27, box 59, FFP.

22. Ibid., April 3, June 16 and June 22, file 27, box 59, FFP.

23. GHF to WBF, undated letter, summer, 1932, file 11, box 13, FFP.

24. William Hodson obituary story, *Minneapolis Tribune*, January 21, 1943.

25. Muriel Nelson and Corrin Hodgson: telephone interview with author, October 24, 1992.

26. Mary Griggs Burke, interview with author, Cable, Wisconsin, September 4, 1994.

27. WBF to GHF, May 8, 1932, file 27, box 59, FFP.

28. Mary Griggs Burke, interview with author, Cable, Wisconsin, September 4, 1994.

29. GHF to WBF, undated letters, November 1931, file 11, box 13, FFP.

30. WBF to GHF, undated, (April ?), 1932, file 27, box 59, FFP.

31. GHF to REM, undated, (July ?), 1932

32. Ibid.

33. GHF to WBF, undated, (fall?) 1932, file 27, box 59, FFP.

34. *St. Paul Dispatch*.

CHAPTER XIII

1. CMF to REM, file 71a, box 5, FFP.

2. GHF to MEP, January 21, 1932, Scribner's archives.

3. MEP to GHF, January 25, 1933, Scribner's archives.

4. GHF to JWR and TPR, undated letter (1933?), file 23, box 68, FFP.

5. WBF to JWR, undated letter, (1933?), file 23, box 68, FFP.

6. GHF to JWR and TPR, undated letter (1933?), box 68, FFP.

7. MEP to GHF, May 8, 1933, Scribner's archives.

8. GHF to MEP, May 20, 1934, Scribner's archives.

9. WBF to GHF, June 22, 1932, file 27; July 19, 1933, file 28, box 59, FFP.

10. CMF to GHF, Aug. 18, 1929, file 2, box 10, FFP.

11. WBF to GHF, Aug. 4, 1933, file 28, box 59, FFP.

12. Ibid., Aug. 29,1933, file 28, box 59, FFP.

13. Ibid.

14. James Gray, *St. Paul Dispatch*, Thursday, July 27, 1933.

15. GHF to MEP, September 7, 1933, Scribner's archives.

16. Meridel Le Sueur, interview with author, July 16, 1990, Hudson, Wisconsin.

17. Ibid.

18. Meridel Le Sueur's postcard to author, February 12, 1990, author's possession.

19. Brenda Ueland Diaries and Logs, MHS collections, March 9, 1935, MHS.

20. James Gray, "Among Those We Know," *Golfer and Sportsman*, May 1934.

21. Meridel Le Sueur, interview with author, July 16, 1990.

22. Meridel Le Sueur to GHF, date unknown, file 69, Box 17, FFP; Ibid., aside, p. 178.

23. GHF to Kyle S. Crichton, (draft) fall, 1933, file 30, box 14, FFP.

24. GHF to WBF, undated letter, winter, 1934 (file 11, box 13, FFP.

25. WBF to GHF, undated letter, winter, 1934, file 28, box 59, FFP.

26. GHF to WBF, undated letter, winter, 1934 , file 11, box 13, FFP.

27. Alfred Dashiell to GHF, November 2, 1934, Scribner's archives.

28. GHF: draft for plot of *Indeed This Flesh*, undated, (summer, 1934?), file 91, box 18.

29. *Indeed This Flesh*, 256-261.

30. *The Daily Oklahoman*, June 8, 1934, file 79, Box 18, FFP.

31. *New Yorker*, date unknown, file 79, box 18, FFP.

32. James Gray, *St. Paul Pioneer Press*, May 4, 1934.

33. Kyle S. Crichton – GHF correspondence, file 30, box 14, FFP.

34. Kay Boyle to GHF, file 42, box 14, FFP.

35. *Indeed This Flesh*, 12.

36. MEP to GHF, Aug. 7, 1934 and November 1, 1934, Scribner's archives.

CHAPTER XIV

1. CMF to GHF, June 8, 1925, file 7, box 2, FFP; L. P. Haeg, "Little Corners of Great Places, The Private Life of Charles Macomb Flandrau," MHS, 278.

2. James Gray to GHF, undated letter, probably October 1934, file 49, box 15, FFP.

3. See Appendix A, author's notes, p. 284.

4. Kay Boyle to GHF, June 10, 1934, and October 26, 1954, file 42, box 15, FFP.

5. Kay Boyle to GHF, October 25, 1936, file 42, box 15, FFP.

6. Kay Boyle to GHF, 1930s, file 42, box 15, FFP.

7. GHF's undated correspondence with MEP and KSC, early 1930s, Scribner's archives.

8. GHF to KSC, undated, 1930's, file I, box 50, Scribner's archives.

9. GHF to MEP, undated letter, 1935, file I, box 50, Scribner's archives.

10. MEP to GHF, February 3, 1936, file II, box 50, Scribner's archives.

11. GHF to WBF, undated letter, file II, box 13, FFP.

12. GHF to MEP, undated letter, winter, 1936, file II, box 50, Scribner's archives.

13. GHF to WBF, undated letter, winter, 1936, file II, box 13, FFP.

14. WBF to GHF, January 30, 1936, file 30, box 59, FFP.

15. WBF to GHF, February 13, 1936, file 30, box 59, FFP.

16. MEP to GHF, Aug. 21, 1936, file II, box 50, Scribner's archives.

17. Jessie G. Ordway to GHF, June 6, 1936, file 86, box 18, FFP.

18. John K. Donohue to KSTP, 1936, file 86, box 18, FFP.

19. John Sherman, *The Minneapolis Star*, October 10, 1936, file 82, box 18, FFP.

20. James Gray, *St. Paul Dispatch*, October 9, 1936, file 82, box 18, FFP.

21. Brenda Ueland, *Golfer and Sportsman*, October (?), 1936, file 82, box 18, FFP.

22. *Philadelphia Inquirer*, October (?), 1936, file 82, box 18, FFP.

23. *Graphic*, Greenwich, CT, December 2, 1936, file 82, box 18, FFP.

24. MEP to GHF, July 17, 1935, file I, box 50, Scribner's archives.

25. GHF to MEP, (Oct. 1936?), file II, box 50, Scribner's archives.

26. MEP to GHF, MEP to GHF, October 13, 1936, file II, box 50, Scribner's archives.

27. GHF to MEP, undated, prob. late October 1936, file II, box 50, Scribner's archives.

28. Drafts for "Child Memories," file 139, box 22; "Memories of a French Convent," files 210 and 211, and "Mexican Reminiscences," file 212, box 26, FFP.

29. MEP to GHF, November 8, 1937, file II, box 50, Scribner's archives

30. GHF to WBF, undated letter, 1936, file 11, box 13, FFP.

31. See note 27, Chap. XV (documents GHF's 1936 visit with AA counselor/ fund raiser E.V. Steele in Farmington).

32. WBF to CMF, October 29, 1991 (eg., at sixteen, drinking a quart of beer at every meal on a hunting trip.), file 3, box 58, FFP.

33. GHF to WBF, undated letter, file 11, box 13, FFP.

34. WBF to GHF, file 30, box 59, FFP.

35. Ibid., undated letter, April, 1937, file 31, box 59, FFP.

36. Ibid., April 13, 1937, file 31, box 59, FFP.

37. Ibid., undated letter, April, 1937, file 31, FFP.

38. GHF to WBF, undated letter, April 1937, file 11, box 13, FFP.

39. CMF to JWR, December 29, 1937, file 64, box 5, FFP.

39. GHF to JWR, November 11, 1937, file 15, box 13, FFP.

40. Milton Griggs to GHF, January 5, 1939, file 95, box 19, FFP.

41. MEP to GHF, December 6, 1938, file 91, box 18, FFP.

CHAPTER XV

1. William J. McNally to GHF, December 19, 1938, file 69, box 17, FFP.

2. GHF to James and Sophie Gray, undated, prob. early 1939, file 22, box 13, FFP.

3. GHF, Notes/Diaries, file 471, box 50, FFP.

4. Brenda Ueland to GHF, June 29, 1939, file 91, box 16, FFP.

5. GHF, Notes/Diaries, summer, 1939, file 471, box 50, FFP.

6. GHF, Notes/Diaries, summer, 1939, file 471, box 50, FFP.

7 . "A Night in Wamba," *Under the Sun* (New York: Charles Scribner's Sons, 1936), 83.

8. GHF, Notes/Diaries, summer 1939, file 471, box 50, FFP.

9. Brenda Ueland to GHF, September 7, 1939, file 59, box 16, FFP.

10. Kate S. Klein to author, June 23, 1993.

11. GHF, Notes/Diaries, summer, 1939, file 471, box 50, FFP.

12. Ibid.

13. Ibid.

14. Ibid.

15. *Minneapolis Times-Tribune*, September 21, 1939.

16. *Minnesota History,* Vol. XXII, March, 1941.

17. Richard E. Myers to GHF, January 14, 1941, file 21, box 16, FFP.

18. Kay Boyle to GHF, early 1942, file 42, box 14, FFP.

19. Author's interviews with Constance S. Otis and Mary Griggs Burke, late 1990s.

20. "Princess," *New Yorker*, May 16, 1942.

21. "What Do You See, Dear Enid?" *New Yorker*, September 26, 1942.

22. GHF, Notes/Diaries, c. 1945, file 471, box 50, FFP.

23. GHF's column, *St. Paul Pioneer Press*, "Fitzgerald Panegyric Inspires Some Queries," September 9, 1945.

24. Joe Macgaheran to GHF, undated, file 89, box 18, FFP; Kate S. Klein to author, June 23, 1993.

25. Franklin P. Adams to GHF, October 1942, file 96, box 19, FFP.

26. *Philosophical Review*, Vol. XLV, March, 1936.

27. Ted Steele (E.V.) to GHF, undated, file 58, box 16, FFP.

28. JSG to author, interviews in Tucson, Arizona, February 1987 and Feb.1988.

29. Ted (E.V.) Steele to GHF, undated, file 58, box 16, FFP.

30. Ibid.

31. Joseph Warren Beach to James S. Gray, Mar. 26, 1942, file 4, box 3, James Gray Papers, Minnesota Historical Society.

32. GHF–Alice O'Brien correspondence, file 26, box 14, and file 53, box 16, FFP.

33. Kay Boyle to GHF, November 13, 1934, file 42, box 14, FFP.

34. Ibid., March 29, 1941, file 42, box 14, FFP.
35. GHF to Kay Boyle, undated, file 17, Box 13, FFP.
36. 37. Earnest Seeman to GHF, file 57, box 16; Frederick Faust to GHF, file 46, box 15; Isabel Paterson to GHF, file 54, box 16, FFP.
38. GHF to Theodate P. Riddle, undated (1940?), file 16, box 13, FFP.
39. GHF, Notes/Diaries, c. 1940, file 471, box 50, FFP.

CHAPTER XVI

1. REM to GHF, undated, early 1940s, file 51, box 16, FFP.
2. William Hodson obituary, *Minneapolis Tribune*, January 21, 1943.
3. Kent Curtiss to GHF, undated, 1940's, file 44, box 15, FFP.
4. GHF to Kent Curtiss, undated, 1940s, file 19, box 13, FFP.
5. Author's interviews and correspondence with Sandra Wheeler and Polly Pasternak, archivists, Hill-Stead Museum, Farmington, CT, June 1988-2003.
6. Kate S. Klein's interviews with author, St. Paul, 1984, 1986, 1989, 1992.
7. Isabel Paterson to GHF, undated (1940s), file 54, box 16, FFP.
8. John S. Greenway's annual interviews with author, Tucson, Arizona, 1987–1993.
9. Ibid.
10. Ibid.
11. Alice O'Brien to GHF, February 27, 1948, file 63, box 16, FFP.
12. Fan letter to GHF, 1948, file 87, box 18, FFP.
13. Edward V. (Ted) Steele to GHF, June 27, 1947, file 58, box 16, FFP.
14. Kay Boyle to GHF, undated, (late 1952 ?), file 42, box 14, FFP.
15.Grace Flandrau to Edward V. Steele, undated, c. 1953, file 29, box 14, FFP.

CHAPTER XVII

1. Anna R. Hodson's date of death was July 25, 1950 (Hennepin County death records).
2. GHF to Edward V. Steele, undated, 1950's, file 29, box 14, FFP.
3. Ibid.
4. GHF to Edward V. Steele, November 10, 1953, file 29, box 14, FFP.
5. Kay Boyle to GHF, Aug. 5, 1950, file 42, box 14, FFP.
6. Kay Boyle to GHF, Aug. 14, 1951, file 42, box 14, FFP
7. Kay Boyle to GHF, Aug. 1, 1954, file 42, box 14, FFP.
8. GHF to Alice M. O'Brien, undated (early 1950's), file 53, box 16, FFP. (Misfiled?)
9. Alice O'Brien to GHF, undated (early 1950's), file 63, box 16, FFP.
10.GHF to Alice M. O'Brien, undated (1953?), file 53, box 16, FFP (Misfiled?).
11. Kate S. Klein to author, interview in St. Paul, June 23, 1993.
12. Meridel LeSeuer to author, interview in Hudson, Wisconsin, July 16, 1990.
13. L. P. Haeg, *In Gatsby's Shadow* (Iowa City: University of Iowa Press, 2004), 168.
14. "Chapter of a Life," file 137, box 22, FFP.
15. GHF to Richard E. Myers, Aug. 6, 1952, file 49, box 4, RE and Alice Lee Myers Papers, YCAL MSS\27, Beinecke Rare Books Library, New Haven, CT (hereafter, Meyers Papers).
16. GHF to Alice M. O'Brien, undated, 1950s, file 26, box 14, FFP.

17. Patricia Hampl, "The Smile of Accomplishment: Sylvia Plath's Ambition," *I Could Tell You Stories* (New York: W.W. Norton & Company, 1999), 129 –165.

18. Based on comments to author by Flandrau friends and associates interviewed in the late 1980s and early 1990s.

19. Simone Weil quote in "Smile of Accomplishment II," from Hampl's *I Could Tell You Stories*, 145-146.

20. Ibid., 145-146.

21. Brenda Ueland to GHF, September 7, 1939, file 59, box 16, FFP.

22. Hampl, "The Smile of Accomplishment: Sylvia Plath's Ambition," 143.

23. GHF to Alice M. O'Brien, file 53, box 16, FFP.

24. Thomond O'Brien (nephew of Alice M. O'Brien) to author, interview in St. Paul, 1987.

25. David Daniels, telephone interview with author, fall, 1998.

26. Alice M. O'Brien to GHF, file 53, box 16, FFP.

27. GHF to Alice M. O'Brien, undated (1950s),file 53, box 16, FFP. (misfiled?)

CHAPTER XVIII

1. GHF to Jack Greenway, undated (1950s), file 13, box 13, FFP.

2. Ibid.

3. Author's annual interviews with JSG at Arizona Inn, 1987–1993, esp. February 2, 1987.

4. JSG to GHF, file 35, box 14, FFP.

5. GHF to JSG, undated, (1958–1960?), file 13, box 13, FFP.

6. Ibid., undated (1962 ?), file 13, box 13, FFP.

7. Ibid., December 7, (1960s?), file 13, FFP.

8. JSG to GHF, 1954, file 35, box 14, FFP.

9. GHF to JSG, undated, file 13, box 13, FFP; GHF to University of Minnesota Press, July 14, 1952, file 91, box 18, FFP.

10. GHF to JSG, undated (1954?), file 35, box 13, FFP.

11. "Random Recollections of Grace Flandrau," unpublished essay by Blair Klein, 1994, author's possession.

12. Kate K. Piper to author, several interviews, 2000–2005.

13. GHF to JSG, undated (1960–1961?), file 13, box 13, FFP.

14. GHF to Alice O'Brien, undated (1953- 1954?), FFP.

15. GHF to John Parsons, trustee, Avon Old Farms School for Boys, April 6, 1950, files 65 and 66, box 17, FFP; author's telephone interview with John Parsons, 92, 1988.

16. GHF correspondence with Wilmarth ("Lefty") Lewis, file 50, box 15, and file 23, box 16, FFP.

17. GHF to JSG, undated (mid-1950's?), file 13, box 13, FFP.

18. Ibid.

19. Charles Breasted to GHF, October 23, 1954, file 31, box 14, FFP.

20. Richard E. Myers to GHF, July 5, 1955, file 51, box 16, FFP.

21. GHF to JSG, undated (early 1960's?), file 35, box 14, FFP.

22. Alice O'Brien–GHF correspondence, 1941–1957, file 53, box 16, FFP;

23. GHF to JSG, undated, (early 1960's?), file 35, box 14, FFP.

24. GHF to Craig Reynold re Lucile Willis, March 24, 1962, file 28, box14, FFP.

25. GHF to John and Katrine Parsons, undated (1955), file 30, box 14, FFP.

26. GHF to Martha Breasted, undated, (1955?), file 3, box 12, FFP.

27. GHF to JSG and Martha Breasted, undated (late 1950s?), file 13, box 13, FFP.

28. Ibid.

29. GHF to Philip Wylie, June 7, (1961?), file 30, box 14, FFP.

30. GHF to Craig Reynold re Lucile, undated (1961?), file 28, box 14, FFP.

31. Alice O'Brien—GHF correspondence, 1941- 1957, file 53, box 16, FFP.

32. GHF to Charles Breasted, undated (late 1950s?), file 3, box 12, FFP.

CHAPTER XIX

1. JSG to author, interview at Arizona Inn, August 25, 1993.

2. "Today's Personality," *Minneapolis Tribune*, interview with Grace Flandrau, August ? 1962.

3. GHF–Patty Ferguson Doar correspondence, late 1950s, file 4, box 12, and file 34, box 14, FFP.

4. Martha Ferguson Breasted, interviews with author, February 14 -15, 1990, Tucson, Arizona.

5. Saranne King Neumann, interview with author, February 16, 1990, Tucson, Arizona.

6. "Today's Personality," *Minneapolis Tribune*, interview with GF (see 2.)

7. GHF to JSG, undated (summer 1962 ?), file 35, box 14, FFP.

8. E. V. Steel to GHF, file 68, box 16, FFP.

9. Ida _____ to GHF, November 1962, FFP.

10. Rochester health report, FFP.

11. GHF–Craig Reynolds correspondence, file 39, box 14, FFP.

12. Ann (Snow) Wooden Rush to author, interviews 1991 and 1992, Tucson.

13. JSG's annual interviews with author, 1987–1991. Arizona Inn, Tucson, Arizona.

14. Author's telephone interview with John Parsons, June, 1988, Farmington, Conn.

15. GHF to John Parsons, April 6, 1950.

16. Ingeborg Carlson to author, interview in Hartford, Conn.., June 1993.

17. JSG to author, 1987–1991, Arizona Inn, Tucson, Arizona.

Bibliography

Published Works Of Grace Hodgson Flandrau
(From Fulton Brylawski's copyright list, expanded by Georgia Ray, 1998)

Books
Cousin Julia. D. Appleton and Company, August 24, 1917.
Being Respectable. Harcourt, Brace and Company, Inc., January 25, 1923.
Entranced. Harcourt, Brace and Company, October 23, 1924.
Then I Saw The Congo. Harcourt, Brace and Company, September 9, 1929.
Indeed This Flesh. Harrison Smith and Robert Haas, May 14, 1934.
Under The Sun. Charles Scribner's Sons, October 9, 1936.

Short Fiction, Historical Journalism, Essays, Travel Writing, Reviews
"Josefina Maria," *Sunset*, 1912 (copy in Grace Flandrau's Papers)
"The Arrangement," *McClure's*, 1916 or 1917
"The Stranger In His House," *McClure's*, September 9, 1918, 50:11.
"Dukes And Diamonds," *Saturday Evening Post*, November 22, 1919, 192:21.
"Making Fine Birds," *Ainslee's*, January, 1920.
"Let That Pass," *Saturday Evening Post*, April 17, 1920, 192:42.
"Who's Who And Why," *Saturday Evening Post*, July 17, 1920, 193:3 (self-written profile;
    photo by Wiebmer, St. Paul).
"Terry Sees Red," *Harper's Monthly Magazine*, Dec. 1920, 142: 847.
"Rubies In Crystal," The *Smart Set*, February 1921, 65:2.
"A Path Of Gold (Aka Ludlow's Luck)," *Hearst's International*, February 1923.
Astor And The Oregon Country. Great Northern Railway, c. 1927
Frontier Days Along The Upper Missouri. Great Northern Railway, c. 1927.
A Glance At The Lewis And Clark Expedition. Great Northern Railway," 1925.
Historic Northwest Adventureland. Great Northern Railway, c. 1927.
Koo-koo-sint, The Star Man. Great Northern Railway, c. 1925.
The Oriental And Captain Palmer. Great Northern Railway, c.1924.
Red River Trails. Great Northern Railway, c. 1925.
Seven Sunsets. Great Northern Railway, c. 1925.
The Story of Marias Pass. Great Northern Railway, c. 1925.
The Verendrye Overland Quest of the Pacific. Great Northern Railway, 1925. (Reprinted
    in *Quarterly Of The Oregon Historical Society*, June 1925)
"St. Paul, The St. Untamable Twin," in *The Taming Of The Frontier*, Duncan Aikman,
    editor. New York: Milton, Balch & Company, October 25, 1925.
"Black Potentates Of Equitorial Africa," *Travel*, September, 1929.
"What Africa Is Not," *Contemporary Review*, December, 1930.
"One Way of Love," *Scribner's*, October, 1930, 88:4.
"Faith," *Scribner's*, February, 1931, 89:2.

"The Happiest Time," *Scribner's*, June 1932, 41:6.

"What Was Truly Mine," *Scribner's*, August, 1932, 42:2.

"She Was Old," *Scribner's*, September, 1932, 42:2.

"Affair of the Senses," *Scribner's*, October, 1932, 40:4.

"Nothing Left," *Collier's*, August 19, 1933.

"Great Life," *Scribner's*, August, 1933, 44:2..

"Giver of the Grape," *Scribner's*, September, 1934, 46:3.

"Return to Mexico," *Scribner's*, December, 1934 And January, 1935; 97:6 and 98:1.

"Gentlefolk," *Scribner's*, Dec. 1935, 48:6.

"Going to the Lake," *Scribner's*, June, 1936, Vol. Xcix, No. 6.

"Bitter Passion," *Scribner's*, July, 1936, 100:1.

"Speaking of Cats And Dogs," *Harper's*, July, 1937.

"Daughter," *Pictorial Review*, March, 1938.

"To Lose One's Life," *Good Housekeeping*, February, 1940.

"Nice Man," *Harper's*, January, 1942.

"Princess," *New Yorker*, May 16, 1942.

"What Do You See, Dear Enid?" *New Yorker*, September 26, 1942.

"All the Modern Conveniences," *New Yorker*, April 3, 1943.

"A Frenchwoman, Too," *Collier's*, April 24, 1943.

"Beyond Price," *Collier's*, February 26, 1944.

"White Horse," *Collier's*, July 14, 1945.

"Week's Work," *Colliers*, July 14, 1945.

"Fiesta in St. Paul," *Yale Review*, September 1943.

"Evil People and the Good," *Scholastic Magazine*, February 21, 1944.

"Palm Beach Soldier," *McCall's*, December 1944

Review of *Glass House* by Carleton Beale: *Saturday Review of Literature*, April 9, 1938, 17:25.

"St. Paul: The Personality of a City," *Minnesota History*, March 1941 (originally a speech at the MHS Annual Meeting in 1941).

"Light on Mexico," *Yale Review*, March, 1948 (Book Review)

"Why Don't We Tell Europe Our Story?" *Saturday Evening Post*, April, 1948

"On What it is to be French," *American Quarterly*, Spring 1949.

"Minnesota," *Holiday*, August 1955.

"Profile of Charles Eugene Flandrau," Speech at rhe MHS Annual Meeting in New Ulm, August, 1962.

Anthologies

O'Brien, Edward, editor. *The Best Short Stories Of 1932*. New York: Dodd and Mead, 1932 (includes F. Scott Fitzgerald's "Crazy Sunday" and Grace Flandrau's "She Was Old.").

O'Brien, Edward J. editor. *The Best Short Stories Of 1933*. New York, Houghton Mifflin Co., 1933. (includes Grace Flandrau's "What Was Truly Mine.")

Uzzell, T. H. editor. *Short Story Hits*, 1932-1933. New York, Harcourt, Brace, Inc., 1933-1934. (includes Grace Flandrau's "She Was Old").

Smart Set Anthology Of World Famous Authors. N.Y., Halcyon House, 1934 (includes Grace Flandrau's "Rubies In Crystal").

Boyle, Kay, and Laurence Vail, editors. *365 Days.* New York: Harcourt, Brace & Company, 1936 (includes "Nine Fictional Sketches on Post-revolutionary Mexico").

Ervin, Jean, editor. *North Country Reader.* Saint Paul: Minnesota Historical Society Press, 2000.

Foley, Martha, editor. *The Best Short Stories Of 1943*: Boston, Houghton Mifflin Co.,1943 (includes Grace Flandrau's "What Do You See, Dear Enid?").

Flanagan, John T. editor. *America is West: An Anthology of Middlewestern Life and Literature.* Minneapolis: University of Minnesota Press, 1945.

Richards, Carmen Nelson, and Genevieve Rose Breen, editors. *Minnesota Writes.* Minneapolis: The Lund Press, 1945.

Publications

Berg, Scott A. *Max Perkins: Editor of Genius.* New York: E. P. Dutton, 1978.

Birkinbine, John. "Our Neighbor, Mexico." *National Geographic* (May 1911).

Bruccoli, Matthew J. *The Short Stories of F. Scott Fitzgerald* (incomplete information)

Bruccoli, Matthew J. *The Correspondence of F. Scott Fitzgerald* (incomplete information)

Christianson, Theodore. *History of Minnesota: A History of the State and Its People*, Vol. IV. Chicago and New York: The American Historical Society, Inc., 1935.

Conn, Peter. *Literature in America.* Cambridge, England: The Press Syndicate of the University of Cambridge, Cambridge University Press, 1989.

Cowley, Malcolm. "Unshaken Friend." The *New Yorker* (April 1944).

Cowley, Malcolm. *Exile's Return.* New York: Viking Press, 1951.

Cowley, Malcolm, ed. *After the Genteel Tradition: American Writers Since 1910.* Gloucester, Massachusetts: Peter Smith, 1959.

Donaldson, Scott. *Fool for Love: F. Scott Fitzgerald.* New York: Congdon and Weed, Inc., 1983.

Dreiser, Theodore. *Jennie Gerhard.* New York and London: World Publishing Company, 1926.

Dreiser, Theodore. *Sister Carrie.* Cleveland: World Publishing Company, 1927.

Fitzgerald, F. Scott. "Echoes of the Jazz Age," in *The Crack Up.* New York: New Directions, 1945.

Flanagan, John T. "Thirty Years of Minnesota Fiction, *Minnesota History,* 31 (September 1950), 129.

Flandrau, Charles M. *Harvard Episodes,* Boston, Copeland and Day, 1897.

————————— *The Diary of a Freshman.* Philadelphia, Curtis Publishing Company, 1900.

————————— *Viva Mexico!* New York: D. Appleton and Company, 1908.

————————— *Prejudices.* New York, D. Appleton and Company, 1912.

————————— *Loquacities.* New York, D. Appleton and Company, 1931.

————————— *Sophomores Abroad.* New York, D. Appleton and Company, 1935.

Francis, Claude and Gontier, Fernande. *Creating Colette.* South Royalton, Vermont: Steerforth Press, 1999.

Fridley, Russell. "Attorney at War." *Minnesota History* (Summer 1962).

Gallagher, Brian. *Anything Goes: A Biography of Neysa McMein.* New York: Times Books, 1987.

Gray, James (books):

_____ *The Penciled Frown.* New York: Scribner's Sons, 1925.

_____ *Shoulder the Sky.* New York: G. P. Putnam's Sons. 1935.

_____ *Wake and Remember.* .

_____ *Wings of Great Desire.* New York: MacMillan Company, 1938.

_____ *Vagabond Path.* New York: MacMillan Company, 1941. A fictionalized biography of Charles M. Flandrau.

Gray, James. (articles)

_____ "Charles Macomb Flandrau," *St. Paul Magazine,* March, 1932, 18.

_____ "Among Those We Know," (profile of Charles M. Flandrau), *Golfer and Sportsman,* December, 1933.

_____ "The Minnesota Muse," (article about Minnesota writers). *Saturday Review of Literature,* 16:7, Ju e12, 1937, 3 — 4.

Haeg, Lawrence Peter. "Little Corners of Great Places," unpublished biography of Charles Macomb Flandrau, Minnesota Historical Society Collections.

Hampl, Patricia. *I Could Tell You Stories,* New York: W.W. Norton, 1999

Hewitt, Mark. "Hill-Stead, Farmington, Connecticut: The Making of a Colonial Revival House." *Antiques* (October 1988).

Hobson, Fred. *Mencken, A Life.* New York: Random House, 1994.

Lynn, Kenneth S. *Hemingway.* New York: Simon and Schuster, 1987.

McCullough, David C. *Mornings on Horseback.* New York: Simon and Schuster, 1981.

Mott, Frank Luther. *A History of American Magazines: Sketches of Twenty-one Magazines,* Vol. V. Cambridge, Massachusetts: The Belknap Press of the Harvard University Press, 1968.

Peterson, Theodore. *Magazines in the Twentieth Century.* Urbana, Illinois: University of Illinois Press, 1964.

Showalter, Joseph. "Mexico and the Mexicans." *National Geographic* (May 1914).

Skrief, D. P. "Viva Flandrau." *Twin Cities* (February, 1956).

Stuhler, Barbara, and Gretchen Kreuter, eds. *Women of Minnesota: Selected Biographical Essays.* St. Paul: Minnesota Historical Society Press, 1977.

Stuhlmann, Gunther, ed. *A Literate Passion: Letters of Anais Nin and Henry Miller.* New York, San Diego, London: Harcourt, Brace, Jovanovich, 1987.

Ueland, Brenda. "Among Those We Know." *Golfer and Sportsman* 15:9 (December 1934).

Weingarten, Renee. *The Double Life of George Sand.* New York: Basic Books, Inc., 1978.

Wharton, Edith. *Ethan Frome.* New York: Charles Scribner's Sons, 1911.

Wharton, Edith. *House of Mirth.* New York: Houghton Mifflin Company, 1905.

Wharton, Edith. *A Backward Glance.* New York: William R. Tyler, 1934, 1935.

Wood, James Playsted. *Magazines in the United States.* New York: The Ronald Press, 1971.

Archival Research

Sylvia Beach Papers, Firestone Library, Princeton, New Jersey (1950s correspondence between Grace Flandrau and Sylvia Beach.)

Beinecke Archive, Yale University, New Haven, Connecticut. (Richard E. and Alice Lee Myers Papers. These papers contain correspondence with Grace Flandrau, Charles M. Flandrau, John Gielgud, Nadia Boulanger, F. Scott Fitzgerald,

Paul Mellon and other prominent figures in artistic circles, 1920—1950)

Flandrau Family Papers, Arizona Historical Society, Tucson, Arizona.

Hamline University Archives, St. Paul (re: Edward J. Hodgson and family).

Minneapolis Public Library, Minneapolis history collection, clipping file on Charles Eugene Flandrau and Grace H. Flandrau.

Minnesota Historical Society Collections, St. Paul, Minnesota.

Charles Scribner's Sons Archive, Firestone Library, Princeton, New Jersey (Containing more than 200 letters between Scribner's editors Maxwell E. Perkins, Kyle S. Crichton, and Alfred Dashiell and Grace Flandrau: excellent source for information on the quality of her writing, their expectations, etc.).

St. Paul Public Library clipping file on Grace Flandrau.

Acknowledgments

THE RECONSTRUCTION of Grace Flandrau's scattered, buried, disputed story would have been impossible without the encouragement and assistance of a number of people and institutions over nearly twenty years. For their help I am very grateful.

Although I first dipped my toe into the almost forgotten author's saga in 1983 after discovering the Grace H. Flandrau Planetarium in Tucson, Arizona, it wasn't until 1987 that I launched the serious investigation that led to ten years of research in eight archival collections in four states. Many interviews helping to restore the author's persona took place with Flandrau and Hodgson descendents and their friends in St. Paul, Cable, Wisconsin, Manhattan, Tucson and in Farmington, Connecticut, where Grace Flandrau lived part-time in the Gundy House for many years. Once the essential facts were in hand, documentation and interpretation of the author's surprisingly impressive but never- recorded literary achievement and touching personal saga required another ten years.

Three publishing products based on my research have preceded this biography into print: "Saving Grace," *Mpls/St. Paul*, 1998; "In Search of the Real Grace Flandrau," *Minnesota History*, 1989; and *Memoirs of Grace Flandrau*, 2003, a book presenting Flandrau's mature prose and her only autobiographical non-fiction account of her youth. Now, with interest in the long-forgotten St. Paul author reviving and evidence of the reality of her writing career reestablished, it is time to present the author's life story for the first time.

I want to acknowledge and give special thanks to archivists and librarians at the Arizona Historical Society in Tucson who assisted me as I plumbed the 9,000-document Flandrau Family Papers on yearly research trips from Minnesota to Arizona for nearly a decade. Adelaide Elm (who first catalogued the Flandrau Family Papers after their final arrival in Tucson in the early 1980s), Rose Byrne, archivist, and Riva Dean, librarian and archivist, and other Arizona Historical Society Historical Society staff have given consistent support. My long distance phone calls to Tucson from Minnesota seeking photo prints, finding aids and information have always been returned, providing the help and materials I sought.

The Minnesota Historical Society made an early grant to support my research and a number of its staff members, active and retired, have provided vital professional skills and insights over two decades to assist my work:

retired MHS Press managing editor, Jean A. Brookins, who guided my work in its early stages and line-edited this biography; Debbie Miller, research assistant; Marilyn Ziebarth and Anne R. Kaplan, *Minnesota History* editors; Steve Nielson, librarian, who has provided reliable and swift assistance in the Research Library; James Fogarty, archivist, and Lucile M. Kane, retired curator of the Minnesota Historical Society's manuscripts collection, who patiently detailed the complicated journey of the Flandrau Family Papers from just before the razing of the Flandrau House in St. Paul in 1955 to their final arrival in Tucson in 1983.

Skilled collaboration of a technical nature has come from Ellen B. Green, book packager/designer for *Memoirs of Grace Flandrau*, and tech support helpers Josh Lethert and Matt Permentier. Chaos would have reined without them.

Grants from a number of local foundations and individuals (including some with old ties to Grace and Blair Flandrau) helped launch and keep aloft the effort to revive Grace Flandrau: the St. Paul Foundation, the Alice M. O'Brien Foundation, the Richard C. Lilly Foundation, the Mary Livingston Griggs and Mary Griggs Burke Foundation, the Northern Star Foundation, the Marbrook Foundation, the Benlei Foundation, Kate S. Klein, Kate K. Piper, Olivia I. Dodge, the late Judson and Barbara White Bemis, Constance S. Otis, Margaret B. Brooks, Markell Brooks, John C. and Janette Burton, Lyman E. Wakefield Jr., W. B. and Patricia R. Saunders, the late Albert W. Lindeke Jr., and Grace Flandrau's cousins Corrin H. Hodgson, Muriel E. Nelson, the late Harold E. Nelson, and the late Ruth H. Cadwell. Most contributed more than once. A select group of loyalists from this group contributed to naming a writing studio for Grace Flandrau at the Open Book in Minneapolis in summer 2000.

Moral support and belief, however, have been of equal importance to funding in bringing about Grace Flandrau's resuscitation. The following people gave unwavering encouragement from the beginning or at least from the moment they read drafts for Grace Flandrau's *Memoirs* in the early 1990s: Constance Shepard Otis, Gail See, Jane Noland (substantive editor for this biography), and John M. Roth, copyright attorney. I hope this book feels like a reward.

Finally, it's wonderful to have an encouraging, unflappable publisher like Daniel Hoisington of Edinborough Press—a true believer. But he might never have met Grace Flandrau and me without the intervention of the late

Virginia Brainerd Kunz, veteran local historian and editor of *Ramsey County History*. Thank you, Virginia.

Georgia Ray
St. Paul
October 16, 2006

Index